Current Progress in Hip and Knee Arthroplasty

Current Progress in Hip and Knee Arthroplasty

Edited by **Robert Berry**

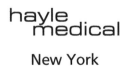

New York

Published by Hayle Medical,
30 West, 37th Street, Suite 612,
New York, NY 10018, USA
www.haylemedical.com

Current Progress in Hip and Knee Arthroplasty
Edited by Robert Berry

International Standard Book Number: 978-1-63241-103-7 (Hardback)

Printed in the United States of America.

Contents

Preface

Over the recent decade, advancements and applications have progressed exponentially. This has led to the increased interest in this field and projects are being conducted to enhance knowledge. The main objective of this book is to present some of the critical challenges and provide insights into possible solutions. This book will answer the varied questions that arise in the field and also provide an increased scope for furthering studies.

The remedial choices in degenerative joint ailments have progressed very quickly. Various surgical methods are available, as opposed to yesteryears. This book brings forth an extensive look at the recent advances in the most performed arthroplasties of large joints of lower parts. Trying to be exhaustive, this book takes up knee arthroplasty with particular accent on advancing minimally invasive surgical procedures. Some difficult subjects have also been discussed. Special concentration is focused on various kinds and types of knee endoprostheses and soft tissue sustenance. Exceptional circumstances in the procedure have been looked into. Latest developments in technology has brought about the chance for the regular use of navigation in knee arthroplasty. This book would serve as an important source of reference for those interested in the field.

I hope that this book, with its visionary approach, will be a valuable addition and will promote interest among readers. Each of the authors has provided their extraordinary competence in their specific fields by providing different perspectives as they come from diverse nations and regions. I thank them for their contributions.

Editor

Part 1

Knee Arthroplasty

History of Condylar Total Knee Arthroplasty

Luca Amendola[1], Domenico Tigani[2],
Matteo Fosco[3] and Dante Dallari[3]
[1]Department of Orthopedic and Traumatology, Maggiore Hospital, Bologna
[2]Department of Orthopaedic Surgery, Santa Maria alle Scotte Hospital, Siena
[3]First Ward of Orthopaedic Surgery, Rizzoli Orthopaedic Institute, Bologna
Italy

1. Introduction

The first attempt of treating patients affected by knee osteoarthritis with arthroplasty go back up to the mid-nineteenth century with the use of either a soft tissue interposed within the joint surface or resection of a different amount of bone of both distal femur and proximal tibia.

However the concept on which total joint replacement is based can be traced only after the 1880 in Berlin with Thermestocles Gluck who gave a series of lectures describing a system of joint replacement by unit made of ivory. The surgeon believed that these unit could be stabilized in bone with cement made of colophony, pumice and plaster of Paris.

The early twentieth saw the return of interposition arthroplasty with the use of autologous tissue or metallic surface and in the 1950s was developed the first surface replacement of the tibia by McKeever (McKeever, 1960). Only during the 1950s and 1960s at last the knee arthroplasty concept diverged into two theories of total joint replacement: the designer focused their effort toward constrained or hinged prosthesis or toward condylar replacement.

Condylar replacement knee prosthesis is defined as one where the femoral and tibial load-bearing surface are replaced with non connected artificial components. Work on the design of an implant that resurfaced the distal femur and proximal tibia without any direct mechanical link between the components began at the end of sixties at the Imperial College in London. The original design known as Freeman-Swanson prosthesis consisted of a metal "roller" placed on the distal femur that articulated with a polyethylene tibial tray and requires resection of both cruciate ligaments.

In other part of the world were developed different experience which carried out to Polycentric, Geomedic, Duocondylar systems (Fig.1).

Even if all of these implants were considered unsatisfactory because of a high percentage of components mobilizations, break of the components and infection the acquired experience permitted the resurfacing prosthesis planning (Insall & Scott, 2001) to occur its successive design phase followed two different ways : the anatomical approach and the functional approach. (Robinson, 2005).

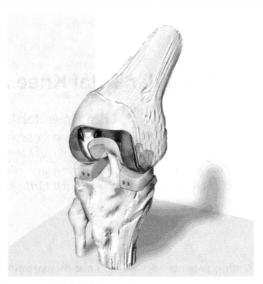

Fig. 1. Duocondylar (courtesy of Prof F. Catani).

2. Anatomical approach

Some designers studied prosthesis that preserve both cruciate ligaments, allowed the femur to roll-back on the tibia.

Yamamoto, from the Okayama University Medical School in Japan, was the first to report on implanting an anatomical femoral component with a minimally constrained single-piece polyethylene tibial component in 1970 (Yamamoto, 1979). The design called the Kodama-Yamamoto knee, consisted of an anatomical femoral mold component, including an anterior femoral flange, made of COP alloy (Co, Cr, Ni, Mo, C, and P). There was a 1-piece, mildly dished polyethylene tibial component that had a central cutout for preservation of both cruciate ligaments.

Others Authors who followed the same approach was Waugh (Waugh et al., 1973) at the University of California UCI, Townley with the cemented Anatomical knee (Townley & Hill, 1974) and Sheedom who designed the Leeds knee. All these prostheses had and horseshoe-shaped tibial component leaving a space behind and centrally for the retention of both anterior and posterior cruciate ligaments.

At the HSS, during the early seventhies, the Duocondylar knee was completely redesigned in an anatomical and symmetrical design: the Duopatellar (Fig.2).

An anterior femoral flange, patellar button, and a more dished tibial surface were added. The tibial component had a fixation peg, identical to the Total Condylar TC, the archetype of the functional approach, and, for the first time, a posterior rectangular cutout—specifically designed for the preserved posterior cruciate ligament.

Although the result of Duopatella were extremely good at the HSS the posterior cruciate-preserving approach would be developed in Boston at the Robert Breck Brigham Hospital (Scott, 1982; Sledge & Ewald, 1979). In Boston the medial tip of the femoral trochlear flange was removed, creating right and left designs based on the asymmetry of the proximal femoral flange.

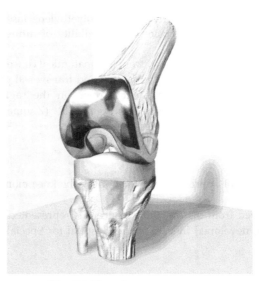

Fig. 2. Duopatellar (courtesy of Prof F. Catani).

This was done to reduce the medial overhang seen in small female rheumatoid patients. The posterior cruciate–sparing version of the Robert Brigham Hospital would later evolved in the PFC knee (Cintor Division of Codman; later, Depuy, Johnson & Johnson). At the same time Peter Walker, Clement Sledge and Fred Ewald, continued the Duopatella concept in the posteriorcruciate–retaining version of the Kinematic knee (Howmedica), which was implanted by Ewald in June 1978. This would evolve into the posteriorcruciate–sparing version of the Kinematic II, Kinemax, and Kinemax Plus systems (Howmedica).

The 80's saw the significant advances in the knee arthroplasty, particularly in the area of surgical technique and instrumentation. Kenna, Hungerford, and Krackow participated in the design of the instruments that were later called the Universal Instruments. Their tools were based on the anatomical concept of measured resection technique rather than the more functional approach of creating equal and parallel flexion and extension gaps which where used until then. The principal aspect of this new conception was that the bone and cartilage removed were to equal the thickness of the prosthetic material replacing them. Up until this time, fixation of the condylar total knee was primarily achieved with cement.

In January 1980 the first Porous-Coated Anatomical Knee (PCA) was inplanted by Hungerford at Johns Hopkins (Hungerford et al., 1982). The implant was anatomical with asymmetric medial and lateral femoral condyles similar to the Leeds and the original Townley designs. However, for the first time, it introduced porous coating in a total condylar knee for a cementless fixation. Each of the 3 components was backed with metal and a 1.5-mm-thick sintered porous coating of cobalt chrome beads.

The Miller-Galante total knee, one of the first knee replacement designed for use with cement or cementless fixation, was first implanted in 1986. The principal innovation of this implant was the choice of a titanium fiber composite for the bony ingrowth surface, because of its well-recognized biocompatibility, and the use of a Titanium Aluminums and Vanadium alloy (Ti6Al4V). The implant is fixed to the tibia with titanium screws and pegs. The uncemented version for patellar resurfacing consists of a metal-backed patella which is fixed with fiber-mesh pegs. Modularity of tibial polyethylene inserts was incorporate in order to allow better ligamentous tension and possibility of future isolated polyethylene replacement.

"Cruciate retaining" prosthesis developed from the anatomical concept were different: some consisted of a relatively flat surface on the sagittal and transversal plane (Kinemax e PCA) while others maintained a more congruent surface on the sagittal plane. Genesis II (Smith&Nephew), Duracon (Howmedica), Nexgen CR (Zimmer), PFC CR (Depuy) represent some actual examples of this conception.

3. Functional approach

Designers of the functional approach tried to simplify the knee biomechanics by removing both cruciate ligaments.

The first system derived from the functional concept is represented by the Total Condylar prosthesis (TC; Fig.3) developed in 1973 at the Hospital for Special Surgery of New York (Insall et al., 1976).

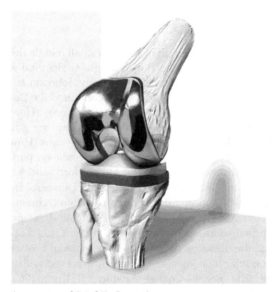

Fig. 3. Total condylar (courtesy of Prof F. Catani).

TC prosthesis consisted of two symmetric condylar surfaces with a posterior decreasing radius of curvature and an articular surface made of polyethylene, perfectly congruent in extension and partially congruent in flexion.

The TC knee would prove to be highly successful, widely used, and would later demonstrate long survival (Vince et al., 1989). Two concerns, however, pointed out the early fases of its clinical use. The femoral component would shift forward, particularly in flexion. In rare cases, this would even result in tibial loosening or anterior dislocation. The second concern was the limited flexion achieved. Average knee flexion with the TC knee was in fact 90° degrees (Robinson, 2005).

In 1978 prosthesis Insall-Burstein was designed to correct these problems by replacing the posterior cruciate ligament with a mechanical lock to reduce posterior translation of the femoral component by using a mechanism of a cam articulated with a post on the tibial component (Fig.4).

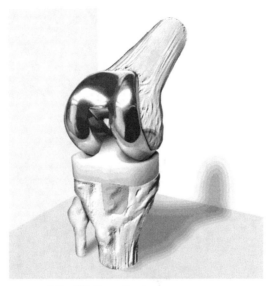

Fig. 4. IB-I allpoly (courtesy of Prof F. Catani).

The cam of the femoral component connected with the tibial central spine at about 70 degrees of flexion and then the femur could roll-back so to increase flexion.
The first IBPS knee was implanted in 1978 by Insall at the HSS.
The IBPS knee become one of the most successful total condylar knee design (Abdeen et al., 2010). Anterior femoral subluxation was eliminated and average flexion would be 115°. A metal-backed monoblock IBPS tibial component with direct-molded polyethylene was introduced in November 1980: the Insall-Burstein Modular (IBPS II) knee (Stern & Insall, 1992).
The HSS posterior-stabilized knee design would evolve into the Insall-Burstein Modular (IBPS II) knee (Zimmer; Fig.5) in 1988, the Optetrak Posterior-Stabilized knee (Exactech; Fig.6) in 1994, and the Advance Posterior- Stabilized knee (Wright Medical) in 1994.
In the 1980s and 1990s, many variations of these functional designs were introduced by different manufacturers. All of them had the characteristic to produce their motion through a so called guided motion, which mean that some characteristics of the motion, such as rollback, are produced by mechanical interaction between the femoral and tibial components.
In the Kyocera Bi-Surface knee (Kyocera Corp, Kyoto, Japan; Fig.7) (Akagi et al., 2000), for the major part of the flexion range, the knee behaves as a standard condylar replacement with moderately conforming bearing surfaces. Beyond that, the load is transferred to a spherical surface protruding behind from the femoral intercondylar region, contacting within a spherical depression at the posterior of the plastic tibial component.

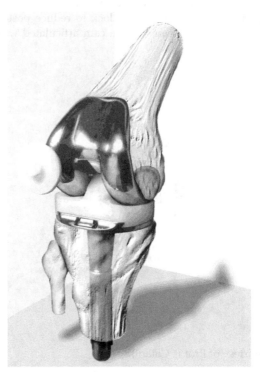

Fig. 5. IB-II PS (courtesy of Prof F. Catani).

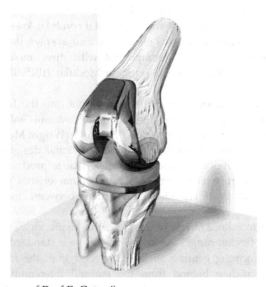

Fig. 6. Optetrak (courtesy of Prof F. Catani).

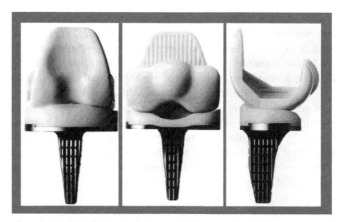

Fig. 7. The Bisurface knee prosthesis (courtesy of Kyocera Corp).

Another example of guided motion knee is represented by The Medial Pivot knee (Wright Mfg Co, Memphis, TN; Fig.8). In that prosthesis the femoral component owns a single radius of femoral curvature and a high level of conformity in the medial compartment where a ball and socket configuration is present. In reason of that configuration the medial side remains in the same position during flexion, but the lateral femoral condyle can displace behind with flexion. The porpoise of the medial pivot design is to reproduce a more physiological kinematics.

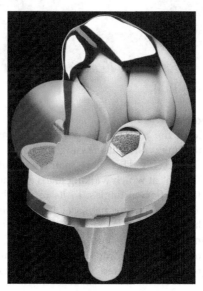

Fig. 8. Spherical condylar surface contacting within a spherical depression at the posterior of the polyethylene (courtesy of Wright Medical).

In contrast with this type of solution more recently has been introduce on the market a new design, the 3D Knee, which provides A/P stability similar to ACL deficient valgus knees through a concave lateral compartment. The lateral compartment is fully congruent in extension and allows 15o of axial rotation. As the knee flexes, a greater range of femoral motion is possible, but is controlled by the concave lateral compartment.

The aim of the 3D Knee is then to accommodate and controls the cruciate deficient patterns of motions without constrain in stripe to reproduce the normal kinematic of the knee.

One of the most innovative functional approaches to condylar total knee design evolved from a collaboration between an orthopedic Surgeon at the New Jersey Medical School Frederic Buechel and a professor of mechanical engineering Michael Pappas. Their project to achieve a low polyethylene contact stresses while maintaining knee flexion and avoiding overload of the implant bone interfaces started in 1977 (Buechel & Pappas, 1986) with the introduction of the Low Contact Stress (LCS) knee system (fig.9). It was the first complete systems approach to total knee replacement using meniscal bearing surfaces.

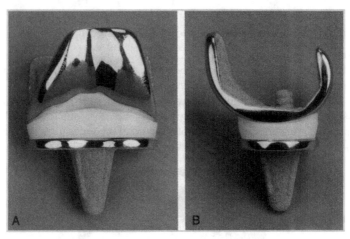

Fig. 9. LCS (courtesy of Depuy J& J).

3.1 Mobile bearing (MB) knee

The principal characteristic of the femoral component was based on the same spherical surface on the mediolateral plane while a decreasing radius of curvature from extension to flexion was present on the lateral side. This shape maintained full area contact on the upper meniscal bearing from the 0 to 45° at which walking loads are encountered, and maintaining at least spherical line at deeper flexion angles. In its origin, the LCS, was proposed as a system inclusive of both cruciate-sparing meniscal bearing and PCL-sacrificing rotating platform variant, with the latter gaining the majority of popular usage over the time.

Afterward the introduction of the LCS system, several types of Mobile bearing knees were produced. They are categorized in according of their conformity: either partially or fully conforming, then a third group is represented by the posterior stabilized MB.

3.2 Partially conforming MB

The LCS other to be the ancestor of all the MB prostheses is also, with its second version featured by a single plastic bearing that freely rotates about its post setaed whitin a hole in the tibial tray, the prototype of the partially conforming one.

Belongs to partially conforming knees the Self Aligning MB (Sulzer) designed by Bourne and Rorabeck in 1987. This prosthesis is characterized by an oval recess in posterior aspect of the polyethylene which allows unlimited rotation and limited AP translation about a tibial tray peg.

The mobile bearing knee produced by the Waldemar Link in Hamburg in 1990, called TACK, is characterized by the presence in the tibial tray of two semicircular guide that engage circular tracks on both sides of the polyethylene platform, permitting wide rotational movement.

The Interax Integrated Secure Asymmetric (Howmedica) prosthesis has nearly fully conformity between femoral condyle and tibial surface in extension and whereas the conformity gradually decrease in flexion. The tibial baseplate has two central posts that engages a curved, t-shaped guide track whitin the meniscal bearing.

In Italy Prof Ghisellini designed the Total Rotating Knee (TRK) (Cremascoli) characterized by a central tibia post projecting from the center of the tibial tray. Two type of plastic bearing were available the R type to allow freedom of rotation was intend to be use incase of PCL excision, whereas the RS allowing 10 mm of AP sliding and freedom of rotation, was indicated when the PCL was retained.

3.3 Fully conforming MB

The progenitor of fully conforming MB knees is certainly the Rotaglide Total knee System (Corin, Cirencester, UK) designed in 1986 by Polyzoides and Tsakonas: the rotaglide femoral component has a constant flexion radius of curvature in the femoro-meniscal articulation, each condyle being part of a sphere of 24 mm radius. This design ensures that congruency is retained throughout the range of flexion. The mobile meniscal bearing has two undercuts which permit up to 5mm of antero-posterior translation and 25° of rotation, 12,5° for each side. The tibial plateau has an anterior bollard that prevents anterior dislocation while restricting the rotation of the platform and another bollard in the middle of the tray that resists posterior dislocation.

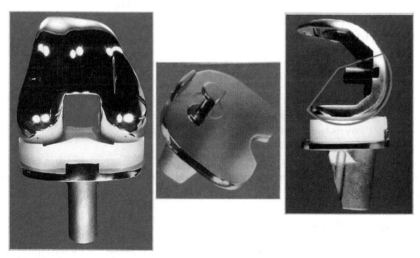

Fig. 10. a) MBK designs (courtesy of Zimmer).

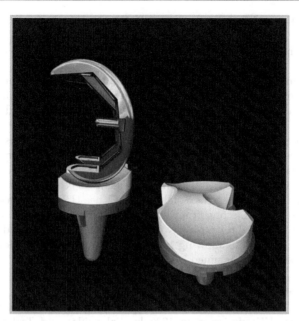

Fig. 10. b) MBK schematic.

The Medially Biased Kinematics Knee (MBK) was developed by J Insall, P Aglietti e P Walker in 1992 (Fig.10a-b). The design concept of this prosthesis is complete conformity between the femoral component and the polyethylene insert at any degree of flexion and during rotation and AP translation of the tibial insert on the tibial tray. The prosthesis design allow a medially biased kinematics guided by the natural knee's stronger medial structures and greater lateral mobility. The polyethylene has approximately 20 degrees of both internal and external rotation on the tibial baseplate about a D-shaped "mushroom" post. The tibial baseplate translates 4,5 mm in an AP direction. An anterior stop prevents the plastic bearing from sliding off the tibial tray.

3.4 Posterior stabilized MB
These design are based on the "cam and post" mechanism on a rotating polyethylene platform. The common feature is the presence of a cam situated between the posterior femoral condyles that engages a post projecting from the mobile polyethylene platform. The "cam and post" mechanism acts as a third weight-bearing condyle to help improve, load transfer and minimize polyethylene stress.
Belongs to this category the Two Radii Area Contact (TRAC, Biomet) which was indroduced in 1997. More recent designs are the P.F.C. Sigma RPF (DePuy) and the LPS mobile Flex (Zimmer).

4. Patellofemoral joint

Symptoms related to the patello-femoral joint have been reported to be a frequent cause of failure following total knee arthroplasty.

During 1980s, up to 30% of patients suffered of complication associated with the patella-femoral joint (Rhoads et al., 1990).

This disappointing feature of what was otherwise a successful procedure led between surgeons to a debate as to whether the articular surface of the patella should be replaced and, in event of the replacement , exactly how this should be performed.

At the some time various authors (Grace & Rand, 1988; Yoshii et al., 1992) pointed out the importance of prosthetic femoral and patella components.

As this problem started off with the improvement of flexion allowed by the second generation of resurfacing condylar knee, so that minimal patellofemoral problems were associate with the TC which permitted at least 90° of flexion, the principal concern of designers was to perform a deeper trochlea which floor could extend behind so as to roof of the intercondylar notch, thereby providing a surface against which the patella can articulate in full extension.

In effort to obtain a suitable designed trochlea Kulkarni and Freeman (Kulkarni et al., 2000) stressed out the importance that the trochlear surface would extended proximally sufficiently to enable even the highest patella to articulate with the femur in full extension. In their philosophy this part of the femoral prosthesis should be provided with a lateral wall and floor to ensure that the patella remains in contact with the floor of the trochlea from 0° to 20° of flexion. Lastly, the Kulkarni and Freeman trochlea surface should have a lateral wall of the trochlear groove sufficiently steep to provide a distinct resistance to lateral subluxation.

According to these criteria most of the design introduced during the nineties have incorporated multiple changes in the geometry of the trochlear groove, which have been shown to have a positive impact on the patellar complication rate (Bindelglass & Dorr, 1998; Kavolus et al., 2008; Mont et al., 1999).

An important contribution to lowering the rate of patello-femoral complication was correlate with greater attention that since that time was given to the rotational alignment of the femoral component (Anouchi et al., 1993; Scuderi et al., 1994).

5. Polyethylene

In spite of the success of designer in solving some the mentioned problems the 90's marked a period of concern regarding the catastrophic failure of the polyethylene.

Polyethylene (UHMW) has been chosen to create articular insert used for knee prosthesis. It's a low friction polymer, very resistant while articulating with metallic and extremely smooth surfaces of prosthesis.

Knee Prosthesis survival curve after 15 years arrives over 94% using this material (Insall & Scott, 2001).

Despite of these characteristics material usury it's a problem especially considering young active patients.

Damage mechanism of polyethylene are: delamination, usury caused by adhesive and abrasive wear mechanism.

Many factors can affect negatively the mechanical properties of polyethylene; some of them are due to type of prosthesis and material, others depend by clinical conditions (post-operatory alignment, weight, age of patient, ecc).

Polyethylene properties can be modified by sterilization by radiation and by exposition to oxidative environment; the effects are increase in density and elasticity of the materials itself.

Since 1995 all the industries virtually modified polyethylene sterilization procedures, by getting rid of gamma ray sterilization.

Sterilization in inert environment, gas plasma, ethylene oxide, represent at the moment the most common sterilization methods. On the same time , packaging and conserving systems has been modified.

Radiation damage on polyethylene underlined cross-link techniques advantages on usury effects.

Cross-linked polyethylene is widely used in hip prosthesis but it didn't reach the same application in knee prosthesis.

In fact a recent study performed on untimely mobilized components of prosthesis do not underlined significant differences concerning usury between conventional polyethylene and cross-linked polyethylene (Muratoglu et al., 2003).

6. High flexion knee and new materials

Some important issues have characterized the beginning of the new millennium as the effort to improve movement and the research for new materials. Both these issues are direct for better-performing prostheses for younger more active patients who wish to run, play tennis, and downhill ski.

Range of motion (ROM) after total knee arthroplasty is an important issue in determining clinical outcome and a better satisfaction from the patient. In association to expanding the indication of total knee arthroplasty to more young and active patients, their demands and expectations have increased including secondary goals other than pain relief, such as restoration of "normal-like" joint function, especially weight bearing range of motion, to suit their desired lifestyle (Noble et al., 2006).

Apart from being influenced by the condition of the patient and surgical technique, the final outcome, at least in part, depends on the implant design. Therefore, more recently, implant manufacturers have attempted to design TKAs that better accommodate knee mechanics in high flexion up to 155°.

Since it has been shown that in general posterior cruciate ligament retaining designs have erratic motion with potential for paradoxical roll forward, most of them belong to the posterior cruciate substituting prostheses (Dennis et al., 1998).

These new high-flexion designs are not radically different from their traditional (non high-flexion designs) counterparts but incorporate subtle changes in the geometry of the components to allow improved contact mechanics in the high-flexion ranges compared to traditional designs.

Regarding the sagittal geometry of the femoral component a reduction of the femoral condyles radii in the mid- and high-flexion ranges has been showed some advantage when compared with the traditional implants. In order to eliminate edge loading on the femoral component, on the posterior tibial articular surface, was necessary to extend the posterior femoral condyles. In addition an extended posterior femoral condyle help to restore the posterior condylar offset which has been previously emphasized (Bellemans et al., 2002) as an important factor in achieving high flexion. In that study the Authors observed that for every 2 mm decrease in posterior condylar offset, the maximal obtainable flexion was reduced by a mean of 12.2°.

Some designers prefer mobile bearings for the assumption that for achieving deep knee flexion is the need for large internal rotation of the tibia, which occurs with extreme posterior shift of the lateral femoral condyle over the posterior tibial plateau increased tibial rotation with deep flexion and the theoretical advantage of improved contact area (Kurosaka et al., 2002; Nakagawa et al., 2000).

These changes are associated to a modified cam/post mechanism which allow a more jump distance and avoids dislocation at deep flexion angles (Fig. 11a-b).

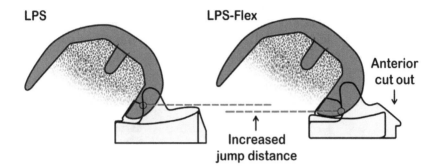

Fig. 11. a) Difference in height distance of the post/cam mechanism between LPS and LPS-Flex designs.

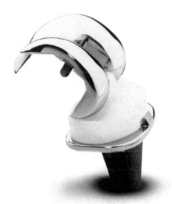

Fig. 11. b) LPS-Flex designs (courtesy of Zimmer).

Other characteristics of high flex design include the patellofemoral joint which should be designed to accommodate high angles of knee flexion. The femoral trochlear articulation should be deep enough to reduce the contact stresses on the patella and the patella should glide smoothly through a full range of motion. These kinds of prostheses in fact, in order to reduce extensor mechanism impingement during deep flexion, the anterior margin of the tibial articular component has been recessed.

In Japan with the aim to accommodate the oriental lifestyle where people sit more often on the floor than on a chair in 1989 was developed a new design originally called KU knee

(Kyoto University knee). The most outstanding feature of this model is that it has an auxiliary joint of a ball and socket at the center of the posterior part not only to facilitate a rollback movement but also to add a rotational function. During a gait under the load, the femorotibial articulation surface in a conventional design works as for standard design, but when the flexion becomes more, the auxiliary joint takes a part as a rotation center in the flexion motion. This auxiliary joint represents a certain type of posterior-stabilized knee and works to achieve a rollback, and when in flexion, rotation of tibia can be also achieved. Because this knee was unique in its biphasic surface structure for the different purposes, weight bearing, and flexion movement, it was later called bisurface knee (BS knee). Another characteristic of this prosthesis is the presence of zirconia ceramics (ZrO2) for femoral component.

Others companies modified design incorporating a lateral compartment which is fully congruent in extension, but relatively lax in flexion (Fig.12) (Mikashima et al., 2010).

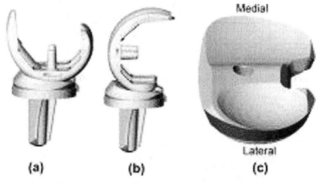

(a)   **(b)**   **(c)**

Fig. 12. From Mikashima: the lateral tibiofemoral joint is completely conforming in extension (a), but less conforming at 90 degrees of flexion (b); the tibial insert has an AP curved medial surface and a spherically recessed lateral surface (c).

This lateral congruency constrains the lateral condyle to a central antero-posterior (AP) position in extension, but allows posterior translation in flexion. This articular geometry provides antero-posterior stability and acts through the lateral femoral condyle, thus there is rough analogy with the location and stabilizing role of the anterior cruciate ligament (ACL). In addition, the modified design has a more posterior tibial sulcus (Banks & Hodge, 2004) and the maximum femoral posterior condylar offset occurs later in the flexion arc (Bellemans et al., 2002).

TKA is an effective, well-established treatment for severe arthrythis of the knee. However, further improvement in the longevity in the longevity of the arthroplasty can be achieved with more durable bearing materials.

Due to the non-conforming shape of the bearing surface, hard-on-hard bearing are unlikely to have a role in TKA and polyethylene (PE) still remain an important bearing surface material.

Despite the improvement in manufacturing and elimination of gamma-irradiation in air have already resulted in fewer wear-related problems, concerns remain about adhesive and abrasive wear caused by the hard counterface of the femoral component.

Previous studies have shown that roughening of the cobalt-chromiun (CoCr) alloy can potentiate wear of the PE (Fisher et al., 2004; White et al., 1994).

This wear can then lead to osteolysis, instability, and loosening of the implants from the underlying bone.

Designers are now concentrated on the research of different alloys for femoral components, alternative to the classic CoCrMo one (Stellite), both for complete ceramic or for ceramic surfaces.

A longer lasting of prosthesis with ceramic femoral components should be useful for younger patients with higher functional demands.

Moreover ceramic is useful when dealing with patients affected by allergies to metallic iones (Stellite) (Spector et al., 2001).

The advantages of ceramic bearing surfaces in terms of superior lubrication, friction, and wear properties compared to cobalt-chrome alloy (CoCr) surfaces in total joint arthroplasty are well recognized (Greenwald et al., 2001; Jacobs et al., 1994).

Laboratory and clinical data have demonstrated that ceramic bearings are associated with fewer wear particles that incite a less intense inflammatory host immune response than the metal-on-polyethylene articulations that are the accepted standard in total hip arthroplasty and total knee arthroplasty (Mont et al., 2003; Spector et al., 2001). The brittle nature of ceramics and the inability of ceramic materials to withstand high-impact tensile forces is of concern in clinical applications.

However, more than 10 years' long-term follow-up of cemented different ceramic knees, were performed in Japan and showed satisfactory results with low rate fractures of ceramic component (Akagi et al., 2000; Koshino et al., 2002).

An important improvement has been recently introduced in Europe by CeramTec (AG, Polchingen, Germany) with the BIOLOX Delta a composite matrix material containing 82% vol. alumina (Al_2O_3) and 17% vol. zirconia (ZrO_2) providing good mechanical characteristics in terms of strength and resistance (Dalla Pria, 2007).

Using this material it was possible to develop a femoral component with a tensile strength that meets the demands for application in TKR (Kluess et al., 2009).

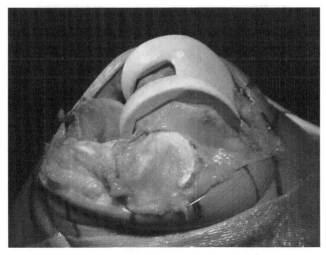

Fig. 13. a) Intraoperative photo of Biolox Delta ceramic femoral component.

A prospective international multicentre study started in 2008 with the aim to evaluate the clinical and radiological outcomes of the unconstrained Multigen Plus total knee system (Lima-Lto) with the new BIOLOX Delta ceramic femoral component (Fig.12a-b).

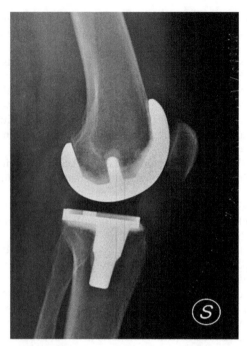

Fig. 13. b) Post-operative x-Ray of Multigen Plus total knee system (sagittal view).

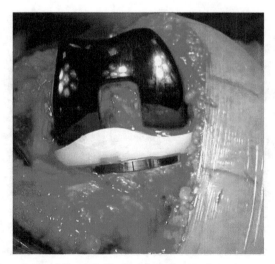

Fig. 14. Intraoperative photo of Genesis II: Oxinium femoral component.

In USA an alternative strategy has been followed to decrease PE wear in THA and TKA, which consists in the surface transformation of metal to oxidized zirconium. A wrought zirconium alloy (Zr-2.5% Niobium) is oxidized by thermal diffusion to create a 5-mm oxidized zirconium layer (Oxinium, Smith & Nephew, Memphis, TN; Fig.14) (Laskin, 2003).

Although existing data are encouraging, with both strategies (Innocenti et al., 2010), further studies are needed to define the precise indications and outcomes of ceramic surfaces in TKA.

7. Conclusions and future perspective

Technological developments in the field of knee replacement continues to increase the range of solutions for the recovery of joint mobility of the painful knee arthritis.

Particularly research and development efforts are focusing on designing effective prosthesis, allowing the movement ever closer to physiological ones, which are well tolerated and long lasting, and are implanted with less invasive interventions.

Explains the considerable attention, first, the morphological aspects of prosthetic components, and second, the quality of materials, with the aim of ensuring greater wear resistance and improved biocompatibility. This is a necessary condition for stability of the prosthetic implant and for the success of the intervention.

8. References

Abdeen, AR., Collen, SB., & Vince, KG. (2010). Fifteen-year to 19-year follow-up of the Insall-Burstein-1 total knee arthroplasty. *J Arthroplasty*, Vol.25, No.2, pp. 173-178.

Akagi, M., Nakamura, T., Matsusue Y., Ueo, T., Nishijyo, K., & Ohnishi, E. (2000). The Bisurface total knee replacement: a unique design for flexion. Four-to-nine-year follow-up study. *J Bone Joint Surg Am*, Vol.82, No.11, pp. 1626-1633.

Anouchi, YS., Whiteside, LA., Kaiser, AD., & Milliano, MT. (1993). The effects of axial rotational alignment of the femoral component on knee stability and patellar tracking in total knee arthroplasty demonstrated on autopsy specimens. *Clin Orthop Relat Res*, Vol.287, pp. 170-177.

Banks, SA., & Hodge, WA. (2004). Implant design affects knee arthroplasty kinematics during stair-stepping. *Clin Orthop Relat Res*, Vol.426, pp. 187-193.

Bellemans, J., Banks, S., Victor, J., Vandenneucker, H., & Moemans, A. (2002). Fluoroscopic analysis of the kinematics of deep flexion in total knee arthroplasty. Influence of posterior condylar offset. *J Bone Joint Surg Br*, Vol.84, No.1, pp. 50-53.

Bindelglass, DF., & Dorr, LD. (1998). Current concepts review: symmetry versus asymmetry in the design of total knee femoral components - an unresolved controversy. *J Arthroplasty*, Vol.13, No.8, pp. 939-944.

Buechel, FF., & Pappas, MJ. (1986). The New Jersey Low-Contact-Stress Knee Replacement System: biomechanical rationale and review of the first 123 cemented cases. *Arch. Orthop Trauma Surg*, Vol.105, No.4, pp. 197-204.

Dalla Pria, P. (2007). Evolution and new application of the alumina ceramics in joint replacement. *Eur J Orthop Surg Traumatol*, 17:253-256 Vol.17, pp. 253-256.

Dennis, DA., Komistek, RD., Stiehl, JB., Walker, SA., & Dennis, KN. (1998). Range of motion after total knee arthroplasty: the effect of implant design and weight-bearing conditions. *J Arthroplasty*, Vol.13, No.7, pp. 748-752.

Fisher, J., McEwen, HM., Tipper, JL., Galvin, AL., Ingram, J., Kamali, A., Stone, MH., & Ingham E. (2004). Wear, debris, and biologic activity of cross-linked polyethylene in the knee: benefits and potential concerns. *Clin Orthop Relat Res*, Vol.428, pp. 114-119.

Grace, JN., & Rand, JA. (1988). Patellar instability after total knee arthroplasty. *Clin Orthop Relat Res*, Vol.237, pp. 184-189.

Greenwald, AS., & Garino, JP. (2001). Alternative bearing surfaces: the good, the bad, and the Ugly. *J Bone Joint Surg Am*, Vol.83, No.2, pp. 68-72.

Hungerford, DS., Kenna, RV., & Krackow, KA. (1982). The porous-coated anatomic total knee. *Orthop Clin North Am*, Vol.13, No.1, pp. 103-122.

Innocenti, M., Civinini, R., Carulli, C., Matassi, F., & Villano, M. (2010). The 5-year Results of an Oxidized Zirconium Femoral Component for TKA. *Clin Orthop Relat Res*, Vol.468, pp. 1258-1263.

Insall, J., Ranawat, CS., Scott, WN., & Walker, P. (1976). Total condylar knee replacement: preliminary report. *Clin Orthop Relat Res*, Vol.120, pp. 149-154.

Insall, J., & Scott WN. (2001). *Surgery of the Knee* (third edition), Churchill-Livingstone, New York.

Jacobs, JJ., Shanbhag, A., Glant, TT., Black, J., & Galante, JO. (1994). Wear debris in total joint replacements. *J Am Acad Orthop Surg*, Vol.2, No.4, pp. 212-220.

Kavolus, CH., Hummel, MT., Barnett, KP., & Jennings, JE Jr. (2008). Comparison of the Insall-Burstein II and NexGen legacy total knee arthroplasty systems with respect to patella complications. *J Arthroplasty*, Vol.23, No.6, pp. 822-825.

Kluess, D., Souffrant, R., Fritsche, A., Mittelmeier, W., & Bader, R. (2009). Explicit Finite-Element-Analysis of the Impaction Behavior of a Ceramic Femoral Component in Total Knee Replacement. *Proceedings 55th Annual Meeting of the Orthopaedic Research Society*, Las Vegas.

Koshino, T., Okamoto, R., Takagi, T., Yamamoto, K., & Saito, T. (2002). Cemented ceramic YMCK total knee arthroplasty in patients with severe rheumatoid arthritis. *J Arthroplasty*, Vol.17, No.8, pp. 1009-1015.

Kulkarni, SK., Freeman, MA., Poal-Manresa, JC., Asencio, JI., & Rodriguez, JJ. (2000). The patellofemoral joint in total knee arthroplasty: is the design of the trochlea the critical factor? *J Arthroplasty*, Vol.15, No.4, pp. 424-429.

Kurosaka, M., Yoshiya, S., Mizuno, K., & Yamamoto, T. (2002). Maximizing flexion after total knee arthroplasty: the need and the pitfalls. *J Arthroplasty*, Vol.17, No.4, pp. 59-62.

Laskin, RS. (2003). An oxidized Zr ceramic surfaced femoral component for total knee arthroplasty. *Clin Orthop Relat Res*, Vol.416, pp. 191-196.

McKeever, DC. (1960). Tibial plateau prosthesis. *Clin Orthop Rel Res*, Vol.192, pp. 3-12.

Mikashima, Y., Tomatsu, T., Horikoshi, M., Nakatani, T., Saito, S., Momohara S., & Banks, SA. (2010). In vivo deep-flexion kinematics in patients with posterior-cruciate retaining and anterior-cruciate substituting total knee arthroplasty. *Clin Biomech (Bristol, Avon)*, Vol.25, No.1, pp. 83-87.

Mont, MA., Yoon, TR., Krackow, KA., & Hungerford, DS. (1999). Eliminating patellofemoral complications in total knee arthroplasty: clinical and radiographic results of 121 consecutive cases using the Duracon system. *J Arthroplasty*, Vol.14, No.4, pp. 446-455.

Mont, MA., Booth, RE. Jr, Laskin, RS., Stiehl, JB., Ritter, MA., Stuchin, SA., & Rajadhyaksha, AD. (2003). The spectrum of prosthesis design for primary total knee arthroplasty. *Instr Course Lect.* Vol.52, pp. 397-407.

Muratoglu, OK., Mark, A., Vittetoe, DA., Harris, WH., & Rubash, HE. (2003). Polyethylene damage in total knees and use of highly crosslinked polyethylene. *J Bone Joint Surg Am*, Vol.85, No.1, pp. 7-13.

Nakagawa, S., Kadoya, Y., Todo, S., Kobayashi, A., Sakamoto, H., Freeman, MA., & Yamano, Y. (2000). Tibiofemoral movement 3: full flexion in the living knee studied by MRI. *J Bone Joint Surg Br*, Vol.82, No.8, pp. 1199-1200.

Noble, PC., Conditt, MA., Cook, KF., & Mathis KB. (2006). The John Insall Award: Patient expectations affect satisfaction with total knee arthroplasty. *Clin Orthop Relat Res*, Vol.452, pp. 35-43.

Rhoads, DD., Noble, PC., Reuben, JD., Mahoney, OM., & Tullos, HS. (1990). The effect of femoral component position on patellar tracking after total knee arthroplasty. *Clin Orthop Relat Res*, Vol.260, pp. 43-51.

Robinson, RP. (2005). The early innovators of today's resurfacing condylar knees. *J Arthroplasty*, Vol.20, No.1, pp. 2-26.

Scott, RD. (1982). Duopatellar total knee replacement: The Brigham experience. *Orth Clinic North Am*, Vol.13, No.1, pp. 89-102.

Scuderi, GR., Insall, JN., & Scott, NW. (1994). Patellofemoral pain after total knee arthroplasty. *J Am Acad Orthop Surg*, Vol.2, No.5, pp. 239-246.

Sledge, CB., & Ewald, FC. (1979). Total knee arthroplasty experience at the Robert Breck Brigham Hospital. *Clin Orthop Relat Res*, Vol.145, pp. 78-84.

Spector, BM., Ries, MD., Bourne, RB., Sauer, WS., Long, M., & Hunter, G. (2001) Wear performance of ultra-high molecular weight polyethylene on oxidized zirconium total knee femoral components. *J Bone Joint Surg Am*, Vol.83, No.2, pp. 80-86.

Stern, SH., & Insall, JN. (1992). Posterior stabilized prosthesis. Results after follow-up of nine to twelve years. *J Bone Joint Surg Am*, Vol.74, No.7, pp. 980-986.

Townley, C., & Hill, L. (1974). Total knee replacement. *Am J Nurs*, Vol.74, No.9, pp. 1612-1617.

Vince, KG., Insall, JN., & Kelly, MA. (1989). The total condylar prosthesis. 10- to 12-year results of a cemented knee replacement. *J Bone Joint Surg Br*, Vol.71, No.5, pp. 793-797.

Waugh, TR., Smith, RC., Orofino, CF., & Anzel, SM. (1973). Total knee replacement: operative technic and preliminary results. *Clin Orthop Relat Res*, 94:196-201 Vol.94, pp. 196-201.

White, SE., Whiteside, LA., McCarthy, DS., Anthony, M., & Poggie, RA. (1994). Simulated knee wear with cobalt chromium and oxidized zirconium knee femoral components. *Clin Orthop Relat Res*, Vol.309, pp. 176-184.

Yamamoto, S. (1979). Total knee replacement with the Kodama-Yamamoto knee prosthesis. *Clin Orthop Relat Res*, Vol.145, pp. 60-67.

Yoshii, I., Whiteside, LA., & Anouchi, YS. (1992). The effect of patellar button placement and femoral component design on patellar tracking in total knee arthroplasty. *Clin Orthop Relat Res*, Vol.275, pp. 211-219.

2

Posterior Stabilized Total Knee Arthroplasty

Fabio Orozco and Alvin Ong

Atlanticare Care Regional Medical Center, Pomona, New Jersey
Joint Replacement, Rothman Institute, Thomas Jefferson
University, Philadelphia, Pennsylvani
USA

1. Introduction

The posterior cruciate ligament (PCL) in total knee arthroplasty (TKA) functions to prevent posterior translation of the tibia and aids in femoral roll-back[1]. Roll-back allows for increased quadriceps lever arm and more efficient use of extensor musculature, permitting more normal stair climbing. Because of this, PCL retaining knees have the advantage of maintenance of ligamentous proprioception, load transfer by the native PCL and anterior-posterior stability. However, retaining the PCL also has several disadvantages. Surgical exposure of the tibia, gap balancing and reliance on diseased ligament morphology make consistent TKA results difficult. The posterior stabilized design in TKA was introduced in the mid-1970s. Surgeons who use this system believed that the results obtained are more consistent because they do not have to rely on abnormal PCL morphology. Consequently, exposure, joint line restoration and appropriate balancing of the knee are easier with PCL stabilized designs. These components are a popular treatment for patients requiring primary TKA. Improvements in implant design, a technically easier procedure in the face of deformity, restoration of knee kinematics and reported very good long-term outcomes may all be reasons for the increased use of this design.

2. History and design rationale

Most of the current total knee implants were derived from the Total Condylar Prosthesis (TCP; Zimmer, Warsaw, Indiana, USA), which was introduced in 1974. This prosthesis was a cruciate sacrificing cemented design. Technique of implantation of the TCP requires excision of the PCL but without substitution. Stability in this implant design was achieved by soft tissue balance in flexion and extension and articular conformity in the coronal and sagittal plane[2]. Consequently, the success of this implant was highly dependent of surgical technique. In 1978, the TCP was modified to the Insall Burstein Posterior Stabilized Prosthesis (IB I) to address posterior subluxation of the tibia and instability. The IB I is the

---

[1] Dorr LD Ochsner JL, Gronley J, Perry J. Functional comparison of posterior curciate-retained versus cruciate-sacrificedot al knee arthroplasty. CORR 1988; 236:36-43.

[2] Scuderi GR, Pagnano MR: Review Article: The rationale for posterior cruciate substituting total knee arthroplasty. J Orthopedic Surgery 2001, 9(2):81-88

first posterior stabilized/substituting TKA design. It incorporated a femoral cam that articulates with a polyethylene tibial post to act as a substitute for the excised native PCL. Most posterior stabilized knee designs evolved from the IB I - incorporating a cam-post mechanism to aid in roll back, increase the amount of distraction tolerated before subluxation occurs, and increase varus-valgus constraint. The cam-post mechanism improves both anterior-posterior and translational stability. Multiply studies have shown that function of the TKA is improved with PCL substitution. PCL substitution allowed for better stability, increased ROM, reduced quadriceps force in extension, improved stair-climbing ability, and improved patellofemoral function.[3][4][5]

3. Advantages of posterior stabilized TKA

There are several advantages with use of posterior stabilized TKA designs. These include: I) easier surgical exposure and ligament balancing, II) predictable restoration of knee kinematics, III) improved range of motion, IV) less polyethylene wear, and V) avoiding the possibility of PCL rupture.

3.1 Easier surgical exposure and ligament balancing
Adequate exposure of the tibia may not be possible with PCL retention. Excision of the PCL aids in exposing the tibia for adequate visualization by releasing the tethering effect of a tight contracted PCL. Moreover, the PCL can be excised from the femoral and tibial attachment in a reproducible way, making the ligamentous balancing and correction of the deformity easier since it is not complicated by the tethering effect of the PCL. Abnormal PCL morphology is often encountered in the diseased knee making predictable gap balancing difficult in PCL retaining designs. If the patient has a "tight", contracted PCL, the knee may be relatively tight in flexion with excessive femoral roll-back. On the other hand, if the PCL is lax or incompetent, the knee may experience posterior sag with no roll-back with knee flexion. Thus, use of posterior stabilized TKA makes balancing more predictable eliminating the reliance on abnormal PCL morphology and function.

3.2 Predictable restoration of knee kinematics
In posterior stabilized TKA, the tibial post articulates with the transverse femoral cam predictably with knee flexion, preventing posterior subluxation of the tibia while maintaining femoral roll back. Many studies report more normal kinematics with the use of posterior stabilized designs.[6][7][8] Fluoroscopic kinematics showed that the posterior

[3] Insall JN, Lachiewicz PF, Burstein AH. The posterior stabilized condylar prosthesis: a modification of the total condylar design. J Bone Joint Surg Am. 1982;64:1317

[4] Scott WN, Rubinstein M, Scuderi G. Results after knee replacement with a posterior cruciate-substituting prosthesis. J Bone Joint Surg Am. 1998;70:1163

[5] Scuderi GR, Insall JN. The posterior stabilized knee prosthesis. Orthop Clin North Am. 1989;20:71

[6] Stiehl JB, Komistek RD, Dennis DA, et al. Fluoroscopic analysis of kinematics after posterior cruciate retaining knee arthroplasty. J Bone Joint Surg Br 1995; 77B:884-889.

[7] Dennis DA, Komistek RD, Hoff WA. In vivo knee kinematics derived using an inverse perspective technique. Clin Orthop 1996; 331:107-117.

[8] Ranawat CS, Komistek RD, Rodriguez JA, et al. In vivo kinematics for fixed and mobile-bearing posterior stabilized knee prostheses. Clin Orthop Relat Res 2004; 418:184-190.

stabilized TKA experienced AP femoro-tibial translation more similar to the normal knee during normal gait and deep knee bend.[9] Moreover, studies have shown no significant difference between posterior stabilized TKA and normal knees with regard to spatio-temporal gait parameters, knee range of motion during stair climbing or in isokinetic muscle strength.[10]

A study comparing cruciate retaining, cruciate sacrificing and posterior stabilized TKA found that posterior stabilized designs produced more roll back and better quadriceps efficiency than cruciate retaining knee designs[11.] Posterior stabilized TKA predictably restores more normal knee kinematics when compared to either PCL substituting or PCL sacrificing designs.

3.3 Improved range of motion

Both cruciate retaining and posterior stabilized TKA designs can provide excellent range of motion. However, range of motion may be better when a posterior stabilized TKA is used to maintain femoral roll back. It appears, according to most comparative studies, that posterior stabilized designs may provide more predictable motion, with greater flexion under fluoroscopic visualization.[12 13] In a very well done meta-analysis Jacobs *et al.* analyzed eight randomized controlled trials comparing posterior stabilized with cruciate retaining TKA and found that the range of motion was 8° higher (105 versus 113°) in the posterior stabilized group than the cruciate retaining group ($P = 0.01$, 95% confidence interval 1.7-15).[14]

3.4 Less polyethylene wear

Retention of the PCL requires that the prosthetic kinematics closely match that of the normal knee. This obligates the implant to have a "flat" polyethylene component relative to the radius of curvature of the femur. This "round on flat" design allows for minimal constraint on tibial component enabling roll back of the femur on tibia with knee flexion. This less forming design can lead to excessive point contact pressure and increase polyethylene wear. In contrast, in posterior-stabilized design, it is possible to use more conforming polyethylene articulation with minimal point contact stress. Increasing the conformity of the implant, increases the contact area, and decreases the stress to which the polyethylene is subjected. This can potentially minimize polyethylene wear and increase the long-term survival of the TKA. Cases of severe polyethylene wear in cruciate retaining implants with less conforming

[9] Udomkiat P, Meng BJ, Dorr LD, Wan Z. Clin Orthop 2000 Sep;(378):192-201

[10] Wilson SA, McCann PD, Gotlin RS, Ramakrishnan HK, Wootten ME and Insall JN. Comprehensive gait analysis in posterior stabilized knee arthroplasty. J Arthroplasty 1996, 11:359–67.

[11] Mahoney OM, Noble PC, Rhoads DD, Alexander JW, Tullos HS. Posterior cruciate function following total knee arthroplasty: A biomechanical study. J Arthroplasty 1994, 9:569-78.

[12] Jacobs WC, Clement DJ, Wymenga AB. Retention versus removal of the posterior cruciate ligament in total knee replacement: a systematic literature review within the Cochrane framework. Acta Orthop 2005; 76:757-768.

[13] Maruyama S, Yoshiya S, Matsui N, Kuroda R, Kurosaka M. Functional comparison of posterior cruciate retaining versus posterior stabilized total knee arthroplasty. J Arthroplasty 2004; 19:349-353.

[14] Jacobs WC, Clement DJ, Wymenga AB. Retention versus removal of the posterior cruciate ligament in total knee replacement: a systematic literature review within the Cochrane framework. Acta Orthop 2005; 76:757-768.

tibial inserts have been reported.[15] [16] Additionally, technical issues may contribute to wear in cruciate retaining TKA if the PCL is left too tight in flexion. This can lead to asymmetric posterior polyethylene wear from posterior femoral subluxation and may predispose to osteolysis.

3.5 Avoiding the possibility of posterior cruciate ligament rupture

The PCL can rupture postoperatively with the use of cruciate retaining TKA. This can occur by trauma or inflammatory disease process. Late flexion instability can occur if the PCL fails over time. This complication can also occur iatrogenically when the PCL it is overzealously recessed intraoperatively or excessive proximal tibial resection is perfomed. When too much proximal tibia is resected, the PCL insertion site can be jeopardized. The PCL can also be is damaged by synovitis from inflammatory arthropathy, resulting in failure.[17] Thus, avoiding the use PCL retaining implants can eliminate failure and instability by avoiding reliance on the integrity of the native PCL.

4. Disadvantages of posterior stabilized TKA

There are several disadvantages with use of posterior stabilized TKA designs. These include: I) tibial post wear and breakage, II) excessive bone resection, III) patellar clunk syndrome, and IV) tibio-femoral dislocations.

4.1 Tibial post wear and breakage

A potential problem with posterior stabilized design is tibial post polyethylene wear from the cam-post articulation. Excessive wear particulate debris can lead to osteolysis. In a wear analysis of retrieved posterior stabilized TKA components, evidence of wear or damage was observed on all specimens of stabilizing posts, including those revised because of infection.[18] Wear caused premature failure and early revision. Moreover, wear can lead to catastrophic failure of the tibial post through fracture. The authors concluded that the cam-post articulation in posterior stabilized implants can be an additional source of polyethylene wear debris. The variability in wear patterns observed among designs may be due to differences in cam-post mechanics, post location, and post geometry. [19]

4.2 Excessive bone resection

It is necessary to remove bone from the intercondylar notch inorder to accommodate the tibial post in most posterior stabilized TKA designs. This obligatory "box" cut can be significant in smaller sized femurs especially is TKA systems where the post remains a

---

[15] Collier JP, Mayor MB, McNamara JL, et al. Analysis of the failure of 122 polyethylene inserts from uncemented tibial knee components. Clin Orthop Relat Res 1991; 273:232-242.

[16] Kilgus DJ, Moreland JR, Finerman GA, et al. Catastrophic wear of tibial polyethylene inserts. Clin Orthop Relat Res 1991; 273:223-231.

[17] Waslewski GL, Marson BM, Benjamin JB. Early, incapacitating instability of posterior cruciate ligament-retaining total knee arthroplasty. J Arthroplasty 1998; 13:763-767.

[18] Puloski SK, McCalden RW, MacDonald SJ, et al. Tibial post wear in posterior stabilized total knee arthroplasty. An unrecognized source of polyethylene debris. J Bone Joint Surg Am 2001; 83A:390-397.

[19] Dolan MM, Kelly NH, Nguyen JT, Wright TM, Haas SB. Implant design influences tibial post wear damage in posterior-stabilized knees. Clin Orthop Relat Res. 2011 Jan;469(1):160-7.

constant size for each femoral component size.[20] The consequence is that there will be a relatively large notch cut for a small femoral component greatly weakening the condyle and increasing the risk of femoral condyle bone loss and periprosthetic fracture. Surgeons who chose to use posterior stabilized TKA should familiarize themselves with relative "box" cut volume to avoid intra-operative and post-operative periprosthetic fractures, especially in small, osteoporotic femurs.

4.3 Patellar clunk

Patella clunk is a complication that is more prevalent in posterior stabilized TKA designs. A prominent fibrous nodule can form at the junction of the proximal patellar pole and the quadriceps tendon. During deep flexion, this fibrous nodule can "catch" in the intercondylar notch of the femoral component causing a catching sensation on the end of the groove as the patella moves back with knee extension. It is this catching and then forceful release with extension that results in the "clunk" and pain characteristic of this condition.[21] Recommended treatment consists of physical therapy and arthroscopic debridement. Arthrotomy and possible revision surgery is reserved for recurrent clunks, malposition or loose components.[22]

4.4 Tibio-femoral dislocations

One of the disadvantages of posterior stabilized TKA is the potential for dislocation in flexion as the tibial post rides underneath the femoral cam. This occurs when there is significant extension-flexion gap mismatch. More specifically, dislocations occur when the flexion gap is larger than the corresponding extension gap, allowing the post to "jump" over the cam. The incidence of dislocation with posterior stabilized TKA is very rare with modern designs (0.2%).[23] To prevent knee dislocation it is mandatory that the surgeon balance the knee both in flexion and extension. When dislocation occurs, closed and sometimes open reduction is required. If recurrent dislocation occurs, revision surgery to correct flexion extension mismatch is imperative.

5. Alternative to cam post design

The "deep-dish" tibial insert, introduced by Hoffman et al in 2000, is an alternative to the cam post posterior stabilized TKA design. This type of design eliminated the need for resection of the intercondylar notch bone stock and use of a tibial post. AP stability is achieved by using highly conforming tibial inserts with anterior build-up[24]. Some advantages of this ultra-congruent design include: bone preservation by eliminating the

[20] Haas S, Nelson C, Laskin R. Posterior stabilized TKA: an assessment of bone resection. The Knee 2000; 7: 25-29.

[21] Hozack WJ, Rothman RH, Booth RE Jr, Balderston RA. The patellar clunk syndrome. A complication of posterior stabilized total knee arthroplasty. Clin Orthop Relat Res 1989; 241:203-208.

[22] Beight JL, Yao B, Hozack WJ, et al. The patellar 'clunk' syndrome after posterior stabilized total knee arthroplasty. Clin Orthop Relat Res 1994; 299:139-142.

[23] Lombardi AV Jr, Mallory TH, Vaughn BK, et al. Dislocation following primary posterior-stabilized total knee arthroplasty. J Arthroplasty 1993; 8:633-639.

[24] Hofmann AA, Tkach TK, Evanich CJ, Camargo MP: Posterior stabilization in total knee arthroplasty with use of an ultracongruent polyethylene insert. J Arthroplasty 2000;15:576-583

need for box cut, elimination of post breakage and wear, elimination of tibio-femoral dislocation and patella clunk syndrome. In addition, the ultracongruent tibial component has the advantage of distributing the loads over a larger surface area of the polyethylene insert, hypothetically limiting and distributing more evenly the loads at the bone—implant interface. Moreover, because femoral box preparation is eliminated, femoral bone stock is preserved, decreasing the potential for fracture and operative time.[25] Several studies comparing the stability, range of motion and stair climbing ability found no significant difference with ultracongruent design TKA when compared to traditional cam post design TKA.

6. Outcomes

Despite the dissimilarities between cruciate retaining and posterior stabilized TKA designs, most comparative studies have found no significant differences in function, patient satisfaction, or survivorship of the two designs in unselected patient cohorts.[26] We have divided the reported results after posterior stabilized TKA into specific outcomes to facilitate the review. Specific outcomes include the performance of posterior stabilized TKA designs in terms of proprioception, wear, loosening, and stability. Also the results with the use of posterior stabilized TKA in two particular subgroups of patients: varus-flexion deformity and postpatellectomy are included in this section.

7. Proprioception

Proprioception after TKA may be improved with the preservation of the native PCL. Mechanoreceptors have been identified in the native posterior cruciate ligament may aid in feedback mechanism improving proprioception.[27] Hystological analysis, however, suggests that marked neurologic degeneration occurs within the posterior cruciate ligament as part of the arthritic process [13]. Clinical studies are not conclusive as to which implant design has better proprioception. Warren et al. [14] observed that proprioception improved after TKA with either a posterior stabilized or cruciate retaining design, but suggested that greater improvement occurred in the cruciate retaining group. In contrast, Simmons et al. [15] noted that in patients with severe arthritis better postoperative proprioception was obtained with a posterior stabilized TKA. Becker et al. [16] compared patients with bilateral paired cruciate retaining and posterior stabilized TKA. Fifty percent of the patients were unable to express a preference for one knee or the other. The other 50% were equally divided between those who preferred the cruciate retaining and those who preferred the posterior stabilized knee. Most recently Swanik et al. [17] performed a prospective, randomized study on 20 patients to assess proprioception, kinesthesia, and balance following TKA comparing posterior stabilized

[25] Laskin RS, Maruyama Y, Villaneuva M, Bourne R. Deep-dish congruent tibial component use in total knee arthroplasty: a randomized prospective study. Clin Orthop Relat Res. 200 Nov;(380):36-44.

[26] Jacobs WC, Clement DJ, Wymenga AB. Retention versus removal of the posterior cruciate ligament in total knee replacement: a systematic literature review within the Cochrane framework. Acta Orthop 2005; 76:757-768.

[27] Warren PJ, Olanlokun TK, Cobb AG, Bentley G. Proprioception after knee arthroplasty: the influence of prosthetic design. Clin Orthop Relat Res. 1993;297:182-187.

versus cruciate retaining designs Joint position sense, the threshold to detect joint motion, and the patient's ability to balance on an unstable platform were assessed prior to and at least 6 months after the operation. They found that after TKA all patients detected motion significantly faster, reproduced joint position with less error and had balance improvement. The group treated with the posterior stabilized TKA more accurately reproduced joint position when the knee was extended from a flexed position. The authors conclude that retention of the PCL does not appear to improve proprioception and balance.

7.1 Loosening
At long-term follow-up there appears to be no significant difference in the aseptic loosening rates of posterior stabilized and cruciate retaining TKA designs. The cemented posterior stabilized TKA has a reported 98.1% survival rate at 14 years [19]. In the most recent study Rasquinha et al. [20••] reported the long-term results of a series of 150 consecutive posterior stabilized TKA that were performed in 118 patients They found a good to excellent result in 90% of patients at mean follow-up of 12 years. At 12 years, the survival rate was 94.6 ± 4.0% with failure for any reason as the end point and 98.3 ± 2.4% with mechanical failure as the end point. Revision surgery was necessary in five cases: two because of infection, one for dislocation and two for polyethylene wear and osteolysis.

7.2 Stability
As mentioned above with posterior stabilized TKA if the knee is not properly balanced dislocation in flexion can occur. This a very rare event, and can be avoided with careful balancing of the flexion and extension gaps. In terms of instability, posterior or flexion instability may in fact be a greater, although less recognized, problem with cruciate retaining TKA designs. Rupture of the PCL after surgery can cause pain and disability. Flexion instability can also result when the flexion space is left too loose, resulting in marked anterior-posterior translation of the tibia on the femur in flexion. Pagnano et al. [21] reported on 25 cruciate retaining TKAs treated for flexion instability. These patients presented with a typical constellation of symptoms that included a sense of knee instability without true give-way, recurrent knee joint effusions, and anterior knee pain. On exam, these knees had obvious anteroposterior instability when tested at 90° of flexion, and even demonstrated a marked posterior sag sign. They all underwent revision surgery to a posterior stabilized design and 22 of the 25 had significant symptomatic improvement after revision surgery.

7.3 Correction of deformity
Most series of patients with varus deformities have shown excellent results after 10-15 years, with either cruciate retaining or posterior stabilized TKA. There is, however, only one comparative study [22] that evaluated the results of cruciate retaining and posterior stabilized implants in the context of severe varus or varus-flexion deformities. In this series, survivorship, range of motion, and pain-related outcomes were worse in patients with fixed varus (or varus-flexion) deformities over 15° who were treated with cruciate retaining devices, compared with patients treated with posterior stabilized implants or with those who did not have such varus deformities and were treated with cruciate retaining devices.

7.4 Postpatellectomy patients

Most authors suggest that a posterior stabilized design is most appropriate in patients with previous patellectomy. The tibial post and femoral cam mechanism limits the posterior translation of the tibia that can occur without the patella. Patellectomy leads to the disruption of the normal kinematics of the knee. In the context of knee replacement, it has been hypothesized that loads on the PCL in the years following surgery may be increased, potentially resulting in late attenuation and instability [23,24]. Patellectomy also can cause decreased extensor mechanism power because of the loss of the fulcrum provided by the intact patella. A retrospective study showed that patellectomized patients treated with posterior stabilized implants had better functional and pain scores than did those treated with cruciate retaining implants [23]. In comparison to cruciate retaining designs, posterior stabilized devices lead to better results when TKA is performed in patients with prior patellectomies [25].

8. Rheumatoid arthritis

Total knee arthroplasty is a proven technique for the management of deformity and unremitting pain in the rheumatoid arthritic knee. Many important considerations must be taken into account in order to maximize the results of total knee replacement in this challenging patient population. In a retrospective study, Laskin et al[28] reported that cruciate retaining implants in patients with rheumatoid arthritis were associated with inferior results compared with posterior stabilized implants, principally because of late instability and progressive recurvatum deformity. The tendency for generalized ligamentous laxity and attenuation and joint deformity in these patients make successful TKA difficult with PCL retaining designs. These patients may present with severe or fixed valgus deformities. Most patients with rheumatoid arthritis typically have poor quality of the soft tissues and the potential for synovitis to cause late attenuation and rupture of the PCL.

9. Conclusion

The use of posterior stabilized TKA has several advantages. Potential benefits of a posterior stabilized TKA over a cruciate retaining TKA include easier surgical exposure and ligament balancing, predictable restoration of knee kinematics, improved range of motion, less wear, and avoiding the possibility of PCL rupture. In addition, the use of posterior stabilized TKA appears to be advantageous in correction of severe varus – valgus deformity. A potential problem with posterior stabilized TKA is tibial post polyethylene wear from the cam-post mechanism. Excessive wear can lead not only to osteolysis but also post fracture. Other disadvantage of posterior stabilized TKA is patellar 'clunk' syndrome, risk of dislocation or flexion instability and bone loss and peri-prosthetic condylar fracture. Despite the dissimilarities between cruciate retaining and posterior stabilized TKA designs, most studies have found no significant differences in function, patient satisfaction, or survivorship of the two designs in unselected patient cohorts. Posterior stabilized TKA outcomes appear to be better in a particular subgroup of patients including patients with patellectomy, large varus or varus-flexion deformity, and rheumatoid arthritis.

---

[28] Laskin RS, O'Flynn HM. The Insall Award. Total knee replacement with posterior cruciate ligament retention in rheumatoid arthritis: Problems and complications. Clin Orthop 1997; 345:24-28.

10. References

[1] Stiehl JB, Komistek RD, Dennis DA, et al. Fluoroscopic analysis of kinematics after posterior cruciate retaining knee arthroplasty. J Bone Joint Surg Br 1995; 77B:884-889.

[2] Dennis DA, Komistek RD, Hoff WA. In vivo knee kinematics derived using an inverse perspective technique. Clin Orthop 1996; 331:107-117.

[3] Ranawat CS, Komistek RD, Rodriguez JA, et al. In vivo kinematics for fixed and mobile-bearing posterior stabilized knee prostheses. Clin Orthop Relat Res 2004; 418:184-190.

[4] Jacobs WC, Clement DJ, Wymenga AB. Retention versus removal of the posterior cruciate ligament in total knee replacement: a systematic literature review within the Cochrane framework. Acta Orthop 2005; 76:757-768.

[5] Collier JP, Mayor MB, McNamara JL, et al. Analysis of the failure of 122 polyethylene inserts from uncemented tibial knee components. Clin Orthop Relat Res 1991; 273:232-242.

[6] Kilgus DJ, Moreland JR, Finerman GA, et al. Catastrophic wear of tibial polyethylene inserts. Clin Orthop Relat Res 1991; 273:223-231.

[7] Waslewski GL, Marson BM, Benjamin JB. Early, incapacitating instability of posterior cruciate ligament-retaining total knee arthroplasty. J Arthroplasty 1998; 13:763-767.

[8] Puloski SK, McCalden RW, MacDonald SJ, et al. Tibial post wear in posterior stabilized total knee arthroplasty. An unrecognized source of polyethylene debris. J Bone Joint Surg Am 2001; 83A:390-397.

[9] Hozack WJ, Rothman RH, Booth RE Jr, Balderston RA. The patellar clunk syndrome. A complication of posterior stabilized total knee arthroplasty. Clin Orthop Relat Res 1989; 241:203-208.

[10] Beight JL, Yao B, Hozack WJ, et al. The patellar 'clunk' syndrome after posterior stabilized total knee arthroplasty. Clin Orthop Relat Res 1994; 299:139-142.

[11] Lombardi AV Jr, Mallory TH, Vaughn BK, et al. Dislocation following primary posterior-stabilized total knee arthroplasty. J Arthroplasty 1993; 8:633-639.

[12] Fantozzi S, Catani F, Ensini A, et al. Femoral rollback of cruciate-retaining and posterior-stabilized total knee replacements: in vivo fluoroscopic analysis during activities of daily living. J Orthop Res 2006; 24:2222-2229.

[13] Kleinbart FA, Bryk E, Evangelista J, et al. Histologic comparison of posterior cruciate ligaments from arthritic and age matched knee specimens. J Arthroplasty 1996; 6:726-731.

[14] Warren PI, Olanlokun TK, Cobb AG, Bentley G. Proprioception after knee arthroplasty: The influence of prosthetic design. Clin Orthop 1993; 297:182-187.

[15] Simmons S, Lephart S, Rubash H, et al. Proprioception after unicondylar knee arthroplasty versus total knee arthroplasty. Clin Orthop 1996; 331:179-184.

[16] Becker MW, Insall JN, Faris PM. Bilateral total knee arthroplasty: one cruciate retaining and one cruciate substituting. Clin Orthop 1990; 271:122-124.

[17] Swanik CB, Lephart SM, Rubash HE. Proprioception, kinesthesia, and balance after total knee arthroplasty with cruciate-retaining and posterior stabilized prostheses. J Bone Joint Surg Am 2004; 86A:328-334.

[18] Scott RD, Thornhill TS. Posterior cruciate supplementing total knee replacements using conforming inserts and cruciate recession: effect on range of motion and radiolucent lines. Clin Orthop 1994; 309:146-149.

[19] Colizza WA, Insall JN, Scuderi GR. The posterior stabilized total knee prosthesis: Assessment of polyethylene damage and osteolysis after a 10-year minimum follow-up. J Bone Joint Surg Am 1995; 77A:1713-1720.

[20] Rasquinha VJ, Ranawat CS, Cervieri CL, Rodriguez JA. The press-fit condylar modular total knee system with a posterior cruciate-substituting design. A concise follow-up of a previous report. J Bone Joint Surg Am 2006; 88A:1006-1010. This was a long-term follow-up study with 118 patients that had a posterior stabilized TKA.

[21] Pagnano MW, Hanssen AD, Stuart MJ, Lewallen DG. Flexion instability after primary posterior cruciate retaining total knee arthroplasty. Clin Orthop 1998; 356:39-46.

[22] Laskin RS. The Insall Award. Total knee replacement with posterior cruciate ligament retention in patients with a fixed varus deformity. Clin Orthop 1996; 331:29-34.

[23] Paletta GA Jr, Laskin RS. Total knee arthroplasty after a previous patellectomy. J Bone Joint Surg Am 1995; 77A:1708-1712.

[24] Cameron HU, Hu C, Vyamont D. Posterior stabilized knee prosthesis for total knee replacement in patients with prior patellectomy. Can J Surg 1996; 39:469-473.

[25] Bayne O, Cameron HU. Total knee arthroplasty following patellectomy. Clin Orthop 1984; 186:112-114.

[26] Laskin RS, O'Flynn HM. The Insall Award. Total knee replacement with posterior cruciate ligament retention in rheumatoid arthritis: Problems and complications. Clin Orthop 1997; 345:24-28.

3

Mobile Bearing Concept in Knee Arthroplasty

Nahum Rosenberg[1,2],
Arnan Greental[1] and Michael Soudry[1,2]
¹Orthopaedic Surgery "A" Dept.,
Rambam – Health Care Campus, Haifa
²Ruth and Bruce Rappaport Faculty of Medicine,
Technion – Israel Institute of Technology, Haifa
Israel

1. Introduction

The rationale for mobile bearing design of knee replacement prosthesis is to increase its survival by reducing the rate of aseptic loosening and to improve the range of movement of the treated knee. The theoretical basis for the achievement of the first goal is the expected lower rates of the polyethylene insert wear in the mobile design in comparison to a fixed design, due to lower contact and constraint forces. A better range of movements following mobile bearing arthroplasty is expected as the result of additional moving surface between to fixed planes at the ends of the articulating bones, allowing mobility with congruency.These expected advantages of the mobile bearing design should be judged cautiously since the initial mobile bearing implants caused higher rates of breakage and disarrangement of the polyethylene inserts, when the implantation method wasn't strictly followed. In order to resolve these technical problems the rotating platform mobile prosthesis was developed.

Mobile bearing concept was implemented in a three compartment replacement prostheses and also in unicompartamental designs, especially for the medial compartment of the knee. Currently, following the more than two decades of the rising experience with implantation of a large number of mobile bearing prostheses, there is a significant amount of data for evaluation of the survival of these prosthetic designs. In order to declare on their higher expected efficiency these implants should show higher than 96-97% of ten year clinical survival, which should remain relatively stable up to 20 years of follow up, as reported in the several of fixed bearing designs. Unfortunately this data is not readily available, because only few well designed survivorship reports on mobile knee implants have been published yet. Furthermore the published data failed to provide a clear evidence of the superiority of mobile bearing design.

The endoprosthetic arthroplasty is the most popular surgical modality for treatment of advanced knee joint disease, either degenerative or inflammatory. The reason for this clinical trend is the ability to reduce pain and to restore the patient's ability to walk.

Although it has been shown that the improvement in ambulation, following knee arthroplasty, is mostly subjective, because other restrictions of a capacity to walk might be revealed following elimination of the pain in the knee (1), the reduction of the pain level while walking is considered by the patients as a significant improvement in the quality of life. For this reason a major effort is exerted by the clinicians and the industry to develop the most effective surgical techniques and prosthetic designs aiming to improve immediate postsurgical outcome of knee prosthetic arthroplasty and the longevity of the implanted prostheses. Several of the currently used prosthetic designs have already reached long term, above 10 years, survivorship of above 95%, therefore the "straggle" for the improvement in the prostheses longevity is aimed to the marginal 5% improvement of long term survivorship following the implantation by reducing the prostheses failure rate in long time scale. The success of this multidisciplinary effort of clinicians and engineers can't be overemphasized because the success will not only eliminate the need for revision surgery in patients, who are mostly in the age above sixty years, because of the expected prostheses' longevity consideration, but also will provide a prosthetic solutions for the younger patients with degenerative knees, who seek for a better treatment modality for their disability.

Therefore logically the widely used generic design of unconstrained knee prosthesis, with metal femoral component and polyethylene insert fixed on metal back-plate on tibia, with cemented or cementless fixation into articulating surfaces, should be improved in one or in several of its components in order to improve its long term clinical performance . Clearly these considerations do not related to the short term prosthetic failures, which are mostly attributed to a basically fault prosthetic design, as observed in the early constrained prostheses (2), to deficient surgical technique or to a complicated general medical condition of the patient that might lead to the prosthesis disarrangement, peri-prosthetic fracture or local infection.

Long standing clinical success of prosthetic knee replacement is dependent on the ability to provide stability with good range of movement, to resist the loosening processes and to provide material longevity of all prosthetic components. Near satisfactory range of movement and stability have been successfully achieved with widely used fixed bearing designs, however, component loosening remains their main long term problem (3,4). Although the early loosening processes, common in the original constrained designs, have been eliminated in the second generation unconstrained prostheses, late loosening, due to osteolysis caused by polyethylene wear of the fixed tibial bearings, remains unresolved (5). Therefore it is logical that the main target that should be addresses in order to reduce the late aseptic loosening of the knee prostheses would be the polyethylene insert and its susceptibility for wear following long standing and continuous exposure to compressing forces from the adjacent metal components. One of the steps for reducing the polyethylene wear was directed to improve the material characteristics of the polyethylene in order to avoid the free radicals release during the gamma sterilization by using a manufacturer process with high temperature towards the melting point with crosslinking induction and generation of ultrahigh molecular weight polyethylene that reduces the plastic insert susceptibility to mechanical wear (6). A high level of crosslinking had been used in several acetabular polyethylene designs in the last decade and showed less surface wear but, on the other hand, presented alteration in the mechanical properties of the bearing insert. For this reason this method is of limited role in the knee prostheses.

Therefore other tribulogical factors should be addressed in order to reduce the cross shear and surface pressure of the polyethylene insert. High conformation between the femoral and tibial surfaces in the prosthesis can reduce the surface pressure and polyethylene wear. But in fixed bearing design the elevation of conformation causes restriction in the range of movement of the knee. Therefore in the fixed bearing prostheses some unconformity is deliberately allowed in order to provide a reasonable range of knee movement.

Another mechanical concept to reduce the bearing component wear, which is mainly induced by the high point and line contact forces between moving metal femoral component and static polyethylene tibial insert, has been developed . By this concept an "area" contact pattern has been introduced (7). The rationale of the "area" contact pattern is based on the assumption that the forces between the prostheses components may be distributed more efficiently by using a mobile bearing polyethylene insert (8). Subsequently the hypothetical advantage is in reduction of material wear and elimination of aseptic loosening (Figure 1).

According to this concept Pappas MJ and Buechel FF developed a total knee prosthesis with mobile bearing (7), and Goodfellow JW and O'Connor J developed the unicompartamental mobile bearing "Oxford Knee" design (9).

The expectation from the later unicompartamental design was to develop a prosthetic method that will replace the technically demanding osteotomies in younger patients with unicompartamental degenerative disease. This goal was achieved only partially, since the unicompartamental design could be successful only in patients who answer to the very strict clinical and radiographic criteria.

The former, LCS® mobile meniscal bearing total knee replacement system, has been designed to lower contact stress with preservation of the crucial low constraint properties. Initially after the introduction of this system for the widespread clinical use in 1977-80 one large multicenter (10) and three independent (11,12,13) middle term follow up studies have been published showing favorable subjective outcome results in 90-97.5% of patients with 94.6 – 95.3% of six to eight years survivorship of cementless LCS® mobile bearing posterior cruciate retaining prostheses. These outcome results are close to the survivorship data reported by the system designers, that showed 97.9% and 95.1% of five and twelve years survivorship rates respectively (14).

Conversely there have been a number of reports of high rate mechanical failures of the LCS® system (8,15). These short term follow up studies showed a tendency for mobile bearing dislocation and breakage. These findings can also be supported by cadaveric biomechanical testing (16). Thus the potential susceptibility of LCS® posterior cruciate retaining design for early mechanical failure may overcome the benefits of long term low loosening rates. In an additional later report on a medium term experience with 35 cementless LCS® mobile meniscal bearing total knee replacements in patients with osteoarthritis there was an evidence of 97.1% five year survivorship (17). This high survival rate, with a satisfactory functional outcome, at middle term follow up, has been achieved by following an optimal technique of implantation, according to the designers recommendations, i.e. the tibial component should be situated perpendicularly to

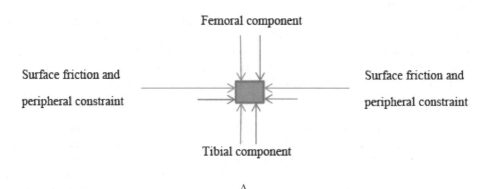

A

A: A schematic representation of vectors of forces on a unit of polyethylene tibial insert in a sagittal plane during knee loading. Blue arrows are the vectors of forces in fixed bearing design and red arrows in a mobile bearing insert, where less magnitude of force from the peripheral constrain should reduce the overall magnitude of force and to reduce the development of the polyethylene insert wear, as represented in B.

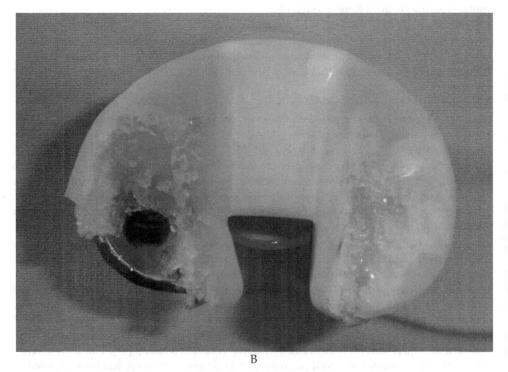

B

B: Reprehensive example of an advanced wear of a polyethylene insert of a fixed bearing design.

Fig. 1. Rationale for mobile bearing concept in knee arthroplasty prosthesis:

longitudinal axis of tibial metaphysis with 5 O - 10 O of posterior inclination relatively to the anatomical axis of tibia in the sagittal plane, the sagittal flexion angle of the femoral component should be close to 5 O relatively to the anatomical axis of femur and overall coronal alignment of the components should be around 5 O of valgus (18). The average three dimensional component alignment in this study group has not deviated more than 3 O from the recommended by the designers' optimal orientation. Therefore it might be suggested that the high survival rates of the prosthesis and good functional outcome in the majority of evaluated patients in this study should be attributed to the effective surgical technique. This was reflected by the satisfactory functional knee scores in 77% and complete pain elimination in 89% of the evaluated knees. Therefore there is evidence that in the middle term the mobile bearing design of total knee replacement can be as effective as the conventional fixed bearing designs. Additional reports on short and middle term outcome of knee replacement with LCS® mobile meniscal bearing cementless design revealed rates of aseptic loosening in the range of 0.4 - 1.8% (8,14), which are compatible with most of the effective fixed bearing designs (19). However, the real advantage of mobile bearing system in reducing the rate of osteolysis should be established in the long term survivorship studies.

The emerged susceptibility of mobile bearing meniscal surfaces to early failure due to dislocation or breakage (8) may provoke a reasonable hesitation to its widespread use. Although the designers of the LCS® mobile meniscal bearing prosthesis claimed that strict operative technique and precise prosthetic placement should avoid its mechanical failure (18), there are only few independent studies that support this claim by showing 0.6% rate of meniscal bearing failure in 2 - 10 years of follow up (13, 17). And on the other hand there is some evidence that greater deviation from the desired three dimensional placement of the mobile bearing prosthesis does not significantly reduce its 10 years survivorship and preferable functional outcome (20). Therefore there is no clear evidence of the precise precise factors contributing to the mobile inserts disarrangement.

In order to reduce the revealed possibility of mechanical failure of meniscal type mobile bearings, a more stable "rotating platform" mobile polyethylene bearing was designed. In this design a single polyethylene insert, without rotational constraint, was used. The rotating platform knee is assumed to follow the normal femoral rotation upon the tibial axis during knee flexion, which is normally between 16⁰-23⁰ degrees (21). But it was found that the measured rotation of the bearing surface in the implanted prostheses is significantly less than expected, e.g. only in 12% of the knees there was more than 10 degrees of rotation.

Additional theoretical advantage of a mobile bearing prosthesis is the expected better patellar tracking due to the self-alignment of the mobile bearing. But this assumption has not been proven in patients, because there was no clinical evidence of a diminished post-operative anterior knee pain even in the first year after surgery (22).

The cautious approach for the efficiency of mobile bearing prostheses is even supported by the results of their biomechanical testing. It has been shown by a simulator based experiment, utilizing six million cycles of repetitive testing of prosthesis movement of mobile bearing designs with rotating platform and one fixed bearing implant, that there was no difference in the amount of in vitro wear (23).

Therefore, according to the published data it is still unclear if the theoretical advantage of the mobile bearing design is reflected in the improved clinical outcome (24,25).

Furthermore a meta-analyses of 33 studies assessing 3532 operated knees failed to present an evidence of a better clinical outcome, including the complication rate, functional and radiological results, of the mobile bearing design for knee arthroplasty in a comparison to standard fixed bearing devices (26).

This disappointing fact is probably related to the original intention to improve the current fixed bearing design survival at its marginal failure occurrence part by addressing mostly the mechanics of the polyethylene bearing insert. It seems that the differences in the bearings' fixation shouldn't be addressed for this purpose, in spite of the theoretical mechanical advantage of the mobile bearing. This suggests that different innovative methods for improvement of the prosthetic longevity should be investigated. These methods will probably be related to the other mechanical or material components of the knee prosthesis design. On this stage there is no clear evidence that the mobile bearing concept of knee prosthesis has justified the advantageous theoretical expectation for its superiority over the fixed bearing implants.

2. References

[1] Rosenberg N, Nierenberg G, Lenger R, Soudry M. Walking ability following knee arthroplasty. A prospective pilot study of factors affecting the maximal walking distance in 18 patients before and six months after total knee arthroplasty. Knee, 2007; 14(6):489-92.

[2] Riley D, Woodyard JE. Long-term results of Geomedic total knee replacement. J Bone Joint Surg, 1985; 67B: 548-50.

[3] Wright TM, Bartel DL. The problem of surface damage in polyethylene total knee components. Clin Orthop, 1986;205: 67-74.

[4] Peters PC, Engh GA, Dwyer KA, Vinh TN. Osteolysis after total knee arthroplasty without cement. J Bone Joint Surg, 1992; 74A: 864-876.

[5] Ayers DC. Polyethylene wear and osteolysis following total knee replacement. Instr Course Lect 1997;46: 205-213

[6] Fisher JD, Jennings LM, Galvin AL, Jin ZM, Stone MH, Ingham E . 2009 Knee Society Presidential Guest Lecture: Polyethylene wear in total knees. Clin Orthop Relat Res, 2010; 468:12–18.

[7] Buechel FF, Pappas MJ. New Jersey low contact stress knee replacement system. Ten year evaluation of meniscal bearings. Orth Clin N Am, 1989;20(2): 147-177.

[8] Weaver JK, Derkash RS, Greenwald AS. Difficulties with bearing dislocation and breakage using a movable bearing total knee replacement system. Clin Orthop Relat Res , 1993; 290: 244-252.

[9] Goodfellow JW, O'Connor J. The mechanics of the knee and prosthesis design. J Bone Joint Surg, 1978; 60B: 864-876.

[10] Sorrells RB, Fenning JB, Davenport JM. Comparison of the clinical results and survivorship of noncemented cruciate sacrificing versus cruciate sparing total knee

replacements. Presented at The American Academy of Orthopaedic Surgeons, San Francisco, California, February 1993.

[11] Huang CH, Lee YM, Su RY, Lai JH. Clinical results of the New Jersey low contact stress knee arthroplasty with two to five years follow-up. J Orth Surg ROC, 1991;8: 295-299.

[12] Jordan LR, Olivo JL, Voorhorst PE. Survivorship analysis of cementless meniscal bearing total knee arthroplasty. Clin Orthop Relat Res, 1997; 338: 119-123.

[13] Keblish PA, Schrei C, Ward M. Evaluation of 275 low contact stress (LCS) total knee replacements with 2- to 8- year follow up. Orthopaedics, 1993;1(2): 168- 173.

[14] Buechel FF, Pappas MJ: Long-term survivorship analysis of cruciate-sparing versus cruciate sacrificing knee prostheses using meniscal bearings. Clin Orthop Relat Res, 1990; 260: 162-169.

[15] Bert JM. Dislocation/subluxation of meniscal bearing elements after New Jersey low-contact stress total knee arthroplasty. Clin Orthop Relat Res ,1990;254: 211-215.

[16] Matsuda S, Whiteside LA, White SE, McCarthy DS: Knee stability in meniscal bearing total knee arthroplasty. J Arthroplasty 1999;14: 82-90.

[17] Rosenberg N, Henderson I. Medium term outcome of the LCS cementless posterior cruciate retaining total knee replacements. Follow up and survivorship study of 35 operated knees. The Knee, 2001; 8(2): 123-128.

[18] Buechel FF. Letters to the editor. Clin Orthop Relat Res ,1991; 264: 309-311.

[19] Lemaire R. Will bearing mobility result in a decreased incidence of TKR loosening? J Bone Joint Surg , 1999; 81B(suppl 2): 127.

[20] Vogt JC, Saarbach C. LCS mobile-bearing total knee replacement. A 10-year's follow-up study. Orthop Traum: Surg Res, 2009;95:177-82.

[21] Wasielewski RC, Komistek RD, Zingde SM, Sheridan KC, Mahfouz MR. Lack of axial rotation in mobile-bearing knee designs. Clin Orthop Relat Res, 2008; 466:2662–8.

[22] Breugem SJM, Sierevelt IN, Schafroth MU, Blankevoort L, Schaap GR, van Dijk CN. Less anterior knee pain with a mobile-bearing prosthesis compared with a fixed-bearing prosthesis. Clin Orthop Relat Res ,2008; 466:1959–65.

[23] Haider H, Garvin K. Rotating Platform versus Fixed-bearing Total Knees. An In Vitro Study of Wear. Clin Orthop Relat Res. 2008; 466:2677–85.

[24] Smith H, Jan M, Mahomed NN, Davey JR,Gandhi R. Meta-analysis and systematic review of clinical outcomes comparing mobile bearing and fixed bearing total knee arthroplasty. J Arthroplasty, 2011 – *in press*

[25] Jacobs W, Anderson PG, van Limbeek J, Wymega AAB. Mobile bearing vs fixed bearing prostheses for total knee arthroplasty for post- operative functional status in patients with osteoarthritis and rheumatoid arthritis (Review). The Cochrane collaboration, 2008;(3):1-15.

[26] Smith TO, Ejtehadi F, Nichols R, Davies L, Donell ST, Hing CB. Clinical and radiological outcomes of fixed- versus mobile-bearing total knee replacement: a meta-analysis. Knee Surg Sports Traumatol Arthrosc, 2010;18(3):325-40.

4

The UniSpacer™: Correcting Varus Malalignment in Medial Gonarthrosis

Joern Bengt Seeger[1] and Michael Clarius[2]
[1]Center for Musculoskeletal Surgery, Charité - Universitätsmedizin Berlin,
Campus Charité Mitte (CCM), Berlin
[2]Department of Orthopaedic and Trauma Surgery,
Vulpius Klinik GmbH, Bad Rappenau
Germany

1. Introduction

The most commonly used operative treatments of osteoarthritis of the medial compartment of the knee joint, especially in younger patients, are arthroscopy, high tibial osteotomy (HTO) and unicompartmental knee arthroplasty (UKA). The last two procedures require resection of bone stock (Iorio & Healy, 2003).

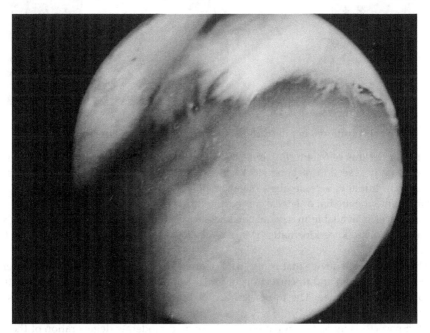

Fig. 1. Typical arthroscopic view of a patient with anteromedial osteoarthritis of the knee and degenerative lesion of the medial meniscus

A less invasive alternative to these procedures has been introduced in 2000 by Rick Hallock and Barry Fell: the UniSpacer™ implant (Zimmer, Inc., Warsaw, IN, USA), which is essentially a modern version of early metallic hemiarthroplasty as described by McKeever (McKeever, 1960) or MacIntosh (MacIntosh, 1958). However, due to a high failure rate between 16 and 44% as described by Bailie and Sisto, the implant is not available any more (Bailie et al., 2008; Sisto & Mitchel 2005).

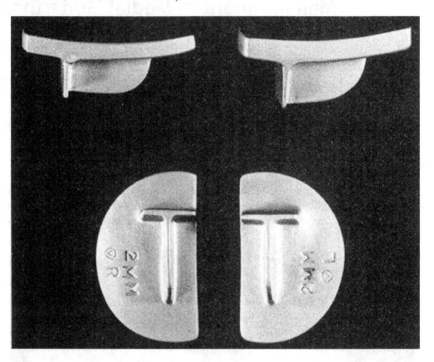

Fig. 2. Early interpositional hemiarthroplasty (Springer et al., 2006)

Implantation of this self-centering, one-piece interpositional device into the knee joint does not require any resection of bone stock and is performed via minimally-invasive surgery (Scott, 2003). Initially, a cementless metal or polyethylene interpositional device has been implanted into the medial or lateral compartment.

The Unispacer is available in several thicknesses (between 2 and 5 mm) and sizes (38 – 58 mm) and adapts to knee kinematics (Marx et al., 2009). There are special models for the left and ride side.

The UniSpacer™ is a device that is not fixed to any structures and therefore self-centering; it is used to relieve pain and to correct or minimize varus malalignment in unicompartmental osteoarthritis of the knee. The upper surface of the implant postoperatively adapts to the femoral condylus (Scott, 2003).

The UniSpacer™ is indicated in patients with isolated moderate degeneration of the medial compartment with minimal degeneration, and no significant loss of joint space in the patellofemoral compartment.

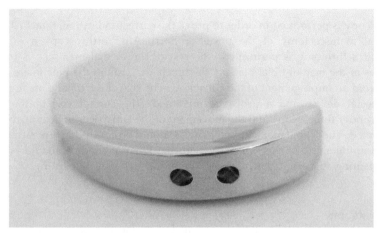

Fig. 3. UniSpacer™ metallic interpositional device

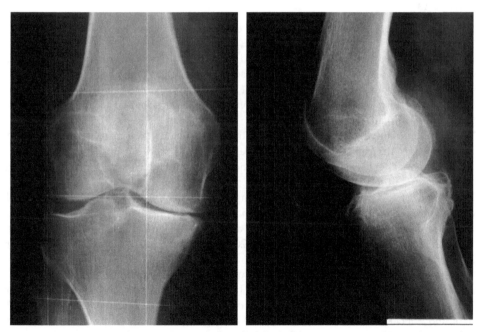

Fig. 4. and 5. Patient with medial osteoarthritis of the knee: a.p. stance and lateral view of the knee

Contraindications are inflammatory arthritis, severe instability due to advanced loss of osteochondral structure or the absence of collateral cruciate ligament integrity, as well as flexion/contracture greater than 15 degrees.

2. Operation technique (Hallock & Fell, 2003)

An arthroscopy is performed in order to prove the correct indication, intact ACL and PCL and medial meniscectomy of the posterior horn. After arthroscopy a 6-7cm medial parapatellar arthrotomy is performed. The rest of the medial meniscus is resected and osteophytes of the medial tibial plateau, the notch and around the patella are removed in order to avoid an impingement of the Unispacer. The size of the tibial plateau is measured with a special device and a probe is implanted. The correct size of the implant is controlled under fluoroscopy and the movement of the Unispacer in flexion and extension is documented. The whole medial tibial plateau should be covered in a.p. radiographs and a ventral impingement of the Unispacer with the femoral condyle should be ruled out. After implanting the original Unispacer, the wound closure is performed under usual conditions.

2.1 Rehabilitation

Weight bearing as tolerated can be performed with the use of crutches. A thrombosis prophylaxis is obligatory.

3. Results

The first results have been published by the designers group on 71 Unispacer knee system implants implanted in 67 patients. (Hallock & Fell, 2003).

The mean Knee Society knee score improved 169% in the 1-year group and 193% in the 2-year group. The mean Knee Society function score improved 31% and 65%, respectively. The mean Lysholm score improved 88% and 140%, respectively. Five implants (7%) were revised to total knee arthroplasty (TKA) and 10 implants (14%) were revised to another Unispacer Knee System implant.

Marx et al. implanted 14 Unispacer in 13 patients (4 women and 9 men). In 8 cases the left and in 6 cases the right knee joint was operated. There were no intra- or postoperative complications. There was no mobilization under anesthesia necessary. A dislocation of the spacer was not observed.

The notion of a self-centering mobile component correcting the varus knee internally without any need for bone resection has been, and still is, appealing. Clarius et al. evaluated clinical and radiological results and whether appropriate alignment change can be achieved by UniSpacer™ implantation (Clarius et al., 2003). In addition they examined the alignment change in the first 5 years after surgery.

In a retrospective study, 18 patients (19 legs) presenting with moderate stage isolated medial gonarthrosis, who had received UniSpacer™ hemiarthroplasty between 2002 and 2004, were assessed (implant thickness: 2, 3 or 4 mm); one patient received bilateral implantation; 12 right and 7 left knees had been treated. The average age of the patients (7 women and 11 men) at the time of surgery was 60.8 (48 to 72) years.

The clinical scores (Lysholm, AKS knee and function) preoperatively and at 1-, 2- and 5 year follow-up are shown in tab. 1.

Only 15 legs could be evaluated, as 4 patients had undergone revision UKA or TKA due to persistent pain. Average time to revision for the knees revised to TKA or UKA was 23.8 (±18.0) months. So far, no dislocations have been observed in this study.

Clinical Scores	preoperative	1 year postop.	2 years postop.	5 years postop
Lysholm	59.1	85.4	90.2	97.2
AKS knee	60.1	87.4	88.7	96.6
AKS function	70.0	93.8	98.5	96.4

Table 1. Clinical scores preoperative, at 1 year-, 2 year- and 5 year follow-up

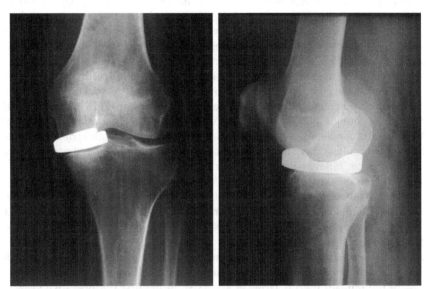

Fig. 6. and 7. Postoperative implant position

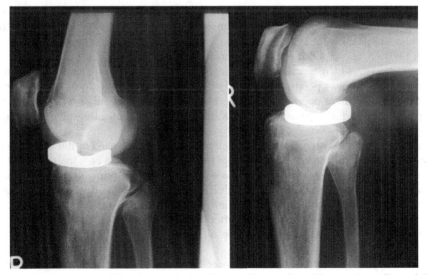

Fig. 8. and 9. Movement of the device during flexion due to the self-centering effect of the Unispacer

4. Conclusion

The use of HTO in the treatment of symptomatic varus malaligned knees has been propagated and thoroughly documented for several decades: it is a well-established therapeutic option (Nelissen et al., 2009). UKA has recently experienced a renewal of interest, with improved prostheses and techniques used. There have been reports of good long-term results for these methods. However, both can lead to distinct issues patients may be troubled with over the course of time. UKA comes with loss of bone matter in the medial compartment and, if conversion to TKA becomes necessary, bone grafts or metal wedge augmentation might be required in some cases (Springer et al., 2006).

Hemiarthroplasty with metallic interpositional devices, while first described over half a century ago, is also currently experiencing a renaissance as a treatment option of varus unicompartmental OA, the idea being to provide a means of treatment that minimizes the disadvantages of other procedures. It is used in cases where HTO is contraindicated or patients are too young for TKA. The ConforMIS iForma™ device, following the MacIntosh and McKeever rationale in being functionally fixed to the tibial surface, has had one favorable review; altogether, there are still few reports examining the use of the self-centering UniSpacer™ device in medial gonarthrosis.

Use of the UniSpacer™ in unicompartmental OA was initially recommended for young and active patients (Hallock & Fell, 2003). The role of this procedure still is not certain as it has been considered suitable for only few patients (1%) (Scott & Deshmukh, 2005) and there have been reports of poor postoperative results due to implant dislocation (up to 44%) (Bailie et al., 2005; Sisto & Mitchell, 2005).

Clarius et al. showed in their study a significant, slightly over-adjusting, correction of moderate varus alignment by UniSpacer™ arthroplasty, which does not correlate with the thickness of the implant used (Clarius et al., 2003). In the first postoperative year, a varus shift into a more neutral position could be observed, which is most likely due to adaptation of the implant to the joint. This effect is partly reversed in the following years by another slight valgus change, resulting, 5 years after surgery, in an average leg axis close to the one first achieved by UniSpacer™ implantation.

A high revision rate of 4 out of 19 UniSpacer™ implants in the first 5 postoperative years has been shown, which is unacceptably high compared to other treatment options. The reason for revision was persistent pain. There were no cases of dislocations. All revisions were technically easy to operate and uncomplicated. In all cases either UKA (2) or TKA (2) was performed and the patients were satisfied with the clinical results achieved after revision.

Looking at the high revision rates of the UniSpacer implant reported in the literature and in our study this metallic interposition arthroplasty does not seem to be a treatment option for patients with medial osteoarthritis of the knee. As there are reproducible good and excellent clinical and functional results reported with UKA after 10-15 years this operation should be preferred. However the clinical results of our remaining 14 patients with 15 operated knees were good and comparable to patients after UKA. Similar to the results of the metallic interpositional device of Mc Keever good results can be possible however the results are not predictable.

As a minimally invasive procedure, UniSpacer™ arthroplasty was seen as an alternative for treatment of varus malaligned knees in isolated medial gonarthrosis, due to good revision and conversion options.

5. References

Bailie AG, Lewis PL, Brumby SA et al (2008) The Unispacer knee implant: early clinical results. *J Bone Joint Surg Br* 90(4), pp. 446-450

Cooke TD, Li J, Scudamore RA (1994) Radiographic assessment of bony contributions to knee deformity. *Orthop Clin North Am* 25(3), pp. 387-393

Cooke TD, Scudamore RA, Bryant JT et al (1991) A quantitative approach to radiography of the lower limb. Principles and applications. *J Bone Joint Surg Br* 73-B(5), pp. 715-720

Cooke TD, Scudamore RA, Li J et al (1997) Axial lower-limb alignment: comparison of knee geometry in normal volunteers and osteoarthritis patients. *Osteoarthritis Cartilage* 5(1), pp. 39-47

Coventry MB, Ilstrup DM, Wallrichs SL (1993) Proximal tibial osteotomy. A critical long-term study of eighty-seven cases. *J Bone Joint Surg Am* 75(2), pp. 196-201

Deshmukh RV, Scott RD (2001) Unicompartmental Knee Arthroplasty: Long-Term Results. *Clin Orthop Relat Res* 392, pp. 272-278

Hallock RH, Fell BM (2003) Unicompartmental Tibial Hemiarthroplasty. Early Results of the UniSpacer(TM) Knee. *Clin Orthop Relat Res* 416, pp. 154-163

Hernigou P, Medevielle D, Debeyre J et al (1987) Proximal tibial osteotomy for osteoarthritis with varus deformity. A ten to thirteen-year follow-up study. *J Bone Joint Surg Am* 69(3), pp. 332-354

Insall JN, Joseph DM, Msika C (1984) High tibial osteotomy for varus gonarthrosis. A long-term follow-up study. *J Bone Joint Surg Am* 66(7), pp. 1040-1048

Iorio R, Healy WL (2003) Unicompartmental Arthritis of the Knee. *J Bone Joint Surg Am* 85(7), pp. 1351-1364

Kennedy WRMD, White RPMD (1987) Unicompartmental Arthroplasty of the Knee Postoperative Alignment and its Influence on Overall Results. *Clin Orthop Relat Res* 221, pp. 278-285

Koeck F, Perlick L, Luring C et al (2009) Leg axis correction with ConforMIS iForma™ (interpositional device) in unicompartmental arthritis of the knee. *Int Orthop* 33(4), pp. 955-960

MacIntosh DL (1958) Hemiarthroplasty of the knee using a space occupying prosthesis for painful varus and valgus deformities. In: of the Joint Meeting of the Orthopaedic Associations of the English-Speaking World. *J Bone Joint Surg Am* 40(6), pp. 1428-1441

McKeever DC (1960) Tibial plateau prosthesis. *Clin Orthop Relat Res* 18, pp. 86-95

Moreland JR, Bassett LW, Hanker GJ (1987) Radiographic analysis of the axial alignment of the lower extremity. *J Bone Joint Surg Am* 69(5), pp. 745-749

Scott RD (2003) UniSpacer: insufficient data to support its widespread use. *Clin Orthop Relat Res* 416, pp. 164-166

Scott RD (2003) UniSpacer(TM): Insufficient Data to Support its Widespread Use. *Clin Orthop Relat Res* 416, pp.164-166

Scott RD, Deshmukh RV (2005) Metallic hemiarthroplasty of the knee. *Curr Opin Orthop* 16(1), pp. 35-37

Sisto DJ, Mitchell IL (2005) UniSpacer Arthroplasty of the Knee. *J Bone Joint Surg Am* 87(8), pp. 1706-1711

Springer BD, Scott RD, Thornhill TS (2006) Conversion of Failed Unicompartmental Knee Arthroplasty to TKA. *Clin Orthop Relat Res* 446, pp. 214-220

Tunggal JA, Higgins GA, Waddell JP (2009) Complications of closing wedge high tibial osteotomy. *Int Orthop* 10.1007/s00264-009-0819-9

Whiteside LA (2005) Making Your Next Unicompartmental Knee Arthroplasty Last: Three Keys to Success. *The Journal of Arthroplasty* 20 (Supplement 2), pp. 2-3

5

Soft Tissue Balance in Total Knee Arthroplasty

Tomoyuki Matsumoto[1], Hirotsugu Muratsu[2], Seiji Kubo[1],
Masahiro Kurosaka[1] and Ryosuke Kuroda[1]
[1]Department of Orthopaedic Surgery, Kobe University Graduate School of Medicine, Kobe
[2]Department of Orthopaedic Surgery, Nippon Steel Hirohata Hospital, Himeji
Japan

1. Introduction

The primary goal of total knee arthroplasties (TKAs) is the achievement of stable tibiofemoral and patellofemoral (PF) joints, which relies on accurately aligning these joint components and balancing the soft tissues. In order to achieve these criteria, it is important to utilize appropriate surgical techniques and well-designed implants [1-3]. To this end, using the more traditional intra- and extra-medullary alignment devices, the proper alignment of each joint component further relies on performing accurate femoral and tibial osteotomies along ideal levels and angles. Recently, computer-assisted and robot-assisted surgeries have been developed and reported to improve the accuracy of osteotomies in TKA [4-7]. We similarly reported on a CT-free navigation system which significantly improved the accuracy of implantations in relation to the mechanical axis, and achieved an early and mid-term clinical outcome equivalent to that of a manual group [8-10].

In contrast, the management of soft tissue balance during surgery remains difficult, leaving much to the surgeon's subjective feel. TKA is a well-established procedure, which generally results in relief of pain, improved physical function, and a high level of patient satisfaction. However, knee instability after primary TKA is considered an important factor for early TKA failure. Fehring et al. studied 279 revision surgeries within 5 years of their index arthroplasty and reported 74 revision cases (27%) caused by instability [11]. In a retrospective study of revision surgery, Sharkey et al. reported instability in 21.2% of their early revision knee arthroplasty failures [12]. They concluded that the instability might be due to inadequate correction of soft tissue imbalances in both the sagittal and coronal planes. As a result, soft tissue balancing has been recognized as an essential surgical intervention for improving the outcomes of TKA.

2. Traditional soft tissue balance assessment

Although several methods and devices for assessing soft tissue balance such as manual distraction [13], traditional tensor [13], space block [14], and lamina spreaders [15] have been described in previous papers, assessment has not been quantitative and has mainly depended on the subjective feeling of the surgeons. The second generation of tensor devices which were quantitatively applied and objective with the measurement under fixed torque or load were commercially available [16-20] or individually developed or modified [21-24].

Asano et al. [25] used a commercially available tensor combined with their original measured torque-driver was and were able to measure the load at every 1 mm interval of gap distance. However, their method could only be used for measurement with an everted, and thereby unphysiological, patellar orientation, without the prosthesis, and only at extension or 90° of flexion.

D'Lima DD et al. developed a knee arthroplasty tibial tray with force transducers and a telemetry system to directly measure tibiofemoral compressive forces in vivo [26, 27]. From 1996, the study group spent time refining manufacturing techniques, improving durability, and safety testing and then reported the first electronic knee prosthesis implant in 2004. Recently, they summarized the design, development, and in vivo use of two generations of electronic knee prosthesis with activities of daily living, rehabilitation, exercise, and athletic activities from their many studies [28]. Although this device provides a lot of useful information on kinematics after TKA, it is too specialized and expensive for routine clinical use. The implantable tibial tray with force transducers and telemetry system is useful for research, but needs a bulky implant with an extension stem-like structure, and cannot be used with other TKA systems, limiting to the population used.

3. New soft tissue balance assessment with offset type tensor

3.1 Design and parameters

In order to permit soft tissue balancing under more physiological conditions, in a surgeon friendly manner, we developed a new third-generation tensor to obtain soft tissue balancing throughout the range of motion with reduced patella-femoral (PF) and aligned tibiofemoral joints [29]. The offset type tensor consists of three parts: an upper seesaw plate, a lower platform plate with a spike and an extra-articular main body (Fig 1). Both plates are placed at the center of the knee, and we apply one of two tensioning devices that are catered to appropriately fit either a cruciate-retaining (CR) or a posterior-stabilized (PS) TKA. The PS TKA tensor consists of a seesaw plate with a proximal post along the center that fits the inter-condylar space, as well as a cam for the femoral trial prosthesis. This post and cam mechanism controls the tibiofemoral position in both the coronal and sagittal planes. The CR TKA tensor consists of a seesaw plate with a proximal convex shaped centralizer that fits the inter-condylar space and controls coronal joint alignment. These mechanisms permit us to reproduce the joint constraint and alignment after implanting the prostheses. This device is ultimately designed to permit surgeons to measure the ligament balance in varus and joint center/joint component gap, while applying a constant joint distraction force. Joint distraction forces ranging from 30lb (13.6 kg) to 80lb (36.3 kg) can be exerted between the seesaw and platform plates through a specially made torque driver which can change the applied torque value. After sterilization, this torque driver is placed on a rack that contains a pinion mechanism along the extra-articular main body, and the appropriate torque is applied to generate the designated distraction force; in preliminary *in-vitro* experiments, we obtained an error for joint distraction within ± 3 %. Once appropriately distracted, attention is focused on two scales that correspond to the tensor: the angle (°, positive value in varus ligament balance) between the seesaw and platform plates, and the distance (mm) between the center midpoints of upper surface of the seesaw plate and the proximal tibial cut (mm, joint center/joint component gap). By measuring these angular deviations and distances under a constant joint distraction force, we are able to measure the ligament balance and joint center/joint component gaps, respectively.

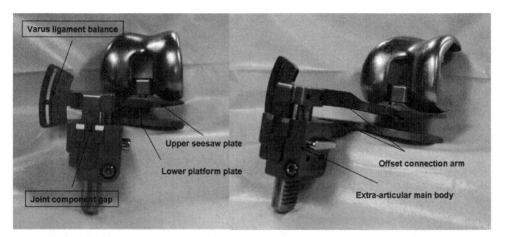

Fig. 1. Offset type tensor
The tensor consists of three parts: upper seesaw plate, lower platform plate and extra-articular main body. Two plates are connected to the extra-articular main body by the offset connection arm.

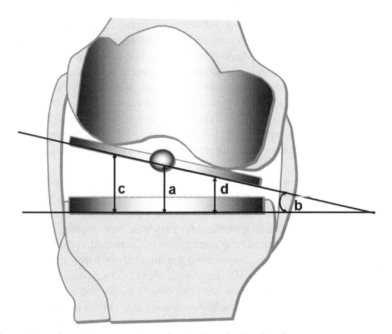

Fig. 2. Illustration showing parameters obtained and calculated.
a. Joint center gap/ joint component gap.
b. Varus ligament balance/ varus angle.
c. Lateral compartment gap
d. Medial compartment gap

Using the tensor, the following parameters can be calculated from the values: *joint component gap (joint center gap)* and *varus ligament balance (varus angle)* (Fig 2).

Joint looseness = "Component gap" – "Insert thickness"

Medial compartment gap = "Component gap" – 0.5× "Width between medial and lateral apex of femoral component representing the contact points to polyethylene insert" ×sin(varus angle)

Lateral compartment gap = "Component gap" + 0.5× "Width between medial and lateral apex of femoral component representing the contact points to polyethylene insert" ×sin(varus angle)

3.2 Soft tissue balance with reduced PF joint

We reported our experience using this device for intra-operative measurement with the PS TKA and further discussed the clinical relevance of this tensor [30-32]. First, we reported joint component gap kinematics in PS TKA with and without patellar eversion. The component gap showed an accelerated decrease during full knee extension. With the PF joint everted, the component gap increased throughout knee flexion. In contrast, the component gap with the PF joint reduced increased with knee flexion but decreased after 60° of flexion [30]. Secondly, we reported that intra-operative joint component gap kinematic assessment with reduced PF joint has the possibility to predict the post-operative flexion angle and thus allows evaluation of the surgical technique throughout the range of knee motion. Both an increased value during the extension to flexion gap and a decreased value during the flexion to deep flexion gap with PF joint reduced, not everted, showed an inverse correlation with the post-operative knee flexion angle, not pre-operative flexion angle [31]. Thirdly, we demonstrated that the correlations between the soft tissue balance assessed by the tensor and the navigation system were higher with reduced PF joint than everted PF joint, suggesting that surgeons should assess soft tissue balance during PS TKA with the PF joint reduced when using a navigation system [32]. In a series of intraoperative soft tissue balance assessments, we emphasized the importance of maintaining a reduced and anatomically oriented PF joint in order to obtain accurate and more physiologically-relevant soft tissue balancing.

Recent studies have emphasized the importance of the physiological post-operative knee condition in assessing soft tissue balance with PF joint reduction and femoral trial replacement in place [33-35]. Using our tensor with a 5-mm-long minute uniaxial foil strain gauge, Gejyo et al. reported a similar kinematic pattern of intra-operative joint component gap; when the patella was reduced, the joint gap was decreased at 90 and 135 degrees of flexion (by 1.9 mm and 5.5 mm, respectively) compared with the gap with the patella everted. Patellar tendon strain at 90 degrees of flexion, increasing with knee flexion, correlated with the joint gap difference with the patella in everted and reduced positions. Based on their study, they concluded the knee extensor mechanism might have an influence on the joint gap and be important in achieving the optimal joint gap balance during TKA [33]. With the use of an original tensor device which can measure the load of the spread joint gap, Yoshino et al. reported a significant difference between the loads in the patella everted position and thr reset position in flexion, not in extension, in PS TKA. However, in CR-TKA, they reported no significant difference between the loads in patella everted position and in patella reset position at either extension or flexion. Therefore, they concluded that the load in the flexion gap will increase in PS TKA or, in other words, the flexion gap distance will decrease by resetting [34]. With the use of an offset type tensor which has been developed based on our tensor, Kamei et al. reported a joint gap size and inclination measured intraoperatively on a knee in 90° flexion, with and without patellar eversion [35]. In the condition after tibial and distal femoral cut, they showed that the joint gap with patella in situ (17.0±3.4 mm) was significantly greater than with patellar eversion (15.4±3.0 mm), as was gap inclination at 90° flexion with the patella in situ (4.9±3.1°) compared to with patellar eversion (4.0±2.9°). Based on the results, they speculated that the steeper flexion gap inclination obtained without patellar eversion than with patellar eversion induced more externally rotated femoral positioning in the absence of patellar eversion. They emphasized that these results ought to be taken into account by surgeons considering switching from conventional to MIS-TKA.

3.3 Soft tissue balance with femoral component in place

The main concepts of measurement using the new tensor are, different from the conventional tensioning devise, with femoral trial component in place as well as a reduced PF joint. As the next step, accordingly, we focused on the difference in soft tissue balancing between the femoral trial component in place and the conventional osteotomized condition. In the intraoperative assessment of soft tissue balance, the joint gap showed significant decrease at extension, not flexion, after femoral trial prosthesis placement, and varus ligament balances were significantly reduced at extension and increased at flexion after femoral trial placement [36]. These changes at extension might be caused by the tensed posterior structures of the knee with the posterior condyle of the externally rotated aligned femoral trial. At knee flexion, a medial tension in the extensor mechanisms might be increased after femoral trial placement with PF joint repaired, and increased ligament balance in varus. We measured the "joint component gap", which is remarkably different from more conventional gap measurement. The joint component gap is measured with the femoral component in place, whereas the conventional gap measurement is made between the cutting surfaces of the femur and tibia. By keeping the femoral component in place, the knee is afforded a greater degree of extension because of its curving arc. In this arrangement, the posterior condyles of the component tighten the posterior capsule, resulting in a smaller joint gap at full extension. In addition, due to the 7 degree posterior slope of the tibia and a slight femoral anterior bowing, we can consider the "conventional extension gap" to be at about 10 degrees of the knee flexion angle. Mihalko et al. stated that the release of more posterior structures had a greater effect on the extension gap than on the flexion gap in explaining the importance of the relationship between posterior structures and the extension gap in a cadaver study [37]. Sugama et al. reported in their operative study that a bone cut from the posterior femoral condyles could change the tension of the posterior soft tissue structures and so alter the width and shape of the extension gap [38]. These previous reports support our hypothetical mechanism.

4. Soft tissue balance in CR and PS TKA

The Our above mentioned series of studies were only implemented with PS TKA. The long term results of CR and PS TKAs have shown an ability to relieve pain and improve function.

Nevertheless, the superiority of the CR or PS TKA remains a source of great controversy in the field of TKA. Proponents of the CR TKA advocate maintaining the PCL in order to increase stability, promote femoral rollback, and thereby enhance the patient's ability to climb stairs [39-43], while proponents of the PS TKA highlight studies in which patients with a resected PCL display a greater post-operative range of motion [43-45]. It is important to note in this debate, however, that investigators have been unable to show a difference in clinical outcome between both types of knees [41, 42, 46]. We have previously shown that among patients undergoing bilateral TKAs performed by the same surgeon, including a CR and PS TKA in alternate knees of the same patient, there was no difference in the post-operative knee score, yet the post-operative range of motion was significantly superior after resecting the PCL [47]. Accordingly, we extended our previous study and report on our experience with this device for the intra-operative soft tissue balance measurements of CR and PS TKAs, performed with both a reduced and everted patella.

While the joint component gap measurements with a reduced patella of PS TKA increased from extension to flexion, these values remained constant for CR TKA throughout the full range of motion. Additionally, the joint component gaps at deep knee flexion were significantly smaller for both types of prosthetic knees when the PF joint was reduced [48]. From our data, the CR TKA had stable joint kinematics from extension into deep flexion, while the joint kinematics for the PS TKA were more dynamic. Our data thereby supports prior studies indicating that the CR TKA affords patients greater stability. Our data further indicate that, compared to a CR TKA, a PS TKA with a reduced patella results in significantly larger gaps when the arc of motion ranges from mid- to deep-flexion.

In the assessment of varus/vagus balance, while the measurements of varus ligament balance with a reduced patella in PS TKA slightly increased from extension to flexion, these values slightly decreased for CR TKA from extension to flexion [49]. The data showed that CR TKA produced constant soft-tissue tension from extension into deep flexion, whereas PS TKA produced soft-tissue tension that tended to be more in varus during flexion. The PCL in knees with osteoarthritis is considered relatively rigid and shortened, despite being relatively macroscopically intact. Our findings indicate that compared with CR TKA, PS TKA with the patella reduced results in a significantly larger varus angle when the arc of motion is between midrange and deep flexion. After performing the independent cut procedure, we applied 3 or 5° of external rotation in the series of studies when setting the femoral component, which may have caused a decreasing varus balance in flexion for those patients who underwent CR TKA. Some studies indicated that the flexion gap in healthy knees is not rectangular and that the lateral joint gap is significantly lax [50-53]. The use of both a traditional soft-tissue release and the measured resection technique for knees with osteoarthritis in varus produces a pattern of soft-tissue tension that may at least partly explain why PS TKA produces a better postoperative range of motion.

Taken together, the kinematic patterns of soft tissue balance differ between the patellae everted and reduced, as well as between PS and CR TKA (Fig. 3). In light of these findings, we should carefully select patients according to the condition of their PCL, set an appropriate angle of external rotation, or do both if we wish to obtain good outcomes in CR TKA.

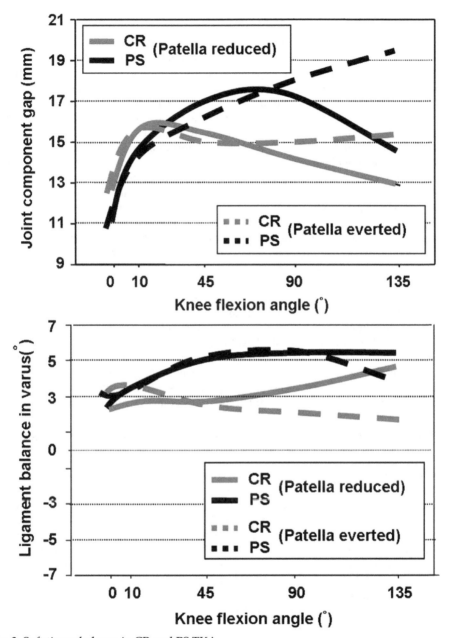

Fig. 3. Soft tissue balance in CR and PS TKA
a. Joint component gap pattern throughout the range of motion differs between CR and PS
TKA as well as between the everted and reduced PF joint condition.
b. Varus ligament balance throughout the range of motion differs between CR and PS TKA
as well as between the everted and reduced PF joint condition.

5. Soft tissue balance in MIS TKA

Recently, minimal incision surgery (MIS) TKA is widely promoted as a possible improvement over conventional TKA. The major advantages of MIS TKA over conventional TKA is the smaller skin incision required, and the avoidance of patellar eversion and quadriceps muscle splitting, leading to reduced blood loss, less perioperative pain, shorter length of hospital stay, and earlier return of knee function [54-61]. Although traditional TKA allow for excellent visualization, component orientation, and fixation, and have been associated with remarkable long-term implant survival, MIS TKA is attractive because of the small incision, and minimal or no pain and discomfort associated with surgery. However, while there is some evidence that these short-term benefits occur with MIS TKA [49-56], there is concern because of an increase in complications using the MIS technique, including vascular injury [62], patellar tendon injury [63, 64], condylar fracture [65], wound dehiscence and necrosis [65, 66], and component malalignment [54, 67-69]. In particular, the quadriceps-sparing (QS) approach has been developed as the least-invasive approach to the extensor mechanism by limiting medial parapatellar arthrotomy to the superior pole of the patella [70]. Although new surgical instrument designs enable surgeons to use this approach, this technique remains challenging to perform without causing damage to the vastus medialis obliquus (VMO) due to the limited working space [71, 72].

Accordingly, we compared intraoperative soft tissue balance measurements of MIS QS and conventional TKA, performed with the patella and femoral component in place. Whereas the joint component gap in MIS QS-TKA was significantly larger through the entire arc of flexion compared with conventional TKA, the pattern of joint looseness (joint component gap-polyethylene insert thickness) showed no difference between the two procedures. The varus ligament balance in MIS QS-TKA was significantly larger than that in conventional TKA at 0, 90, and 135 degrees of knee flexion [73]. The study suggested that MIS-TKA may lead to ligament imbalance due to the difficulties induced by a limited working space.

6. Influence of intra-operative soft tissue balance on post-operative flexion angle

Factors influencing the range of flexion after TKA can mainly be classified as intra-capsular or extra-capsular factors. Among extra-capsular factors the importance of pre-operative motion for post-operative results has been previously recognized [74-78]. Similarly, the pre-operative tightness of the extensor mechanism is an important factor influencing the post-operative knee flexion angle [79]. In contrast, intra-capsular factors, including implant design, ligament balancing, flexion-extension gap balance, height of the joint line, and patella resurfacing, have also been discussed by many authors [80-85]. Among such factors, although soft tissue balancing has been recognized as the essential surgical intervention for improving the outcome of TKA, the direct relationship between soft tissue balance and postoperative outcomes has never been clarified. As another concept of the joint condition, posterior condylar offset has recently been described as a determinant for flexion [86-88]. A mean reduction in flexion of 12° was reported to be found with every 2 mm decrease in offset [86]. Although posterior condylar offset is thought to be related to flexion gap, this relationship has not been discussed.

In the series of studies in PS TKA, joint gap change value (90-0°) with PF joint reduced, not everted, showed inverse correlation with post-operative knee flexion angle (R=-0.484, p=0.019) and posterior condylar offset (R=-0.62, p=0.002) [31]. However, in another series of studies in CR TKA, the post-operative flexion angle was positively correlated with the joint gap change value (90-0°). In either case, multivariate regression analysis among various values including various joint gap change values, ligament balance, and pre-operative knee flexion angle demonstrated the pre-operative knee flexion angle and the joint gap change value (90-0°) had a significant independent result on post-operative knee flexion angle [89]. One of the reasons for this discrepancy may be the different patterns of soft tissue balance between PS and CR TKA [48, 49]. In that report, CR TKA showed significantly smaller gaps when the arc of movement ranged from mid- to deep flexion, compared to PS TKA [48]. The posterior cruciate ligament in osteoarthritic knee is considered relatively rigid and shortened despite being relatively macroscopically intact. When we consider flexion gap tightness, Ritter et al. reported that 30% of CR TKA required ligament balancing to obtain a smooth flexion arc [90]. If the PCL was too tight, excessive femoral rollback resulted in anterior lift-off of the tibial trial in flexion, leading to a limitation of flexion [91]. To make a better post-operative flexion angle, balancing the flexion gap can result in a satisfactory range of motion [92, 93]. In our series of studies in CR TKA, it was identified that 16% more flexion gap tightness (smaller flexion gap than extension gap) resulted in a smaller flexion angle. Similarly, using a commercially available knee balancer with the measurement under 80 N distraction force, Higuchi et al reported flexion medial/lateral gap tightness led to restriction of the flexion angle [94]. Therefore, in these cases, surgeons are advised to avoid flexion gap tightness by soft tissue release such as PCL [90, 91, 95].

7. Influence of preoperative deformity on intra-operative soft tissue balance

Pre-operative deformity of the knee differs from patient to patient. In the varus knee especially, many surgeons recognize that progressive shortening or contraction of soft tissue structures on the medial side may occur, whereas the lateral structures may become stretched [96-99]. Although severe intra-operative varus deformity needs substantial soft tissue release on the medial side during TKA, the ideal amount of medial release is still controversial; two strategies exist for soft tissue balancing in the varus knee. Some surgeons believe it is best to create equal medial and lateral gaps even in severely deformed knees [2, 100, 101]. Others accept some degree of lateral laxity is permissible, as long as proper alignment is maintained, based on evidence showing post-operative diminishment with time of lateral laxity after TKA [102, 103].

Accordingly, we compared intra-operative soft tissue balance measurements in various grades of preoperative varus deformity (10° < varus deformity, 10° < varus deformity < 20°, varus deformity >20°) during PS TKA, performed with a reduced patella. In the comparison of the changing pattern of joint component gap among the three different pre-operative deformity groups, we observed similar kinematic patterns showing an increase until 90° of knee flexion and a decrease towards deep knee flexion, and no difference among the groups throughout the flexion angle of the knee. In the comparison of medial-lateral ligamentous balance, on the other hand, the varus angle showed significant larger values in the varus alignment > 20° group compared to that of the other two groups throughout knee flexion in spite of similar patterns showing slight increases in the varus angle to 90° of knee flexion and constant balance after that. These results indicate that appropriate medial-lateral balancing is difficult in knees with severe pre-operative varus deformity, especially with varus alignment > 20° [104].

Even in normal knees, lateral ligamentous laxity and medial ligamentous laxity are not balanced and more lateral ligamentous laxity than medial ligamentous laxity has been observed [105-107]. To restore the joint line, we believe lateral laxity of less than 5 degrees is permissible in the varus alignment < 20° groups as long as proper alignment is maintained [102, 103, 108]. In such severely deformed varus knees, some surgeons may recommend the complete release of medial-sided structures including an MCL cut for achievement of a well-balanced knee [109]. However, we avoided this procedure due to the potential widening of the joint gap with elongation of the lower extremity, and subsequent patella baja as a result of joint line elevation due to a thicker polyethylene insert. Therefore, results in this series may be based on these operative procedures.

8. Soft tissue balance in gap technique

In the above mentioned study, soft tissue balance measurements were only performed in posterior-stabilized (PS) or cruciate-retaining (CR) TKAs using the measured resection technique. However, the best method of obtaining rotational alignment of the femoral component in flexion remains controversial. Some investigators favor a measured resection technique in which bony landmarks (femoral epicondyles, posterior femoral condyles, or the anteroposterior axis) are the primary determinants of femoral component rotation [110-115]. Others recommend a gap-balancing methodology in which the femoral component is positioned parallel to the resected proximal tibia with each collateral ligament equally tensioned [116-118]. Under such debate, several surgeons recently reported more consistent equalization of extension and flexion gaps with the use of computer-assisted gap balancing technique, compared with conventional measured resection technique [119, 120]. In contrast, in the comparison between the navigation-assisted measured resection and navigation-assisted gap balancing technique, some surgeons reported a better restoration of the joint line position in the navigation-assisted measured resection technique despite no differences in short-term clinical outcomes [120, 121].

Using the offset type tensor, which can be used in the gap technique [123], we performed soft tissue balance assessment during CR TKA using the tibia first gap technique with navigation system. With the tibia first gap technique, the kinematics of the component gap showed a similar pattern to the measured resection technique during CR TKA; following a significant increase during the initial 30° of knee flexion, the joint component gap showed a gradual decrease toward 120° of flexion [48, 89]. After that, soft tissue balance was assessed at extension and flexion between the basic value after tibial cut and the final value following femoral cut and with femoral component in place. The basic value of the joint gap before femoral osteotomy reflected the final value following femoral cut and with femoral component in place (unpublished data). Accordingly, the tibia first gap technique may have the advantage that surgeons can predict the final soft tissue balance from that before femoral osteotomies.

9. Summary

In the series of study using offset type tensor with PF joint reduced and femoral component in place, the kinematic pattern of intraoperative joint gap and ligament balance can be observed in TKA when they are performed while preserving a more physiological condition of the knee. Additionally, various factors influencing soft tissue balance such as patellar orientation, PS/CR type of prosthesis design, MIS/conventional technique, grade of preoperative deformity, and operation procedures, measured resection or gap technique can be examined. We believe the information provided by the use of the offset type tensor is useful and essential for providing insight into true post-operative kinematics, and thus by maintaining a reduced patella for each intra-operative measurement, the surgeon will be able to adjust the soft tissue balance more accurately and thereby expect a better post-operative outcome.

10. References

[1] Insall JN, Tria AJ, Scott WN. The total condylar knee prosthesis: the first 5 years. *Clin Orthop Relat Res.* 1979; 145: 68

[2] Insall JN, Binazzi R, Soudry M, Mestriner LA. Total knee arthroplasty. *Clin Orthop Relat Res.* 1985; 192: 13

[3] Dorr LD, Boiardo RA. Technical consideration in total knee arthroplasty. *Clin Orthop Relat Res.* 1986; 205: 5

[4] Stulberg SD, Loan P, Sarin V. Computer-assisted navigation in total knee replacement: results of an initial experience in thirty-five patients. J Bone Joint Surg Am 2002;84-A Suppl 2:90-8.

[5] Sparmann M, Wolke B, Czupalla H, Banzer D, Zink A. Positioning of total knee arthroplasty with and without navigation support. A prospective, randomised study. J Bone Joint Surg Br 2003;85:830-5.

[6] Laskin RS, Beksac B. Computer-assisted navigation in TKA: where we are and where we are going. Clin Orthop Relat Res 2006;452:127-31.

[7] Lutzner J, Krummenauer F, Wolf C, Gunther KP, Kirschner S. Computer-assisted and conventional total knee replacement: a comparative, prospective, randomised study with radiological and CT evaluation. J Bone Joint Surg Br 2008;90:1039-44.

[8] Matsumoto T, Tsumura N, Kurosaka M, Muratsu H, Kuroda R, Ishimoto K, Tsujimoto K, Shiba R, Yoshiya S. Prosthetic Alignment and Sizing in Computer-Assisted Total Knee Arthroplasty. *Int Orthop.* 28: 282-285, 2004

[9] Matsumoto T, Tsumura N, Kurosaka M, Muratsu H, Yoshiya S, Kuroda R. Clinical Values in Computer-Assisted Total Knee Arthroplasty. *Orthopedics.* 29(12): 1115-1120, 2006

[10] Ishida K, Matsumoto T, Tsumura N, Kubo S, Kitagawa A, Iguchi T, Kurosaka M, Kuroda R. Clinical Outcomes of Computer-assisted Total Knee Arthroplasty: Mid-term Results of Minimum 5 Years. *Knee Surg Sports Traumatol Arthrosc.* [Epub ahead of print]

[11] Fehring TK, Odum S, Griffin WL, Mason JB, Nadaud M. Early failures in total knee arthroplasty. *Clin Orthop Relat Res* 392: 315-318, 2001

[12] Sharkey PF, Hozack WJ, Rothman RH, Shastri S, Jacoby SM. Insall award paper. Why are total knee arthroplasties failing today? *Clin Orthop Relat Res* 404: 7-13, 2002

[13] Griffin FM, Insall JN, Scuderi GR. Accuracy of soft tissue balancing in total knee arthroplasty. *J Arthroplasty.* 15: 970-973, 2000

[14] Insall JN (1984) Total knee replacement. In: Insall JN (ed) Surgery of the knee. Churchill-Livingstone, New York

[15] Freeman MAR, Todd RC, Bamert P, Day WH (1978) ICLH arthroplasty of the knee: 1968–1977. J Bone Joint Surg 60-B:339–344

[16] Attfield SF, Warren-Forward M, Wilton T, Sambatakakis A (1994) Measurement of soft tissue imbalance in total knee arthroplasty using electronic instrumentation. Med Eng Phys 16:501–505

[17] Booth RE (2003) Tensioners: essential for accurate performance of TKA. Orthopedics 26:962–964

[18] Winemakaer MJ (2002) Perfect balance in total knee arthroplasty. J Arthroplasty 17:2–10

[19] Sambatakakis A, Attfield SF, Newton G. Quantification of soft-tissue imbalance in condylar knee arthroplasty. *J Biomed Eng*. 15: 339-343, 1993

[20] Unitt L, Sambatakakis A, Johnstone D, Briggs TW; Balancer Study Group. Short-term outcome in total knee replacement after soft-tissue release and balancing. *J Bone Joint Surg Br*. 90:159-65, 2008

[21] Viskontas DG, Skrinskas TV, Johnson JA, King GJ, Winemaker MJ, Chess DG (2007) Computer-assisted gap equalization in total knee arthroplasty. J Arthroplasty 22:334–342

[22] Wasielewski RC, Galat DD, Komistek RD (2005) Correlation of compartment pressure data from an intraoperative sensing device with postoperative fluoroscopic kinematic results in TKA patients. J Biomech 38:333–339

[23] Yagishita K, Muneta T, Ikeda H (2003) Step-by-step measurement of soft tissue balancing during total knee arthroplasty for patients with varus knees. J Arthroplasty 18:313–320

[24] Zalzal P, Papini M, Petruccelli D, de Beer J, Winemaker MJ (2004) An in vivo biomechanical analysis of the soft-tissue envelope of osteoarthritis knees. J Arthroplasty 19:217–223

[25] Asano H, Hoshino A, Wilton T (2004) Soft-tissue tension total knee arthroplasty. J Arthroplasty 19:558–561

[26] D'Lima DD, Patil S, Steklov N, Slamin JE, Colwell CW Jr (2006) Tibial force measured in vivo after total knee arthroplasty. J Arthroplasty 21:255–262

[27] Morris BA, D'Lima DD, Slamin J, Kovacevic N, Arms SW, Townsend CP, Colwell Jr CW (2001) e-Knee: evolution of the electronic knee prosthesis. J Bone Joint Surg 83-A(supplement 2, Part 1):62–66

[28] D'Lima DD, Patil S, Steklov N, Colwell CW Jr. The 2011 ABJS Nicolas Andry Award: 'Lab'-in-a-Knee: In Vivo Knee Forces, Kinematics, and Contact Analysis. Clin Orthop Relat Res. 2011 May 20. [Epub ahead of print]

[29] Muratsu H, Tsumura N, Yamaguchi M, Mizuno K, Kuroda R, Harada T, Yoshiya S, Kurosaka M. Patellar eversion affects soft tissue balance in total knee arthroplasty. *Trans Orthop Res Soc*. 28: 242, 2003

[30] Matsumoto T, Muratsu H, Tsumura N, Mizuno K, Kuroda R, Yoshiya S, Kurosaka M. Joint gap kinematics in posterior-stabilized total knee arthroplasty measured by a new tensor with the navigation system. *J Biomech Eng*. 128 (6): 867-871, 2006

[31] Matsumoto T, Mizuno K, Muratsu H, Tsumura N, Fukase N, Seiji K, Yoshiya S, Kurosaka M, Kuroda R. Influence of Intra-operative Joint Gap on Post-operative Flexion Angle in Osteoarthritis Patients Undergoing Posterior-Stabilized Total Knee Arthroplasty. *Knee Surg Sports Traumatol Arthrosc*. 15(8): 1013-1008, 2007

[32] Matsumoto T, Muratsu H, Tsumura N, Mizuno K, Kurosaka M, Kuroda R. Soft tissue balance measurement in posterior-stabilized total knee arthroplasty with a navigation system. *J Althroplasty*. 24(3): 358-64, 2009

[33] Gejo, R., Y. Morita, I. Matsushita, K. Sugimori, and T. Kimura. Joint gap changes with patellar tendon strain and patellar position during TKA. *Clin Orthop Relat Res.* 466:946-51, 2008

[34] Yoshino, N., N. Watanabe, Y. Watanabe, Y. Fukuda, and S. Takai. Measurement of joint gap load in patella everted and reset position during total knee arthroplasty. *Knee Surg Sports Traumatol Arthrosc.* 17:484-90, 2010

[35] Kamei G, Kamei G, Murakami Y, Kazusa H, Hachisuka S, Inoue H, Nobutou H, Nishida K, Mochizuki Y, Ochi M. Is patella eversion during total knee arthroplasty crucial for gap adjustment and soft-tissue balancing? *Orthop Traumatol Surg Res.* 97(3):287-91, 2011.

[36] Muratsu H, Matsumoto T, Maruo A, Miya H, Kurosaka M, Kuroda R. Femoral component placement chnges soft tissue balance in posterior-stabilized total knee arthroplasty. *Clin Biomech.* 25(9): 926-30, 2010

[37] Mihalko, W.M., L.A. Whiteside, and K.A. Krackow. 2003. Comparison of ligament-balancing techniques during total knee arthroplasty. *J Bone Joint Surg Am.* 85-A Suppl 4:132-5.

[38] Sugama, R., Y. Kadoya, A. Kobayashi, and K. Takaoka. 2005. Preparation of the flexion gap affects the extension gap in total knee arthroplasty. *J Arthroplasty.* 20:602-7.

[39] Andriacchi TP, Andersson GB, Fermier RW, Stern D, Galante JO. A study of lower-limb mechanics during stair-climbing. *J Bone Joint Surg Am.* 1980; 62(5); 749-757.

[40] Andriacchi TP, Galante JO, Fermier RW. The influence of total knee-replacement design on walking and stair-climbing. *J Bone Joint Surg Am.* 1982; 64(9): 1328-1335.

[41] Becker MW, Insall JN, Faris PM. Bilateral total knee arthroplasty. One cruciate retaining and one cruciate substituting. *Clin Orthop Relat Res.* 1991; 271: 122-124.

[42] Dorr LD, Ochsner JL, Gronley J, Perry J. Functional comparison of posterior cruciate-retained versus cruciate-sacrificed total knee arthroplasty. *Clin Orthop Relat Res.* 1988; 236: 36-43.

[43] Maloney WJ, Schurman DJ. The effects of implant design on range of motion after total knee arthroplasty. Total condylar versus posterior stabilized total condylar designs. *Clin Orthop Relat Res.* 1992; 278: 147-152.

[44] Hirsch HS, Lotke PA, Morrison LD. The posterior cruciate ligament in total knee surgery. Save, sacrifice, or substitute? *Clin Orthop Relat Res.* 1994; 309: 64-68.

[45] Insall JN, Hood RW, Flawn LB, Sullivan DJ. The total condylar knee prosthesis in gonarthrosis. A five to nine-year follow-up of the first one hundred consecutive replacements. *J Bone Joint Surg Am.* 1983; 65(5): 619-628.

[46] Udomkiat P, Meng BJ, Dorr LD, Wan Z. Functional comparison of posterior cruciate retention and substitution knee replacement. *Clin Orthop Relat Res.* 2000; 378:192-201.

[47] Maruyama S, Yoshiya S, Matsui N, Kuroda R, Kurosaka M. Functional comparison of posterior cruciate-retaining versus posterior stabilized total knee arthroplasty. *J Arthroplasty.* 2004; 19(3): 349-53.

[48] Matsumoto T, Kuroda R , Kubo S, Muratsu H, Mizuno K, Kurosaka M. The intra-operative joint gap in cruciate-retaining compared with posterior-stabilizsed total knee replacement. *J Bone Joint Surg Br.* 91(4): 475-80, 2009

[49] Matsumoto T, Muratsu H, Kubo S, Matsushita T, Kurosaka M, Kuroda R. Soft-tissue tension in cruciate-retaining and posterior-stabilized total knee arthroplasty. *J Arthroplasty*. [Epub ahead of print]

[50] Malkolf KL, Mensch JS, Amstutz HC. Stiffness and laxity of the knee—the contributions of the supporting structures. A quantitative in vitro study. J Bone Joint Surg Am 1976;58:583

[51] Seering WP, Piziali RL, Nagel DA, Schurman DJ. The function of the primary ligaments of the knee in varus-valgus and axial rotation. J Biomech 1980;13:785

[52] Moore TM, Meyers MH, Harvey JP Jr. Collateral ligament laxity of the knee. Long-term comparison between plateau fractures and normal. J Bone Joint Surg Am 1976;58:594

[53] Tokuhara Y, Kadoya Y, Nakagawa S, Kobayashi A, Takaoka K. The flexion gap in normal knees. An MRI study. J Bone Joint Surg Br 2004;86:1133

[54] Chen AF, Alan RK, Redziniak DE, Tria AJ Jr (2006) Quadriceps sparing total knee replacement. The initial experience with results at two to four years. J Bone Joint Surg Br 88: 1448-1453

[55] Hass SB, Cook S, Beksac B (2004) Minimally invasive total knee replacement through a mini midvastus approach: A comparative study. Clin Orthop Relat Res 428: 68-73

[56] Kashyap SN, Van Ommeren JW (2008) Clinical experience with less invasive surgery techniques in total knee arthroplasty: a comparative study. Knee Surg Sports Traumatol Arthrosc 16: 544–548

[57] Laskin RS, Beksac B, Phongjunakom A, Pittors K, Shim JC, Pavlov H, Petersen M (2004) Minimally invasive total knee replacement through a mini-midvastus incision; an outcome study. Clin Orthop Relat Res 428: 74-81

[58] Lombardi AV Jr, Viacava AJ, Berend KR (2006) Rapid recovery protocols and minimally invasive surgery help achieve high knee flexion. Clin Orthop Relat Res 452:117–122

[59] Luring C, Beckmann J, Haibo"ck P, Perlick L, Grifka J, Tingart M (2008) Minimal invasive and computer assisted total knee replacement compared with the conventional technique: a prospective, randomized trial. Knee Surg Sports Traumatol Arthrosc 16: 928–934

[60] Schroer WC, Diesfeld PJ, Reedy ME, Lemarr AR (2010) Isokinetic strength testing of minimally invasive total knee arthroplasty recovery. J Arthroplasty 25: 274–279

[61] Tria Jr AJ, Coon TM (2003) Minimal incision total knee arthroplasty: early experience. Clin Orthop Relat Res 416: 185-190

[62] Tria Jr AJ. Advancements in minimally invasive total knee arthroplasty (2003) Orthopedics 26: s859

[63] Aglietti P, Baldini A, Sensi L (2006) Quadriceps-sparing versus mini-subvastus approach in total knee arthroplasty. Clin Orthop Relat Res 452: 106-111

[64] Boerger TO, Aglietti P, Mondanelli N, Sensi L (2005) Mini-subvastus versus medial parapatellar approach in total knee arthroplasty. Clin Orthop Relat Res 440: 82-87

[65] Kolisek FR, Bonutti PM, Hazack WJ, Purtill J, Sharkey PF, Zelicof SB, Ragland PS, Kester M, Mont MA, Rothman RH (2007) Clinical experience using a minimally invasive approach for total knee arthroplasty: early results of a prospective randomized study compared to a standard approach. J Arthroplasty 22: 8-13

[66] Pagnano MW, Meneghini RM (2006) Minimally invasive total knee arthroplasty with an optimized subvastus approach. J Arthroplasty 21: 22-26

[67] Dalury DF, Dennis DA (2005) Mini-incision total knee arthroplasty can increase risk of component malalignment. Clin Orthop Relat Res 440: 77-81

[68] Lin WP, Lin J, Horng LC, Chang SM, Jiang CC (2009) Quadriceps-sparing, minimal-incision total knee arthroplasty. A comparative study. J Arthroplasty 24: 1024-1032

[69] Yau WP, Leung A, Liu KG, Yan CH, Wong LS, Chiu KY (2008) Errors in the identification of the transepicondylar and anteroposterior axes of the distal femur in total knee replacement using minimally-invasive and conventional approaches. J Bone Joint Surg Br 90: 520-526

[70] Tria Jr AJ, Coon TM (2003) Minimal incision total knee arthroplasty: early experience. Clin Orthop Relat Res 416: 185-190

[71] Pagnano MW, Meneghini RM, Trousdale RT (2006) Anatomy of the extensor mechanism in reference to quadriceps-sparing TKA. Clin Orthop Relat Res 452: 102-105

[72] Robert VI, Mereddy PKR, Donnachie NJ, Hakkalamani S (2007) Anatomical variations in vastus medialis obliquus and its implications in minimally invasive total knee replacement. J Bone Joint Surg Br 89: 1462-1465

[73] Matsumoto T, Muratsu H, Kubo S, Mizuno K, Kinoshita K, Ishida K, Matsushita T, Sasaki K, Tei K, Takayama K, Sasaki H, Oka S, Kurosaka M, Kuroda R. Influence of minimum invasive approach of total knee arthroplasty on the soft tissue balance. *Knee Surg Sports Traumatol Arthrosc.* 19(6): 880-6, 2011

[74] Anouchi YS, McShane M, Kelly F Jr, Elting J, Stiehl, J. Range of motion in total knee replacement. *Clin Orthop Relat Res* 1996; 331: 87-91.

[75] Lizaur A, Marco L, Cebrian R. Preoperative factors influencing the range of movement after total knee arthroplasty for severe osteoarthritis. *J Bone Joint Surg [Br]* 1997; 79-B: 626-9.

[76] Harvey IA, Barry K, Kirby SP, Johnson R, Elloy MA. Factors affecting the range of movement of total knee arthroplasty. *J Bone Joint Surg [Br]* 1993; 75-B: 950-5.

[77] Parsley BS, Engh GA, Dwyer KA. Preoperative flexion. Dose it influence postoperative flexion after posterior-cruciate-retaining total knee arthroplasty? *Clin Orthop Relat Res* 1992; 275: 204-10.

[78] Ritter MA, Stringer EA. Predictive range of motion after total knee replacement. *Clin Orthop Relat Res* 1999; 143: 115-9.

[79] Matsumoto T, Tsumura N, Kubo S, Shiba R, Kurosaka M, Yoshiya S (2005) Influence of hip position on knee flexion angle in patients undergoing total knee arthroplasty. J Arthroplasty 20:669-673

[80] Dennis DA: *Problems After Knee Arthroplasty.* The Stiff Total Knee Arthroplasty: Causes and Cures. *Orthopedics* 2001; 24: 901-2.

[81] Harvey IA, Barry K, Kirby SPJ, Johnson R, Elloy MA: Factors affecting the range of movement of total knee arthroplasty. *J Bone Joint Surg [Br]* 1993; 75-B: 950-5.

[82] Kawamura H, Bourne RB. Factors affecting range of flexion after total knee arthroplasty. *J Orthop Sci* 2001; 6: 248-52.

[83] Schurman DJ, Matityahu A, Goodman SB, Maloney W, Woolson S, Shi, H, Bloch DA: Prediction of postoperative knee flexion in Insall-Burstein II total knee arthroplasty. *Clin Orthop Relat Re* 1998; 353: 175-84.

[84] Schurman DJ, Parker JN, Orstein D: Total condylar knee replacement. A study of factors influencing range of motion as late as two years after arthroplasty. *J Bone Joint Surg [Am]* 1985; 67-A: 1006-14.

[85] Joshi AB, Lee CM, Markovic L, Murphy JCM, Hardinge K: Total knee arthroplasty after patellectomy. *J Bone Joint Surg [Br]* 1994; 76-B: 926-9.

[86] Bellemans J, Banks S, Victor J, Vandenneucker H, Moemans A. Fluoroscopic analysis of the kinematics of deep flexion in total knee arthroplasty. Influence of posterior condylar offset. *J Bone Joint Surg [Br]* 2002; 84-B:50-3.

[87] Victor J, Bellemans J. Physiologic Kinematics as a Concept for Better Flexion in TKA. *Clin Orthop Relat Res* 2006 Aug 17; [Epub ahead of print]

[88] Kim YH, Sohn KS, Kim JS. Range of motion of standard and high-flexion posterior stabilized total knee prostheses. A prospective, randomized study. *J Bone Joint Surg [Am]* 2005; 87-A: 1470-5.

[89] Takayama K, Matsumoto T, Kubo S, Muratsu H, Ishida K, Matsushita T, Kurosaka M, Kuroda R. The Influence of Intra-operative Joint Gap on Post-operative Flexion Angle in Cruciate-retaining Total Knee Arthroplasty. Knee Surg Sports Traumatol Arthrosc [Epub ahead of print]

[90] Ritter MA, Faris PM, Keating EM (1988) Posterior cruciate ligament balancing during total knee arthroplasty. J Arthroplasty 3:323-326

[91] Kim H, Pelker RR, Gibson DH, Irving JF, Lynch JK (1997) Rollback in posterior cruciate ligament-retaining total knee arthroplasty. A radiographic analysis. J Arthroplasty 12:553-561

[92] Arima J, Whiteside LA, Martin JW, Miura H, White SE, McCarthy DS (1998) Effect of partial release of the posterior cruciate ligament in total knee arthroplasty. Clin Orthop Relat Res 353:194-202

[93] Lombardi AV, Jr., Berend KR, Aziz-Jacobo J, Davis MB (2008) Balancing the flexion gap: relationship between tibial slope and posterior cruciate ligament release and correlation with range of motion. J Bone Joint Surg Am 90 Suppl4. 121-132

[94] Higuchi H, Hatayama K, Shimizu M, Kobayashi A, Kobayashi T, Takagishi K. Relationship between joint gap difference and range of motion in total knee arthroplasty: a prospective randomised study between different platforms. Int Orthop. 2009;33(4):997-1000.

[95] Yamakado K, Kitaoka K, Yamada H, Hashiba K, Nakamura R, Tomita K (2003) Influence of stability on range of motion after cruciate-retaining TKA. Arch Orthop Trauma Surg 123:1-4

[96] Krackow KA, Mihalko WM. The effect of medial release on flexion and extension gaps in cadaveric knees: implications for soft-tissue balancing in total knee arthroplasty. *Am J Knee Surg.* 1999; 12(4) : 222

[97] Mihalko WM, Miller C, Krackow KA. Total knee arthroplasty ligament balancing and gap kinematics with posterior cruciate ligament retention and sacrifice. *Am J Orthop.* 2000; 29(8): 610

[98] Siston RA, Goodman SB, Delp SL, Giori NJ. Coronal plane stability before and after total knee arthroplasty. *Clin Orthop Relat Res.* 2007; 463: 43

[99] Mihalko WM, Saleh KJ, Krackow KA, Whiteside LA. Soft-tissue Balancing During Total Knee Arthroplasty in the Varus Knee. *J Am Acad Orthop Surg.* 2009; 17(12): 766

[100] Teeny SM, Krackow KA, Hungerford DS, Jones M. Primary total knee arthroplasty in patients with severe varus deformity. A comparative study. *Clin Orthop Relat Res.* 1991; 273: 19

[101] Winemaker MJ. Perfect balance in total knee arthroplasty: the elusive compromise. *J Arthroplasty.* 2002; 17(1): 2

[102] Lotke PA. Primary total knees: standard principles and techniques. In: Lotke PA, Lonner JH, eds. *Knee Arthroplasty.* Philadelphia, PA: Lippincott Williams & Wilkins; 2003: 49

[103] Sculco TP. Soft tissue balancing in total knee arthroplasty. In: Goldberg VM, ed. *Controversies of Total Knee Replacement.* New York, NY: Raven Press; 1991: 167

[104] Matsumoto T, Muratsu H, Kubo S, Matsushita T, Kurosaka M, Kuroda R. The Influence of Pre-operative Deformity on Intra-operative Soft Tissue Balance in Posterior-Stabilized Total Knee Arthroplasty. *J Arthroplasty.* [Epub ahead of print]

[105] Okazaki K, Miura H, Matsuda S, Takeuchi N, Mawatari T, Hashizume M, Iwamoto Y. Asymmetry of mediolateral laxity of the normal knee. *J Orthop Sci.* 2006; 11(3): 264

[106] Tokuhara Y, Kadoya Y, Nakagawa S, Kobayashi A, Takaoka K. The flexion gap in normal knees. An MRI study. *J Bone Joint Surg Br.* 2004; 86(8): 1133

[107] Nagamine R, Kondo K, Nomura H, Kanekasu K, Sonohata M, Sugioka Y. Shape of the joint gap for 90 degrees and 120 degrees knee flexion after total knee arthroplasty. *J Orthop Sci.* 2008; 13(4): 354

[108] Sekiya H, Takatoku K, Takada H, Sasanuma H, Sugimoto N. Postoperative lateral ligamentous laxity diminishes with time after TKA in the varus knee. *Clin Orthop Relat Res.* 2009; 467(6): 1582

[109] Mihalko WM, Saleh KJ, Krackow KA, Whiteside LA. Soft-tissue Balancing During Total Knee Arthroplasty in the Varus Knee. *J Am Acad Orthop Surg.* 2009; 17(12): 766

[110] Berger RA, Rubash HE, Seel MJ, Thompson WH, Crossett LS.Determining the rotational alignment of the femoral component in total knee arthroplasty using theepicondylar axis. Clin OrthopRelat Res. 1993;286:40–47.

[111] Griffin FM, Math K, Scuderi GR, Insall JN, Poilvache PL. Anatomy of the epicondyles of the distal femur: MRI analysis of normal knees. J Arthroplasty. 2000;15:354–359.

[112] Mantas JP, Bloebaum RD, Skedros JG, Hofmann AA. Implications of reference axes used for rotational alignment of the femoral component in primary and revision knee arthroplasty. J Arthroplasty. 1992;7:531–535.

[113] Poilvache PL, Insall JN, Scuderi GR, Font-Rodriguez DE. Rotational landmarks and sizing of the distal femur in total knee arthroplasty. Clin Orthop Relat Res. 1996;331:35–46.

[114] Schnurr C, Nessler J, Ko¨nig DP. Is referencing the posterior condyles sufficient to achieve a rectangular flexion gap in total knee arthroplasty? Int Orthop. 2008 Oct 28. [Epub ahead of print].

[115] Whiteside LA, Arima J. The anteroposterior axis for femoral rotational alignment in valgus total knee arthroplasty. Clin Orthop Relat Res. 1995;321:168–172.

[116] Dennis, DA. Measured resection: An outdated technique in total knee arthroplasty. Orthopedics. 2008;31:940, 943–944.

[117] Fehring TK. Rotational malalignment of the femoral component in total knee arthroplasty. Clin Orthop Relat Res. 2000;380: 72–79.

[118] Katz MA, Beck TD, Silber JS, Seldes RM, Lotke PA. Determining femoral rotational alignment in total knee arthroplasty: reliability of techniques. J Arthroplasty. 2001;16:301–305.

[119] Pang HN, Yeo SJ, Chong HC, Chin PL, Ong J, Lo NN. Computer-assisted gap balancing technique improves outcome in total knee arthroplasty, compared with conventional measured resection technique. Knee Surg Sports Traumatol Arthrosc. 2011 Mar 30. [Epub ahead of print]

[120] Seon JK, Song EK, Park SJ, Lee DS. The use of navigation to obtain rectangular flexion and extension gaps during primary total knee arthroplasty and midterm clinical results. J Arthroplasty. 2011 Jun;26(4):582-90. Epub 2010 Jun 26.

[121] Tigani D, Sabbioni G, Ben Ayad R, Filanti M, Rani N, Del Piccolo N. Comparison between two computer-assisted total knee arthroplasty: gap-balancing versus measured resection technique. Knee Surg Sports Traumatol Arthrosc. 2010 Oct;18(10):1304-10.

[122] Lee HJ, Lee JS, Jung HJ, Song KS, Yang JJ, Park CW. Comparison of joint line position changes after primary bilateral total knee arthroplasty performed using the navigation-assisted measured gap resection or gap balancing techniques. Knee Surg Sports Traumatol Arthrosc. 2011 Mar 23. [Epub ahead of print]

[123] Tanaka K, Muratsu H, Mizuno K, Kuroda R, Yoshiya S, Kurosaka M. Soft tissue balance measurement in anterior cruciate ligament-resected knee joint: cadaveric study as a model for cruciate-retaining total knee arthroplasty. J Orthop Sci. 2007 Mar;12(2):149-53. Epub 2007 Mar 30.

6

The Role of Drainage After Total Knee Arthroplasty

Ta-Wei Tai, Chyun-Yu Yang and Chih-Wei Chang
Department of Orthopedics,
National Cheng Kung University Hospital,
Tainan
Taiwan

1. Introduction

Total knee arthroplasty (TKA) is associated with significant postoperative blood loss for which blood transfusion might be necessary. The role of wound drainage is controversial. The use of drainage was believed to be effective in decreasing hematoma formation (Drinkwater and Neil 1995; Holt et al. 1997; Martin et al. 2004), which has been theoretically thought to decrease postoperative pain, swelling, and incidence of infection(Kim et al. 1998). However, a closed suction drainage system inevitably increases bleeding because the tamponade effect of a closed and undrained wound is eliminated. Though some studies have shown that drainage after TKA is not necessary(Adalberth et al. 1998; Niskanen et al. 2000; Esler et al. 2003; Parker et al. 2004; Jones et al. 2007), it is still widely used by orthopedic surgeons(Canty et al. 2003).

Surgeons who routinely drain total knee replacements may also use adjunctive measures such as autologous blood transfusion, use of fibrin tissue adhesive, compression bandaging and local ice packing(Gibbons et al. 2001; Kullenberg et al. 2006; Radkowski et al. 2007) to reduce the excessive blood loss from the drain. Recently, drain clamping has received increasing attention. Since most of the blood loss in TKA occurs during the first few postoperative hours (37% in 2 hours and 55% in 4 hours)(Jou IM 1993; Senthil Kumar et al. 2005), it seems reasonable to clamp the drain tube in the first few hours after TKA to temporarily create a tamponade effect for bleeding control. Various methods of clamping drain have been reported in the literature. However, no consensus has been achieved to date.

To clarify the role of drainage system after total knee arthroplasty, we conduct a review process in the present project. A comprehensive search was carried out and the articles regarding the drainage after surgery were reviewed. This review article focused on:

1. Effectiveness of postoperative drainage in TKA.
2. Safety and complications of postoperative drainage in TKA.
3. Effect of temporary drain clamping.

The purpose of this article is to analyze the pros and cons in using the drainage system after total knee arthroplasty and to provide practical information for orthopedic surgeons and medical care givers.

2. Search of literature

Our review team completed the search of electronic databases, including the Cochrane Central Register of Controlled Trials (2010), PubMed Medline (1966 to May 2011), and Embase (1980 to May 2011). We used the following search terms and Boolean operators: (drain OR drainage) AND (knee OR arthroplasty OR joint replacement). We also searched the reference lists of the relevant articles for any further associated studies. The criteria for inclusion in our study were: 1) reports dealing with patients undergoing primary TKA, 2) studies about postoperative drainage. After reviewing the titles and abstracts of the studies, we then determined if the study was appropriate for retrieval. These retrieved articles were reviewed by our review team. A consensus about the content of this review article was reached through out series of discussion.

3. Postoperative drainage

The effectiveness of wound drainage following TKA is still controversial. Some authors believed drains would reduce postoperative hematoma formation.(Drinkwater and Neil 1995; Holt et al. 1997; Martin et al. 2004) Postoperative drainage have been shown to provide a better wound outcome in orthopedic surgery.(Berman et al. 1990) Serous discharge from the wounds in TKA without drainage was a major concern of postoperative care.(Ovadia et al. 1997) Using a drain theoretically decreased postoperative pain, swelling, and incidence of infection(Kim et al. 1998).

Using a drain would facilitate the postoperative wound management. It is probably the most established benefit of the drainage in TKA. The number of dressing reinforcement was reported to be less in the drainage group.(Holt et al. 1997; Ovadia et al. 1997; Kim et al. 1998) Some other articles assessed the volume of blood in the dressing by measuring the weight of the dressing and found less weight in the drainage group.(Esler et al. 2003; Tao et al. 2006) In addition, Holt et al and Kim et al found that the area of ecchymosis is significant less in the drainage group.(Holt et al. 1997; Kim et al. 1998) Omonbude et al applied musculoskeletal ultrasound to measure the formation of hematoma and effusion on the fourth post-operative day and reported that the range of hematoma was less in the drainage group than the non-drainage group.(Omonbude et al. 2010) The above results of reinforcement of dressings and degree of ecchymosis and hematoma indicated the using a drain may reduce the leakage of blood from the joints and wounds.

According to a previous survey, most surgeons used closed suction drainage and believed that it would prevent from infection.(Canty et al. 2003) Many articles addressed this issue but failed to prove its effectiveness in the prevention of infection.(Holt et al. 1997; Ovadia et al. 1997; Kim et al. 1998; Esler et al. 2003; Tao et al. 2006; Cao et al. 2009; Lin et al. 2009; Tai et al. 2010a) A recent meta-analysis showed that the incidence of infection was 0.5% in the drainage group and 1.2% in the non-drainage group, but pooled data demonstrated no significant difference.(Zhang et al. 2011)

Thromboembolism is one of the most common complications after TKA, and is of great concern because of the associated increases in morbidity and mortality reported in the literature. To date, no approach to venous thromboembolic prophylaxis has been universally accepted by orthopedic surgeons. The methods of prophylaxis varied among the included studies. Using a drain in TKA theoretically reduces postoperative knee swelling and may reduce the risk of thromboembolism. However, the evidence provided in the literature seems not to support this claim. Several studies compared the incidence of deep vein thrombosis between the drainage and non-drainage groups and all of them found no significant difference.(Holt et al. 1997; Adalberth et al. 1998; Mengal et al. 2001)

Dose using a drain increase the postoperative range of motion through reducing swelling? Several studies mentioned this issue but the results were disappointed.(Ovadia et al. 1997; Adalberth et al. 1998; Tao et al. 2006; Lin et al. 2009) All reports stated no significantly better range of motion after application of drainage. We believe that postoperative range of motion is influenced by many perioperative factors. Using a drain cannot alter the long-term range of motion.

Recently, more and more articles against the use of the drain in TKA have been published. (Adalberth et al. 1998; Crevoisier et al. 1998; Niskanen et al. 2000; Esler et al. 2003; Parker et al. 2004; Jones et al. 2007) These articles compared the outcomes of the conventional continuing drainage and non-drainage and showed that the drain system not only had no major benefits but also increased blood loss.

The number of patients requiring homologous blood transfusion was provided in several studies. Compared to the non-drainage group, the patients of the drainage group showed higher risk for excessive blood loss which required blood transfusion.(Ovadia et al. 1997; Esler et al. 2003; Cao et al. 2009) The postoperative drop of hemoglobin was also more severe in the drainage group.(Tai et al. 2010a) Longer hospital stay of the drainage group has also been reported in the same article. One possible reason was that the patients were unwilling to do physical activities with a drain inserted in their knees. Delayed rehabilitational programs kept them in the hospital for a longer time. However, this is still a controversial issue because hospital stay is affected by many confounding factors.

4. Make balance between pros and cons of drainage

According to the current evidence, we could not make a conclusion to either support using drainage or non-drainage strategies. The literature indicated that drainage after TKA reduced soft tissue ecchymosis and requirement for dressing reinforcement, but caused more blood loss and increased the blood transfusion rate. The literature also failed to support that drainage could reduce incidence of infection, deep venous thrombosis, or increase postoperative range of motion. Whether using drainage or not depends on each patient's clinical condition, surgeon's preference and consideration.

5. Effect of temporary drain clamping

Several reports regarding the delayed release of the drain have been published in the last decade. After surgery, reactive blood flow increases, with the peak flow appearing within five minutes once the tourniquet is deflated(Larsson et al. 1977). Most of the blood loss in TKA occurs during the first few postoperative hours.(Jou IM 1993; Senthil Kumar et al. 2005) Control of the bleeding is very important during this period. This may be the reason that temporary clamping of the drain tube can significantly reduce the volume of the drained blood.

The ideal drainage system would decrease hematoma formation and not cause excess blood loss. Some blood-saving strategies such as the autologous blood reinfusion, fibrin sealant, pharmacological intervention, or other additional management have been reported to achieve this goal. The drain clamping method, if it is effective, is a much easier way to reduce blood loss compared to these interventions. The initial clamping provides a temporary tamponade effect, as well as the delayed release prevents hematoma formation.

An earlier study(Kiely et al. 2001) about the clamping drainage was reported in 2001 and it claimed that there was no significant difference between the clamping and non-clamping drainage groups in volume of drained blood, transfusion requirements, knee motion or wound status. However, several following studies(Shen et al. 2005; Tsumara et al. 2006; Raleigh et al. 2007; Stucinskas et al. 2008) showed that the drained volume was decreased by temporarily clamping the drain tubes. The other one(Eum et al. 2006) involving the 1-hour clamping method demonstrated a significant decrease in the drained volume in the clamping group during the postoperative 24 hours, but not 48 hours. The total drained blood volume ranged from 297 to 807 ml in the clamping group and 586 to 970 ml in the non-clamping group in the literature.

No matter clamping or not, most of the patients showed similar postoperative hemoglobin levels.(Kiely et al. 2001; Shen et al. 2005; Eum et al. 2006; Tsumara et al. 2006; Stucinskas et al. 2008) Only one study revealed higher postoperative hemoglobin level in the clamping group.(Raleigh et al. 2007) The number of patients requiring transfusion was provided in four studies(Shen et al. 2005; Eum et al. 2006; Tsumara et al. 2006; Stucinskas et al. 2008). One study(Eum et al. 2006) claimed that no transfusions were administered in either group. Shen et al.(Shen et al. 2005) reported similar transfusion rates in the both group. The other two articles(Tsumara et al. 2006; Stucinskas et al. 2008) showed slightly lower transfusion rates with clamped drains. Recently, administration of tranexamic acid and carbazochrome sodium sulfonate hydrate in the drain-clamping method was reported to reduce bleeding after TKA without increasing the risk of deep venous thrombosis.(Onodera et al. 2011)

It seemed that the results about blood loss were heterogeneous. One of the main reason might be the various clamping time in these trials. The debate on the length of time for which the drain should be clamped is still going on. Periods of between 1 and 24 hours have been reported.(Ryu et al. 1997; Kiely et al. 2001; Yamada et al. 2001; Prasad et al. 2005; Shen et al. 2005; Roy et al. 2006; Tsumara et al. 2006; Raleigh et al. 2007; Stucinskas et al. 2008) Some intermittent clamping methods have also showed their effectiveness in bleeding control(Prasad et al. 2005; Tsumara et al. 2006). A meta-analysis of the randomized controlled trials showed that the clamping methods could reduce the true blood loss only when the drain was clamped for four hours or more.(Tai et al. 2010b) We found three trials dealing with the two-hour, one-hour, and half-hour clamping methods and then showing no reduction in true blood loss.(Kiely et al. 2001; Eum et al. 2006; Tsumara et al. 2006) These findings suggest that when using the clamping methods to manage the drainage system after TKA, the ideal clamping period should be four hours or more. However, the patients managed with the longer duration of drain-clamping may have less blood loss but may also eliminate the potential advantages of the drainage. In addition, the situation of long clamping is similar to that of non-drainage; therefore, it is not logical for clinical practice.

Some studies(Kiely et al. 2001; Shen et al. 2005; Tsumara et al. 2006; Stucinskas et al. 2008) mentioned the effect of clamping drainage on postoperative range of motion of the knee. In these studies, the timing of measuring the range of motion varied from 6 to 83 days postoperatively. However, no significant difference was found in this issue. This finding suggested that although clamping the drain might potentially keep the knee swollen and reduce the range of motion shortly after operation, the influence did not persist.

For incidence of thromboembolic events, the previous trials demonstrated no difference in the between of the clamping and non-clamping groups. The pooled results of a recent meta-analysis also suggested that the temporary clamping methods did not significantly increase the risk of thromboembolic events. The symptomatic events occurred in 2.9% (7/244) of patients in the clamping group and 1.2% (3/259) in the non-clamping group (relative risk: 2.25, p = 0.17). The reported wound problems of these trials included severe oozing, bruising, blistering, partial breakdown, wound infection, and cellulitis. Another study reported an episode of transient hypotension upon release of the drain that resolved spontaneously.(Kiely et al. 2001) Again, no significant difference was found between the clamping and non-clamping groups regarding these complications.

In summary, the available evidence indicated that temporarily clamping the drains after TKA decreased the volume of drainage, but only clamping for not less than four hours decreased the reduction in hemoglobin levels. Although clamping does not increase the complication rate, its effectiveness and necessity is still questionable.

6. Authors' preference

For the past decade, we have focused on the studies about the role of the drainage system after total knee arthroplasty. In the first observational study, we found then most of the blood loss in TKA occurs during the first four postoperative hours.(Jou IM 1993; Senthil Kumar et al. 2005) Then we conducted a randomized controlled trial to check the effectiveness of four-hour temporary clamping drainage and found it is an effective method to reduce postoperative blood loss after total knee arthroplasty.(Shen et al. 2005) We also published a meta-analysis of the randomized controlled trials comparing outcomes between the various drain-clamping methods and immediately open drainage after TKA.(Tai et al. 2010b) We focused on blood loss and complications to evaluate the pros and cons of drain clamping. A trial comparing four-clamping drainage and non-drainage was conducted and revealed the role of drainage is still questionable after total knee arthroplasty.(Tai et al. 2010a) Despite clamping the drain for the first four hours after TKA, we found that the patients with drainage showed more blood loss and gained no other benefit compared with those without a drain. Although the clamping drainage was superior to the conventional drainage according to previous literature, we found no advantage of using this method compared with non-drainage. Thus, we did not routinely use the drainage system in primary total knee arthroplasty in our daily practice.

7. References

Adalberth G, Bystrom S, Kolstad K, Mallmin H, Milbrink J. Postoperative drainage of knee arthroplasty is not necessary: a randomized study of 90 patients. Acta Orthop Scand 1998;69:475-8.

Berman AT, Fabiano D, Bosacco SJ, Weiss AA. Comparison between intermittent (spring-loaded) and continuous closed suction drainage of orthopedic wounds: a controlled clinical trial. Orthopedics 1990;13:309-14.

Canty SJ, Shepard GJ, Ryan WG, Banks AJ. Do we practice evidence based medicine with regard to drain usage in knee arthroplasty? Results of a questionnaire of BASK members. Knee 2003;10:385-7.

Cao L, Ablimit N, Mamtimin A, Zhang KY, Li GQ, Li G, Peng LB. [Comparison of no drain or with a drain after unilateral total knee arthroplasty: a prospective randomized controlled trial]. Zhonghua Wai Ke Za Zhi 2009;47:1390-3.

Crevoisier XM, Reber P, Noesberger B. Is suction drainage necessary after total joint arthroplasty? A prospective study. Arch Orthop Trauma Surg 1998;117:121-4.

Drinkwater CJ, Neil MJ. Optimal timing of wound drain removal following total joint arthroplasty. J Arthroplasty 1995;10:185-9.

Esler CN, Blakeway C, Fiddian NJ. The use of a closed-suction drain in total knee arthroplasty. A prospective, randomised study. J Bone Joint Surg Br 2003;85:215-7.

Eum DS, Lee HK, Hwang SY, Park JU. Blood loss after navigation-assisted minimally invasive total knee arthroplasty. Orthopedics 2006;29:S152-4.

Gibbons CE, Solan MC, Ricketts DM, Patterson M. Cryotherapy compared with Robert Jones bandage after total knee replacement: a prospective randomized trial. Int Orthop 2001;25:250-2.

Holt BT, Parks NL, Engh GA, Lawrence JM. Comparison of closed-suction drainage and no drainage after primary total knee arthroplasty. Orthopedics 1997;20:1121-4; discussion 4-5.

Jones AP, Harrison M, Hui A. Comparison of autologous transfusion drains versus no drain in total knee arthroplasty. Acta Orthop Belg 2007;73:377-85.

Jou IM LK, Yang CY. Blood loss associated with total knee arthroplasty. J Orthop Surg (ROC) 1993;10:213.

Kiely N, Hockings M, Gambhir A. Does temporary clamping of drains following knee arthroplasty reduce blood loss? A randomised controlled trial. Knee 2001;8:325-7.

Kim YH, Cho SH, Kim RS. Drainage versus nondrainage in simultaneous bilateral total knee arthroplasties. Clin Orthop Relat Res 1998;188-93.

Kullenberg B, Ylipaa S, Soderlund K, Resch S. Postoperative cryotherapy after total knee arthroplasty: a prospective study of 86 patients. J Arthroplasty 2006;21:1175-9.

Larsson J, Lewis DH, Liljedahl SO, Lofstrom JB. Early biochemical and hemodynamic changes after operation in a bloodless field. Eur Surg Res 1977;9:311-20.

Lin J, Fan Y, Chang X, Wang W, Weng XS, Qiu GX. [Comparative study of one stage bilateral total knee arthroplasty with or without drainage]. Zhonghua Yi Xue Za Zhi 2009;89:1480-3.

Martin A, Prenn M, Spiegel T, Sukopp C, von Strempel A. [Relevance of wound drainage in total knee arthroplasty--a prospective comparative study]. Z Orthop Ihre Grenzgeb 2004;142:46-50.

Mengal B, Aebi J, Rodriguez A, Lemaire R. [A prospective randomized study of wound drainage versus non-drainage in primary total hip or knee arthroplasty]. Rev Chir Orthop Reparatrice Appar Mot 2001;87:29-39.

Niskanen RO, Korkala OL, Haapala J, Kuokkanen HO, Kaukonen JP, Salo SA. Drainage is of no use in primary uncomplicated cemented hip and knee arthroplasty for osteoarthritis: a prospective randomized study. J Arthroplasty 2000;15:567-9.

Omonbude D, El Masry MA, O'Connor PJ, Grainger AJ, Allgar VL, Calder SJ. Measurement of joint effusion and haematoma formation by ultrasound in assessing the effectiveness of drains after total knee replacement: A prospective randomised study. J Bone Joint Surg Br 2010;92:51-5.

Onodera T, Majima T, Sawaguchi N, Kasahara Y, Ishigaki T, Minami A. Risk of Deep Venous Thrombosis in Drain Clamping With Tranexamic Acid and Carbazochrome Sodium Sulfonate Hydrate in Total Knee Arthroplasty. J Arthroplasty 2011;

Ovadia D, Luger E, Bickels J, Menachem A, Dekel S. Efficacy of closed wound drainage after total joint arthroplasty. A prospective randomized study. J Arthroplasty 1997;12:317-21.

Parker MJ, Roberts CP, Hay D. Closed suction drainage for hip and knee arthroplasty. A meta-analysis. J Bone Joint Surg Am 2004;86-A:1146-52.

Prasad N, Padmanabhan V, Mullaji A. Comparison between two methods of drain clamping after total knee arthroplasty. Arch Orthop Trauma Surg 2005;125:381-4.

Radkowski CA, Pietrobon R, Vail TP, Nunley JA, 2nd, Jain NB, Easley ME. Cryotherapy temperature differences after total knee arthroplasty: a prospective randomized trial. J Surg Orthop Adv 2007;16:67-72.

Raleigh E, Hing CB, Hanusiewicz AS, Fletcher SA, Price R. Drain clamping in knee arthroplasty, a randomized controlled trial. ANZ J Surg 2007;77:333-5.

Roy N, Smith M, Anwar M, Elsworth C. Delayed release of drain in total knee replacement reduces blood loss. A prospective randomised study. Acta Orthop Belg 2006;72:34-8.

Ryu J, Sakamoto A, Honda T, Saito S. The postoperative drain-clamping method for hemostasis in total knee arthroplasty. Reducing postoperative bleeding in total knee arthroplasty. Bull Hosp Jt Dis 1997;56:251-4.

Senthil Kumar G, Von Arx OA, Pozo JL. Rate of blood loss over 48 hours following total knee replacement. Knee 2005;12:307-9.

Shen PC, Jou IM, Lin YT, Lai KA, Yang CY, Chern TC. Comparison between 4-hour clamping drainage and nonclamping drainage after total knee arthroplasty. J Arthroplasty 2005;20:909-13.

Stucinskas J, Tarasevicius S, Cebatorius A, Robertsson O, Smailys A, Wingstrand H. Conventional drainage versus four hour clamping drainage after total knee arthroplasty in severe osteoarthritis: a prospective, randomised trial. Int Orthop 2008;

Tai TW, Jou IM, Chang CW, Lai KA, Lin CJ, Yang CY. Non-Drainage Is Better Than 4-Hour Clamping Drainage in Total Knee Arthroplasty. Orthopedics 2010a;156-60.

Tai TW, Yang CY, Jou IM, Lai KA, Chen CH. Temporary drainage clamping after total knee arthroplasty: a meta-analysis of randomized controlled trials. J Arthroplasty 2010b;25:1240-5.

Tao K, Wu HS, Li XH, Qian QR, Wu YL, Zhu YL, Chu XB, Xu CM. [The use of a closed-suction drain in total knee arthroplasty: a prospective, randomized study]. Zhonghua Wai Ke Za Zhi 2006;44:1111-4.

Tsumara N, Yoshiya S, Chin T, Shiba R, Kohso K, Doita M. A prospective comparison of clamping the drain or post-operative salvage of blood in reducing blood loss after total knee arthroplasty. J Bone Joint Surg Br 2006;88:49-53.

Yamada K, Imaizumi T, Uemura M, Takada N, Kim Y. Comparison between 1-hour and 24-hour drain clamping using diluted epinephrine solution after total knee arthroplasty. J Arthroplasty 2001;16:458-62.

Zhang QD, Guo WS, Zhang Q, Liu ZH, Cheng LM, Li ZR. Comparison Between Closed Suction Drainage and Nondrainage in Total Knee Arthroplasty A Meta-Analysis. J Arthroplasty 2011;

7

Proximal Tibiofibular Joint in Knees with Arthroplasty

Hakan Boya
Başkent University, Faculty of Medicine,
Department of Orthopaedics and Traumatology,
Zübeyde Hanım Hospital, İzmir
Turkey

1. Introduction

Because proximal tibiofibular joint (PTFJ) is a diarthrodial joint encased in a synovial-lined articular capsule, it is possible to observe disorders at synovial joints, such as traumatic dislocation, osteoarthritis, inflammatory arthritis, ganglion cysts, pigmented villonodular synovitis, and infection.

Because of its close proximity to the knee joint, PTFJ may be the cause of lateral knee pain. This issue is important, especially in knees with arthroplasty. However, knee arthroplasty may exacerbate PTFJ. Consequently, the joint should be examined in detail before and after knee arthroplasty operations.

2. Embryology and postnatal development

Before 12 weeks of fetal age, PTFJ does not create a cavity (Bozkurt et al., 2003; Resnick et al., 1978). Subsequently, narrow cavities, which may be separated from the lateral femorotibial joint by a small amount of loose fibrous or areolar tissue, are apparent (Resnick et al., 1978). Subsequent development of the PTFJ includes the formation of articular cartilage, synovial tissue, synovial recesses, and a fibrous capsule (Resnick et al., 1978). Ossification usually begins in the proximal tibia within the first three months following birth. The tibiofibular joint morphology has considerable morphologic variation, and the joint may communicate with the knee joint (Ogden, 1984).

3. Anatomy

PTFJ is a diarthrodial joint between the lateral tibial condyle and fibular head; it is located posterolaterally on proximal tibia (Bozkurt et al., 2003). PTFJ has certain characteristics of synovial joints, such as synovial membrane, hyaline cartilage, and a fibrous capsule (Bozkurt et al., 2003; Resnick et al., 1978). The stability of the joint is provided by anterosuperior and posterosuperior capsular ligaments (Ogden, 1974; Resnick et al., 1978; Gray, 1977). The tendon of the biceps femoris muscle inserts into the anterior part of the fibular head and enforces the anterosuperior ligament of the joint (Bozkurt et al., 2003; Marshall et al., 1972).

Communication between the knee joint and PTFJ is reported to be 10-63% (Bozkurt et al., 2003; De Franca, 1992; Eichenblat et al., 1983, Veth et al., 1984). Communication between the proximal tibiofibular and the knee joint occurs via the subpopliteal recess-associated defect in the posterior ligament of the fibular head (Dirim et al., 2008). The relation of the defect to trauma or developmental deficiency is unclear (Dirim et al., 2008).

Two types of PTFJ were defined according to joint line inclination; oblique (inclination > 20⁰) and horizontal (inclination < 20⁰) (Ogden, 1974). Moreover, planar, trochoid and double trochoid types of PTFJ have been reported (Espregueira-Mendes & Vieira, 2006).

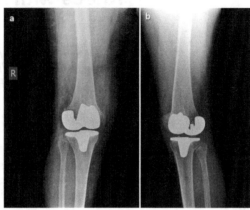

Fig. 1. Horizontal (a) and oblique (b) type PTFJ

3.1 Functional anatomy
Primary functions of PTFJ include the following:
1. Dissipation of torsional stresses applied at the ankle. With external rotation of the fibula about its longitudinal axis during dorsiflexion of the ankle joint, the proximal fibula rotates a few degrees externally (Barnett & Napier, 1952). The amount of external rotation is much greater in horizontal-type PTFJs (Barnett & Napier, 1952).
2. Dissipation of lateral tibial bending movements. Tensile and torsional forces influence the proximal-middle fibula in contrast to the distal fibula, which is affected by compressive forces (Ogden, 1974).
3. Transmitting axial loads in weight-bearing. Approximately one-sixth of the static load is applied at the ankle being transmitted to the PTFJ (Lambert, 1971).

4. Pathologies of PTFJ

It is possible to observe all disease at the PTFJ, similar to other synovial joints. Pathologies of this joint include primary osteoarthritis (Bozkurt et al., 2004; Öztuna et al., 2003; Özcan et al., 2009), trauma (Ogden, 1974; Resnick et al., 1978), infection, and inflammatory arthritis (Resnick & Niwayama,1995), synovial osteochondromatosis (Bozkurt et al., 2007; Heybeli et al., 2009; Weiss et al., 1975), neoplasms (Forster et al., 2007), ganglion cysts (Miskovsky et al., 2004; Mortazavi et al., 2006; Ward & Echardt, 1994), and pigmented villonodular synovitis (Ryan et al., 2004).

4.1 PTFJ in knees with severe primary osteoarthritis
PTFJ can be affected by primary osteoarthritis (Öztuna et al., 2003). The degree of osteoarthritis of the proximal tibiofibular joint strongly correlates with the degree of arthritis

in tibiofemoral joints (TFJ) that have severe degenerative joint disease (Boya et al., 2008). Inflammatory enzymes passing between the joint spaces through possible anatomical communication between the TFJ and PTFJ may contribute to the advancement of arthritis in the respective compartments (Boya et al., 2008; Bozkurt et al., 2003). As with other joints, osteophytes, subchondral cysts, subchondral sclerosis, and joint-space narrowing are typical imaging findings (Forster et al., 2007).

Although primary degenerative disease of the PTFJ is commonly associated with primary degenerative disease of the knee joint, radiographic findings of the PTFJ in patients with severe degenerative knee osteoarthritis and varus misalignment do not correlate with clinical findings (Özcan et al., 2009).

4.2 PTFJ in other pathologies

Various neoplasms can affect the proximal tibiofibular joint, including osteochondroma, osteoblastoma, osteosarcoma, and nerve sheath tumors (Schwannomas and neurofibromas) (Forster et al., 2007).

Tuberculosis lesions at the fibular head can destroy PTFJ and mimic tumoral lesions (Abdelwahab et al., 2003-2004).

Synovial chondromatosis is a chronic, progressive disease of the synovial tissue in which free chondral loose bodies are formed after metaplasia (Bozkurt et al., 2007; Heybeli et al., 2009; Weiss et al., 1975).

A ganglion is a tumorlike, cystic lesion that arises from the joint, tendon sheath, or muscle (Miskovsky et al., 2004). It is a rare pathology at the PTFJ but can cause three different pathologies: asymptomatic mass, symptomatic fluctuant mass, and mass with peroneal nerve dysfunction (Forster et al., 2007).

PTFJ is affected similarly to other synovial joints in rheumatoid arthritis. Peroneal nerve dysfunction due to subluxation, dislocation of dextruted PTFJ is a pathologic entity of the joint with RA (Ishikawa & Hirohata, 1984). Moreover, it is possible to observe radiological deterioration of the PTFJ in patients with ankylosing spondylitis (Hong et al., 2009).

Pigmented villonodular synovitis (PVNS) is an uncommon proliferative disease of the synovium, which is usually monoarticular, presenting as chronic monoarthritis of the knee (Forster et al., 2007). PVNS is characterized by synovial hypertrophy with diffuse or focal hemosiderin deposition in the joint (Ryan et al., 2004). The disease can affect the PTFJ similarly to other synovial joints.

5. Importance of PTFJ in knees with arthroplasty

The PTFJ can be considered the fourth compartment of the knee joint because of its communication with the knee joint cavity (Bozkurt et al., 2003). PTFJ can be a source of lateral knee pain because of its pathologies. However, frequently it is overlooked because of its lack of emphasis in the literature (Forster et al., 2007). For this reason, the PTFJ should be carefully evaluated for osteoarthritis in patients being considered for a total knee arthroplasty operation. If it is overlooked as an etiology of a patient's lateral knee pain, pain from the diseased PTFJ may continue post-operatively. Furthermore, pathologies of the PTFJ may cause peroneal nerve dysfunction in patients with knee arthroplasty (Gibbon et al., 1999). PTFJ stability is important in cases with knee arthroplasty, especially in patients with rheumatoid arthritis. In those patients, the PTFJ may became unstable. Because of proximal movement of the fibular head, it may impinge to extruded bone cement under the tibial base plate posterolaterally (Otani et al., 1998). This possibility should be considered during cementing of the tibial base plate; posterolateral cement excursion should be avoided in patients with inflammatory arthritis.

PTFJ pathologies can affect the arthroplasty results. Conversely, knee arthroplasty can produce PTFJ pathologies. It is possible to inadvertently destroy the PTFJ during an erroneous lower-level tibial cut; this may produce joint-related symptoms after a knee arthroplasty operation. Knees with aseptic loosening of the prosthesis produce inflammatory mediators and polyethylene particles can migrate to the PTFJ via communication between the knee and proximal tibiofibular joints. This can result in deterioration of the PTFJ and subsequent symptoms (Crawford et al., 1998).

6. Conclusion

The degree of osteoarthritis of the proximal tibiofibular joint strongly correlates with the degree of arthritis in tibiofemoral joints that have severe degenerative joint disease. Although primary degenerative disease of the PTFJ is commonly associated with primary degenerative disease of the knee joint, radiographic findings of the PTFJ in patients with severe degenerative knee osteoarthritis and varus misalignment do not correlate with clinical findings. It is possible to observe all disease at the PTFJ, similar to other synovial joints. Because of its close proximity to the knee joint, PTFJ may be the cause of lateral knee pain. This issue is important, especially in knees with arthroplasty. However, knee arthroplasty may exacerbate PTFJ. Consequently, the joint should be examined in detail before and after knee arthroplasty operations.

7. References

Abdelwahab, IF., Poplaw, S., Abdul-Quader, M. & Naran, D. (2003). Tuberculous pseudotumor of the proximal end of the fibula. A case report. *Bull Hosp Jt Dis*, Vol.61, No.3-4, pp. 145-147, ISSN 0883-9344

Barnett, CH. & Napier, JR. (1952) The axis of rotation of the ankle joint in man. Its influance upon the form of the talus and mobility of the fibula. *J Anat*, Vol.86, No.1, (January1952), pp. 1-9, ISSN 1136-4890

Boya, H., Ozcan, O. & Oztekin, HH. (2008). Radiological evaluation of the proximal tibiofibular joint in knees with severe primary osteoarthritis. *Knee Surg Sports Traumatol Arthrosc*, Vol.16, No.2, (February 2008), pp. 157-159, ISSN 0942-2056

Bozkurt, M., Yılmaz, E., Atlihan, D., Tekdemir, I., Havitçioğlu, H. & Günal, I. (2003). The proximal tibiofibuar joint: An anatomic study. *Clin Orthop Relate Res*, Vol.406, No.1 (January 2003), pp. 136-140, ISSN 0009-921X

Bozkurt, M., Yılmaz, E., Akseki, D., Havıtcıoğlu, H. & Günal, I. (2004). The evaluation of the proximal tibiofibular joint for patients with lateral knee pain. *The Knee*, Vol.11, No.4, (August 2004), pp. 307-312, ISSN 0968-0160

Bozkurt, M., Uğurlu, M., Doğan, M. & Tosun, N. (2007) Synovial chondromatosis of four compartments of the knee: medial and lateral tibiofemoral spaces, patellofemoral joint and proximal tibiofibular joint. *Knee Surg Sports Traumatol Arthrosc*, Vol.15, No.6, (June 2007), pp. 753-755, ISSN 0942-2056

Crawford, R., Sabokbar, A., Wulke, A., Murray, DW. & Athanasou, NA. (1998). Expansion of an osteoarthritic cyst associated with wear debris: a case report. *J Bone Joint Surg Br*,Vol.80, No.6, (November 1998), pp. 990-993, ISSN 0301-620X

De Franca, GG. (1992). Proximal tibiofibular joint dysfunction and chronic knee and low back pain. *J ManipPhysiol Ther*, Vol.15, No.6, (July-August 1992), pp. 382–387, ISSN 0161-4754

Dirim, B., Wangwinyuvirat, M., Frank, A., Cink, V., Pretterklieber, ML., Pastore, D. & Resnick, D.(2008). Communication between the proximal tibiofibular joint and knee via the subpopliteal recess: MR arthrography with histologic correlation and stratigraphic dissection. *AJR Am J Roentgenol*, Vol.191, No.2, (August 2008), pp. W44-51, ISSN 1546-3141

Eichenblat, M. & Nathan, H. (1983). The proximal tibiofibular joint. An anatomical study with clinical and pathological considerations. *Int Orthop*, Vol.7, No.1, pp. 31–39, ISSN 0341-2695

Espregueira-Mendes, JD. & da Silva, MV. (2006). Anatomy of the proximal tibiofibular joint. *Knee Surg SportsTraumatol Arthrosc*, Vol.14, No.3, (March 2006), pp. 241-249, ISSN 0942-2056

Forster, BB., Lee, JS., Kelly, S., O'Dowd, M., Munk, PL., Andrews, G. & Marchinkow, L. (2007) Proximal tibiofibular joint: an often-forgotten cause of lateral knee pain. *AJR Am J Roentgenol*, Vol.188, No.4, (April 2007) pp. W359-366, ISSN ISSN 1546-3141

Gibbon, AJ., Wardell, SR. & Scott, RD. (1999). Synovial cyst of the proximal tibiofibular joint with peroneal nerve compression after total knee arthroplasty. *J Arthroplasty*, Vol.14, No.6, (September 1999), pp. 766-768, ISSN 0883- 5403

Gray, H. (1977). *The classic Collector's Edition. Gray's Anatomy*, Churchill Livinstone Inc, ISBN 978-051-7223-65-9, New York, USA

Heybeli, N., Ozcan, M., Copuroğlu, C. & Yalniz, E. (2009). Isolated synovial chondromatosis of the proximal tibiofibular joint. *Acta Orthop Traumatol Turc*, Vol.43, No. 5, (November-December 2009), pp. 448-452, ISSN 1017-995X

Hong, HP., Chung, HW., Choi, BK., Yoon, YC. & Choi, SH. (2009) Involvement of the proximal tibiofibular joint in ankylosing spondylitis. Acta Radiol, Vol.50, No.4, (May 2009), pp. 418-422, ISSN 0284-1851

Ishikawa, H. & Hirohata K. (1984). Bilateral peroneal nerve palsy secondary to posterior dislocation of the proximaltibiofibular joint in rheumatoid arthritis. *Rheumatol Int*, Vol.5, No.1, pp. 45-47, ISSN 0172-8172

Lambert KL. (1971). The weight-bearing function of the fibula. A strain gauge study. *J Bone Joint Surg Am*, Vol.53, No.3, (April 1971), pp. 507-513, ISSN 0021-9355

Marshall, JG., Girgis, FG. & Zelko, RR. (1972). The Biseps Femoris tendon and its functional significance. *J Bone Joint Surg Am*, Vol.54, No.7, (October 1972), pp. 1444-1450, ISSN 0021-9355

Miskovsky, S., Kaeding, C. & Weis, L. (2004) Proximal tibiofibular joint ganglion cysts: excision, recurrence, and joint arthrodesis. *Am J Sports Med*, Vol.32, No.4, (June 2004), pp.1022-1028, ISSN 0363-5465

Mortazavi, SM., Farzan, M. & Asadollahi, S. (2006). Proximal tibiofibular joint synovial cyst-one pathology with three different presentations. *Knee Surg Sports Traumatol Arthrosc*, Vol.14, No.9, (September 2006), pp. 875-879, ISSN 0942-2056

Ogden, JA. (1974). The anatomy and function of the proximal tibiofibular joint. *Clin Orthop,* Vol.101, No.6, (June 1974), pp. 186-191, ISSN 0009-921X

Ogden, JA. (1984). Radiology of postnatal skeletal development. IX. Proximal tibia and fibula. *Skeletal Radiol,* Vol.11, No.3, pp. 169-177, ISSN 0364-2348

Otani, T., Fujii, K., Ozawa, M., Kaechi, K., Funaki, K., Matsuba, T. & Ueno, H. (1998). Impingement after total knee arthroplasty caused by cement extrusion and proximal tibiofibular instability. *J Arthroplasty,* Vol.13, No.5, (August 1998), pp. 589-591, ISSN 0883-5403

Özcan, O., Boya, H. & Oztekin, HH. (2009) Clinical evaluation of the proximal tibiofibular joint in knees with severe tibiofemoral primary osteoarthritis. *The Knee,* Vol.16, No.4, (August 2009), pp. 248-250, ISSN 0968- 0160

Öztuna, V., Yıldız, A., Özer, C., Milcan, A., Kuyurtar, F. & Turgut, F. (2003). Involvement of the proximal tibiofibular joint in osteoarthritis of the knee. *The Knee,* Vol.10, No.4, (December 2003), pp. 347-349, ISSN 0968-0160

Resnick, D., Newell, JD., Guerra, J Jr., Danzing, LA., Niwayama, G. & Goergen, TG. (1978) Proximal tibiofibular joint: Anatomic-pathologic-radiographic correlation. *Am J Roentgenol,* Vol.131, No.1, (July 1978), pp. 133-138, ISSN 0361-803

Resnick, D. & Niwayama, G. (1995). Anatomy of individual joints, In: *Diagnosis of bone and joint disorders,* Resnick, D. & Niwayama, G. pp. 741-750, WB Saunders, ISBN 072165066X, 9780721650661, Philadelphia

Ryan, RS., Louis ,L., O'Connell, JX. & Munk, PL. (2004). Pigmented villonodular synovitis of the proximal tibiofibular joint. *Australas Radiol,* Vol.48, No.4, (December 2004), pp. 520-522, ISSN 0004-8461

Ward, WG. & Eckardt, JJ. (1994) Ganglion cyst of the proximal tibiofibular joint causing anterior compartment syndrome. A case report and anatomical study. *J Bone Joint Surg Am,* Vol.76, No.10, (October 1994), pp. 1561- 1564, ISSN 0021-9355

Weiss, C., Averbuch, PF., Steiner, GC. & Rusoff, JH. (1975). Synovial chondromatosis and instability of the proximal tibiofibular joint. *Clin Orthop Relat Res,* Vol.108, No.5, (May 1975), pp. 187-190, ISSN 0009-921X

Veth, RP., Kingma. LM. & Nielsen, HK. (1984). The abnormal proximal tibiofibular joint. Arch Orthop Trauma Surg, Vol.102, No.3, pp. 167-171, ISSN 0936-8051

Part 2

Special Topics in Knee Arthroplasty

8

Special Situations in Total Knee Arthroplasty

Orlando M. de Cárdenas Centeno and Felix A. Croas Fernández
"Frank País" International Scientific Orthopedic Complex
Medical Sciences University, Havana
Cuba

1. Introduction

Total Knee Arthroplasty TKA has become a highly successful joint reconstruction procedure.

Surgical outcomes, patients satisfaction and implant survival have improved, and the operation has become widely accepted to afford relief pain, restoration of range motion and function. TKA has been shown to have durable and predictable results in elderly patients.

The principals indications for TKA are severe pain and functional disability. Others indications include deformity, instability and loss of motion.

The diagnosis associated with this features for which TKA has been successfully performed include osteoarthritis, rheumatoid arthritis, inflammatory arthritis, osteonecrosis, and others disability disorders, including tumors and fractures.

The indications and contraindications to perform a TKA have been well established and documented.

Nevertheless there are situations well-known as special or complex, where sometimes could be considered controversial or relative contraindications, and require a deep analysis and take difficult decision.

Up today, specials situations are not presented in elderly patient only. These situations occur in young patient less than 55 or 40 years old too. (De Cárdenas et al 2009) at present, on the basis of obtained results and different reported, the indications for TKA have been expanded eventually to younger people.

Total Joint Arthroplasty continues to confer immense benefits upon patients with joint disease, and it is considered as one of the most cost-effective surgical procedures (Dunbar et al 2009).

In special situations, TKA may be performed in patients in any age to salvage a knee or even to restore motion and relief pain where other procedures are not possible. This indication, however, remains controversial and could be considered relatives contraindications.

The aim of this study is present our modest experience and valuate a group of patients with different situations to whom were performed a complex TKA in specials situations using a Kalisté Knee System.

1.1 Special situations

Complex TKA in specials situations have been presented and development by differents Orthopaedics Surgeons and although controversial criterions have been collected, the concept and the outcomes has been well accepted by orthopedic community.

While the literature does not resolve all the controversies in TKA, sometimes we will encounter apparently disparate advice in some areas; some of which is due to honest differences in opinion and personal experiences and some related to the type of implants.

Based in the evidence of scientific papers, literature, experts opinion and by consensus, we would like to present our modest experience and results.

Different representative patients with specials situations: Fig. 1

- Stiff and ankylosed Knee
- Knee angular deformity: Varus / Valgus (figure 1.a / figure 1.b)
- High Tibial Osteotomy HTO (after) (figure 1.c)
- Patellar problems (after Maquet osteotomy or patellectomy)
- Rheumatoid Arthritis (Total Joint Collapsed) (figure 1.d)
- Post-traumatic Osteoarthritis
- Arthrodesed Knee
- Achondroplasic

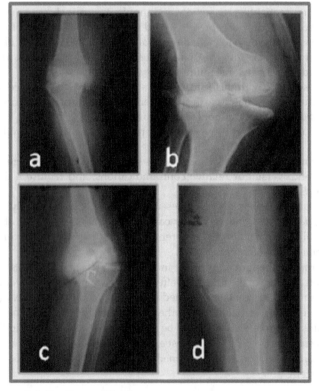

Fig. 1. Different special situations of the knee.

Many of these conditions are associated or combined with:

Instability, flexed or extended painful rigid knee and/or bone defect.

In summary all this patients have diagnosis of Severe Osteoarthritis of the Knee. (figure 2.)

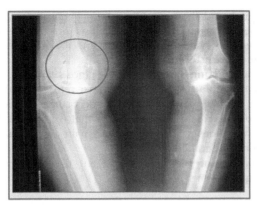

Fig. 2. Severe Bilateral Osteoarthritis of the Knee

2. Material and method

This is a longitudinal, prospectively and follow-up study. Between January 2004 and January 2010 the authors did 636 consecutive Total Knee Arthroplasty in 582 patients with moderate to severe Osteoarthritis of the Knee. They were treated using Kalisté Knee System (FHorthopedic. France).

From this group were selected 132 patients (146 TKA) to be included in this study. They were 14 Bilateral in two stage and 118 Unilateral, 69 left Knee and 49 right Knee. 81patients (61,4 %) were female and 51 (38,6 %) male, with a mean age of 62.5 years old (range 25 to 82 years old).

2.1 Patient selection

The patient selected to be included in this study has been patients with specials situations as was descripted.

All of them has severe primary knee osteoarthritis IV-V Alback's radiographic classification or secondary to others conditions like post-traumatic, rheumatic arthritis with total joint collapse, angular deformity: varus / valgus.

Stiff or ankylosed knee, patellar problems as after Maquet osteotomy or patellectomy, history or failured high tibial osteotomy, arthrodesed knee and achondroplasic.

Gender, race or age not were criteria to exclude. The authors excluded patients with ligth or moderate primary knee osteoarthritis and varus / valgus/ flexed deformity less than 10 degrees, additional exclusion criteria included history of septic arthritis of the knee, neuropathic knee, and hemophilic arthritis not was criteria to be included.

2.2 Ethical considerations

The study was approved by the institutional review board.

All the patients were well informed and documented about the methodology, purpose and procedure of this study, and have given their consent in writing.

2.3 Clinical assessment

Pre-operative clinical evaluation include detailed medical history, full name, identification card number, gender, race, age and all dates according to the standard file to all patients admitted in this hospital, and thorough clinical-functional and radiographic examination using the Knee Society Scoring KSS, because it is one of the more acceptable and standardized instruments to evaluation of results, and it is a powerful tool for comparing specific dynamics of the knee arthroplasty.

The Knee Society Clinical Rating System available since 1989 (Insall et al.1989), have been the preferred method of outcome assessment after knee replacement for many surgeons.

The new KSS is being validated and updated to reflect current trend in Knee Arthroplasty and contemporary expectation and activities levels that were not well addressed in earlier assessment models. It includes visual analog and pain assessment, as well as objective measures of knee motion and stability.

The functional component of the KSS is relevant to contemporary patients of any demographic background (Lonner JH, 2009).

2.4 Radiographic evaluation

Pre-operative image evaluation includes standard differents Knee radiographs:

Comparative anterior-posterior AP standing view (if the patient could be stand) or in supine position, lateral view in 25-30 flexion degree (each one) and patella axial view (all of this, if it was possible according to the knee joint condition).

Additionally radiographic studies of the both hip and both ankle were taken to know the conditions of these joints.

Pangonogramme not was possible, and anterior-posterior radiographic views were done standing or supine position with 14" x 17" cassettes.

Radiographic analysis permitted the determination of the preoperative knee osteoarthritis classification (Alback S, 1968) and included measurement of the mechanical axis, measurement of the femorotibial axis and assessment of the degree of correction.

On standing AP radiographic view, were measured the varus or valgus deformity.

On lateral radiographic view, were measurement the posterior slope of the tibia and observed the posterior knee aspect and the patella localization.

On axial radiographic view were observed patellofemoral alignment, joint space and joint surface.

All this measurements were done using a goniometer.

To the determination of the preoperative osteoarthritis classification an co-author (RJTR) who did not do surgeries reviewed all available radiograph taken before surgery, and at the most recent follow-up for evidence of component loosening, radiolucencies, and overall alignment, using the Knee Society total knee roentgenographic evaluation and Scoring System (Ewald FC, 1989).

Using the X-Ray template (transparences) of the Kalisté components systems were calculated the size of the each component during pre-operative plannification.

2.5 Surgical technique
2.5.1 Kalisté Total Knee System

Kalisté Total Knee System (FHorthopedic.France) is a tricompartmental resurfacing prosthesis.

The femoral and tibial resections are independent.

This design allows the surgeons to begin with either the tibial stage or the femoral stage.

It is mainly based on intramedullary femoralalignment. Pre-operative control of the femoral guide alignment is performed with the help of extramedullary rods.

The pre-operative plannification (radiographic studies) allow the surgeon to calculate the anatomical axis of the leg, in order to calculate the angle o femoral valgus.

The resections (distal femoral and proximal tibial) are perpendicular to the mechanical axis of the leg. Tibial viewing in intramedullary, if the entry point used is located at the level of the insertion of the anterior cruciate ligament or external (tibia varus). Definition of the axes and estimation of the size of the implants are determined thanks to X-Rays template at a 1.15 scale.

The Kalisté Total Knee System was designed to admit posterior cruciate ligaments PCL-retaining or posterior stabilized PS Knee prosthesis. (Fig. 3.a, 3.b)

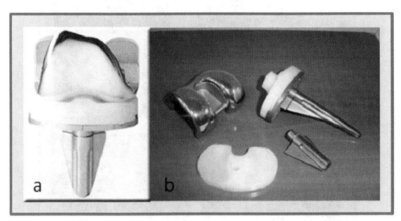

Fig. 3. a. Kaliste Total Knee System (PCL retaining), b. Kaliste Total Knee System (Posterior Stabilized) (with permission FHorthopedic. France)

The accessories, augmentation devices, and short or long stem for the operative technique are available in the instrumentation sets.

The surgeon decides if use or not use the patellar prosthesis component and it is available too.

2.5.2 Surgical protocol

All surgeries were done by one surgeon (OMCC), the same surgical team and at one institution (CCOI Frank Pais, La Habana, Cuba) all procedures followed a standard operative protocol. Surgeries were done with the patient in supine position.

All surgical procedures were performed in a standard operation theatre with standard air conditions (not ultra-clean air, not laminar flow). Standard clothing was used by the surgical team. 87% of the surgeries were with spinal, epidural anesthesia using intravenous sedation too, and only in selective patients with specific clinical conditions were under general anesthesia as anesthesiologist advised. Pneumatic tourniquet not were used in nobody case. Hemostasis achieved with use of cauterization and diathermy.

The limb washed and draping technique for TKA was done as usually. Ancilliary leg-holding device was placed on the limb and operating table to provide stable and gradual positioning of the Knee during surgery.

In all cases of this study were used posterior-stabilized Kalisté Knee System cemented with Polymethylmethacrylat.

The procedure to implant the components was according to the standards total knee arthroplasty, using the instrumentation designed to it. Variants were used as advisable in each special situation (Lotke PA, 1999, 2002, Nelson CL 2002, Scuderi GR 2002, Padgell D. 2002, Griffin FM 2002, Lombardi AV et al. 2009).

In general, a straight anterior longitudinal (midline) skin incision was the most appropriate performed when skin condition was possible, followed by a medial parapatellar capsular arthrotomy (Fig. 4).

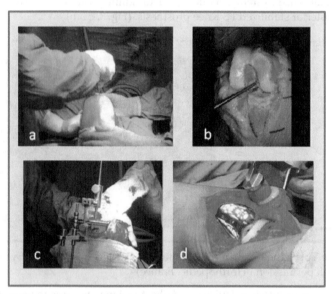

Fig. 4. a. b. c. d. Different phases of the surgical procedure to implant the knee prosthesis.

It provides adequate access to medial or lateral aspect of the limb. In some cases was necessary a variant, selected of classical approach options according the need.

All patients had placement of drain 24-48 hours post-operation according to standard practice peri-operative prophylaxis consisted of intravenous cephalosporin (Cephazoline 1 gr) starting one hour prior to surgery and continue for 24 to 72 hours. Patients also received subcutaneous low molecular weight heparin LMWH for prophylaxis again deep vein thrombosis DVT started in the evening of the operation day till 10 days according to the conditions of the patients.

2.6 Rehabilitation protocol

All the patients were assigned to regimen for post-operative early mobilization.

Day of the operation: Following skin closure and wound dressing, the knee was placed straight on the bed until early next morning, in an extension splint, with a pillow under the foot, in order to increase the venous backflow and decrease edema. An ice bag over the knee is allowed for the reduction of the hyperemia, the edema and the inflammation.

Post-operative day 1: The regime of rehabilitation program consists in "to leave make" or "allow make" by him/her self (patient) under physiotherapist guide.

We never used continues passive motion CPM machine.

The physiotherapist passively and actively moved the Knee and taught the patient to repeat different exercises during the day alone (5 times daily, at least 3 times), and after each, ice bag over Knee. (figure 5 a, b, c, d)

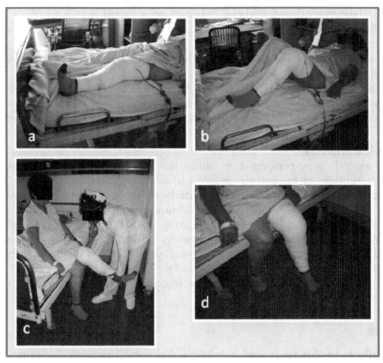

Fig. 5. a. b. c. d. The patient in the postoperative first day, doing exercises intensive rehabilitation program under the guidance of the physiotherapist.

The patient is allowed to sit on the bed or on a seat, bending the knee as tolerated, isometric strengthening of the quadriceps and concentric dynamic exercises of periarticular hip and ankle muscles were encouraged. The knee was placed in the extension splint again overnight.

Post-operative day 2: Continue the same as day 1, increasing the range of motion ROM. The patient started to walk with walker and muscular strengthening recovery was intensified.

Post-operative day 3: The same as day 2, but increasing the ROM, bending the knee to 90° and started to walk with two crutches.

Between the post-operative days 3 to day 5, the patient can go at home with Doctor's orderly and exercises program written and follow-up by outpatient department OPD.

2.7 Evaluation and follow-up

To evaluate the patients, they were checked and recorded according to the KSS all categories were collected in data base and processed in the Med Cal program.

Clinical and functional assessment was performed pre-operatively and post-operative at 3, 6, 12 months and yearly. Patients were evaluated prospectively by means of the Knee

Society Scoring System KSSS and by Analogical Visual Scale AVS to the Health Perception Criteria.

A locally-designed patient satisfaction questionnaire was also given to all patients before operation and yearly after operation, asking them to rate their replacement on a scale from 0 to 10, with 0 being very dissatisfied and 10 being very satisfied.

A deep infection was any infection that concurred inside the knee joint, requiring prosthesis removal.

A superficial infection was any infection of the skin that responded well to antibiotic with not residual problems.

Aseptic loosening was considered to be the presence of a radiolucent line larger than 2 mm around the entire prosthesis which was not related to infection.

Fatal deep venous thrombosis was an acute thromboembolism episode that ended in death.

2.8 Statistical analysis

Statistical analysis was performed to study the possible differences between clinical-functional conditions of the patients before and after operation and radiographic changes for evidence of component loosening, radiolucencies and overall alignment. Before operation each patient was valuated clinical-functionally according KSS. Postoperative were repeated the valuation with the same Scoring System (KSS) at 3, 6 months and yearly. The obtained results were compared. The primary information was recorded in data base elaborated for this study. The results were presented in tables and graphics performed using Microsoft Office Excel and Word program, Window seven operative systems.

Statistical technique of absolute and relative frequency were applied, odds ratio and p-value.

3. Results

All the patients in this study had substantial pain and functional limitation before the surgery. Some of them used wheelchair and many used walker, crutches or cane (support dependence).

This study is one of the largest series of specials situations in TKA. Several authors has reported on the results of total knee arthroplasty in patients with specials situations and reported significant improvement in KSS and ROM.

The study population of this series composed by 132 patients (100%) are summarized in the table 1, and were according gender 81 (61,4%) female and 51 (38.6) male and the age distribution were 38 (28.8%) less than 50 years old and 94 (71,2%) more than 50 years old.

| GENDER | AGE (Years Old) | | | | | |
| | < 50 | | > 50 | | TOTAL | |
	N	%	N	%	N	%
Female	29	22.0	52	39.4	81	61.4
Male	9	6.8	42	31.8	51	38.6
TOTAL	38	28.8	94	71.2	132	100

Table 1. Study population between age and gender distribution (Sources: Data Base)

The primary diagnosis distributions have been summarized in table 2.

"Special Situations" Diagnosis	PATIENTS	
	N	%
After High Tibial Osteotomy	42	31.8
Rheumatoid Arthritis (Joint Collapsed)	14	10.6
Post-traumatic Osteoarthritis	19	14.4
After Patellectomy	5	3.8
Severe Knee deformity Varus/Valgus	31	23.5
Stiff and Ankylosed Knee	18	13.6
After Maquet Osteotomy	3	2.3
TOTAL	132	100

Table 2. "Special Situations". Diagnosis Distribution

In our series study, the side distribution of the knees operated was as showed the Table 3 and Graphic 1.

Number operated knee								
Bilateral		Unilateral						
		Left		Right		Total		
N	%	N	%	N	%	N.	%	
14	10,6	67	56,8	51	42,2	118	89,4	
Odds ratio	1,0742	Odds ratio	2,4219	Odds ratio	2,3355			
p value	0,0593	p value	0,0374	p value	0,0453			

Table 3. Number of Knee operated with "Special Situations" CCOI Frank País. January 2004 – January 2010. (Source: Data Base)

In the sample, 118 patients were operated unilaterally on one knee to 56.8% and 42.2% distributed left knee and right knee respectively. As the number of patients who underwent bilateral knee represent 10.6% of the total. Patients undergoing unilateral knee had both left and right odds ratio of 2.4219 and 2.3355 respectively, indicating that there are two times more likely a patient could be operated on one knee than both, particularly, the left knee.

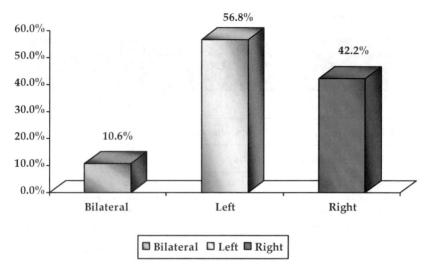

Graphic 1. Number of knees operated according to location

The clinical and functional pre-operative (1 year to follow-up) results according KSS were summarized in the Table 4 and Graphic 2.

Indicator	Clinical				Functional			
	Pre operative	Post operative	Odds ratio	P - value	Pre operative	Post operative	Odds ratio	P - value
Mean	29	89	3,4673	0,0321	23	88	4,0284	0,0382
Range	14 - 49	64 - 100	3,1632	0,0493	0 - 58	62 – 100	4,4570	0,0302

Table 4. Clinical and Functional pre-operative and post-operative (1 year follow-up) Results according KSS. CCOI "Frank País" January 2004 – January 2010 (**Source: Data Base**).

The mean preoperative scale application in clinical phase KSS was 29, indicating that there is a limited deterioration in the knee as a result of joint degeneration, a year is a significant improvement of this parameter as it close to 100 which is the optimum value (89), indicating a favourable clinical evolution of these patients after total knee arthroplasty. According to the level in the preoperative stage, it is appreciated that there was a path of the mean values in the clinical assessment between 14 and 49 points, and in the postoperative phase was reached 64 to 100 points, which is evidence of clinical improvement of patients after surgery. For the value that represents the odds ratio 3.1632 of the clinical phase is to infer that a patient operated year total knee arthroplasty has 3 times more likely to improve in the KSS scale score that if does not apply this surgical procedure.

As for the functional parameter the patients were on average 23 points which shows result in loss of function after knee surgery, and in the postoperative phase is reached near 88 to 100, showing a significant recovery in the functional state of the knees operated patients. The functional range of this phase before the operation is relatively moderate to low once the replacement will elevate this range from 62 to 100 which show functional improvement in knee patients after surgery. For the value 4.4570 represents the odds ratio in this functional setting. We must infer that a patient per year to operate for total knee arthroplasty has 4 times more probabilities to improve his-her functionality according to the KSS scale score that if does not apply this surgical procedure.

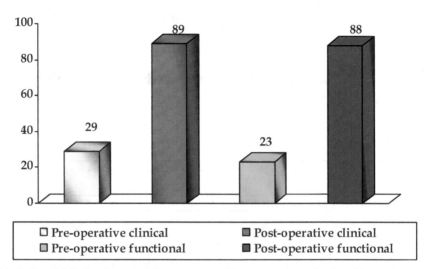

Graphic 2. Graphic behaviour and the year according to preoperative level in patients with knee osteoarthritis KSS operated by ATR.

And finally clinical-functional pre-operative and post-operative, evolution according KSS during 6 years follow up study were showed as a total mean punctuation in the Table 5 and Graphic 3.

Indicator	Pre-operative total mean punctuation	Post-operative total mean punctuation	Follow-up (months)	Odds ratio	P – value
		166	3		
		176	6		
		177	12		
	51	174	24		
		176	36	4,0932	0,0352
		180	48		
		182	60		
		180	72		
Reference Value	200	200	.		
Mean	51	177			

Table 5. Clinical – functional pre-operative and post-operative. Evolution according KSS during 6 years follow-up study. **(Source: Data base).**

It is observed in the preoperative average score achieved on average in the six years was 51 points, and in the postoperative period shows that every year the score is close to 200, the average score is 177, significantly favourable outcome once the total knee arthroplasty. For the odds ratio value reached 4.0932 as can be inferred that a patient operated for total knee arthroplasty from 3 months of surgery is four times more likely to improve their clinical and functional rating scale that a patient KSS not yet been operated with this procedure.

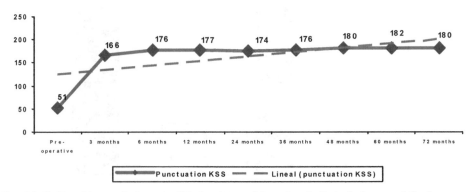

Graphic 3. Graphic trends in overall behavior and functional clinical phases, of the knee as punctuation in the KSS scale.

The graph shows trends as there is a significant evolution (P <0.05) clinical and functional satisfactory phases in the recovery of patients undergoing knee for knee replacement as early as three months after surgery, where this evolution remains a tendency to increase average scale score as KSS.

The final radiographic evaluation showed that 138 (94,5%) of the 146 (100%) operated knee were in neutral alignment, 4 were in valgus and 4 flexed less than 10 degrees each one.

About complications, were 2 deep infection that required revision, prosthesis removed and arthodesis. 3 were superficial infection, 3 mechanical problems: 1 patellar tendon rupture (revision and reconstruction) and 2 patella dislocation (1 arthroscopy to release and 1 revision and realignment).About death (before 90 days post-operative): 1 multiple organic failure in a 78 years old man with high risk and 1 fatal deep venous thrombosis DVT (suddenly).

Our results showed not significant differences in complications between others reported in the medical literature in terms of death, infections, dislocations or revision.

None of the knees had evidence of aseptic loosening, radiolucent or implant migration at the time of the lasted follow up. It may be that a longer follow-up will be required to reveal any difference in outcome.

An efficient surgery, with an aggressive post-operative rehabilitation program and a proper patient selection should maximize favorable results and limit perioperative morbidity.

Every surgeon must evaluate the risk-to-benefit ratio for each individual patient; by the way, the management of these specials conditions has changed over the last years.

Up-today TKA is considered "high tech" procedures.

All patients in our study had functional improvement at the time of latest follow-up. There was a substantial improvement in pain relief and in the range of motion of the knees after TKA in specials situations and the degree of satisfaction of patients significantly improved according to criteria autopersección as shown in Table 6 according to the visual analog scale and of course, improved the quality of life.

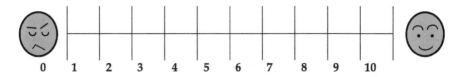

PRE-OP	VS	POST-OP
MEAN: 1.5	VS	MEAN: 8.7
RANGE: 0 – 3	VS	RANGE: 7 - 10

Table 6. Analogical visual scale avs. (Source: Data Base)

3.1 Evolutive cases presentation.

Finally, as evidence of the results were showed some evolutive cases off this study.

The first case, was 64 years old, female, with that diagnosis severe bilateral osteoarthritis of the knee, combined with genus varus and flexion contracture, she has history of high tibial osteotomy in her left knee eight years ago. A sequence evolutive was showed in the figure 6. a, b, c, d, e, f, g, h.

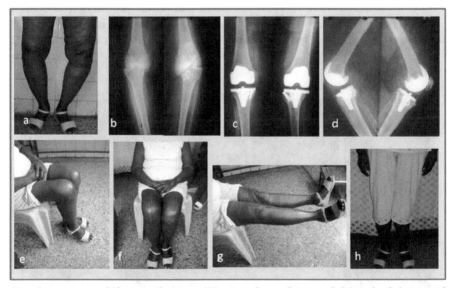

Fig. 6. a. Genus varus deformity, b. X-ray AP view showed severed OA in both knee with HTO in the left, c. X-ray AP view showed bilateral TKA implanted in both knee with two screw reinforced the medial side of the tibial to solve the bone loose and corrected deformity, d. Lateral view of both knee whit TKA implanted, e. f. g. h. the patient rehabilitated with range of motion and full stability.

The second case showed was a 34 years old, female with diagnosis of Rheumatoid arthritis and total joint collapse of both knee in wheelchair the last 3 years, and of course both knee were in fixed flexion the figure 7 a, b, c, d, e, f, g, h showed the sequence of follow – up.

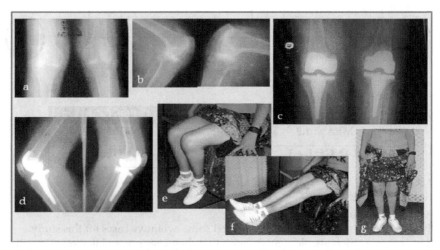

Fig. 7. a. b. Pre-operative AP and Lateral view X-ray of both knee showed the total joint collapse and fixed flexion deformity, c. d. Post-operative bilateral TKA implanted, and e. f. g restored the patient, showing full extension.

The last case presented was a 32 years old, male, with history of multiple injured patient involved in route traffic accident RTA 2 years ago, that actually has diagnosis of post traumatic severe ostearthritis , with stiff and posterior subluxated left knee. The figure 8 a. b. c. d. e. f. g. h. showed the sequence of pre and post operative results to recovery assessed at one year of evolution.

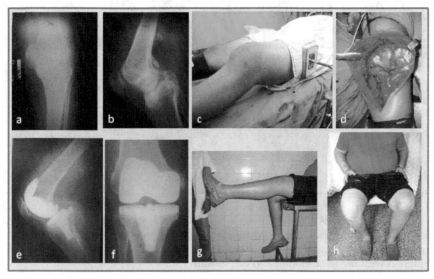

Fig. 8. a. b. c. Evident deformity of the left knee sequel of trauma that required extensive soft tissue release (d.) and TKA implanted (e. f.) and final recovery of the patient with excellent range of motion.

4. Conclusion

In this study about complex Total Knee Arthroplasty in special situation according to our results an outcome, till now the evidence permitted arrive to the following conclusions: patients with specials situations in the knee may look complex or difficult, but the Total Knee Arthroplasty using Kalisté System has been a very successful operation with a high level of patient satisfaction and functional improvement like others reports.

Best results were achieved when the surgeon has carefully evaluated all the factors influencing in each individual special situation and did a preoperative plannification according to it.

The selections of patient and prosthesis design were very important, but we believe that efficient surgery and overall the experience and skill of the surgeon could be more important.

At one to six years follow-up postoperative, the functional outcome between before and after operation appears to be significant different, nevertheless we considered the weakness of this study is the short-mid time's follow-up and need further investigation and follow-up at least ten to fifteen years after implantation.

We believe that the use of Kalisté Knee System improved our results and we can advice this design as an excellent system of TKA.

Finally, our study showed the aim of the evaluation and the evidence: improved the Quality of Life of the Patient in Relation with Health QLPRH.

5. Acknowledgment

The first acknowledgment and gratitude is to Professor Sc. Dr. Rodrigo J.Alvarez Cambras, my mentor, and to Dr. Ricardo J. Tarragona too,for their participation in this study.

I gratefully acknowledge Margarita Garcia, Mayra Leon, Emma Sanchez, Isabel Vega and Gonzalez Liuba for your time, patience and support during the writing, language, as well as making the graphs, tables and photos. And special thanks to Ms Adriana Pecar for her invitation to submit this chapter.

6. References

Agencia de Evaluación Tecnologías Sanitarias (AETS) (2002). Índice y escalas utilizadas en ciertas tecnologias de la prestación ortoprotésica. (Protetización del Sistema Osteoarticular). AETS Instituto de Salud Carlos III. Ministerio de Sanidad y Consumo. Madrid. Noviembre. pp. 5.8, 55-64, 120-28 ISBN 84-95463-14-8

Aglietti P.; Windsov RE.; Buzzi R. and Insall JN (1989). Arthroplasty for stiff or ankylosed Knee. J. Arthroplasty. 41(1):1-5

Aglietti P.; Buzzi R.; Segoni F., et al (1995). Insall-Burstein posterior-stabilized Knee prosthesis in rheumatoid arthritis. J. Arthroplasty; 10:217-25

Alhback S (1968). Osteoarthritis of the Knee. A radiographic investigation. Acta Radiol Diagn. (Suppl) 27:77-82

Ayers DC, Dennis DA, Johanson NA, Pellegrini VD (1997). Instructional Course Lectures. The American Academy of Orthopaedic Surgeons. Common Complication of Total Knee Arthroplasty. J. Bone Joint Surg; 79-A(22):278-331

Bayne O & Camero HV (1984). Total Knee Arthroplasty following patellectomy. Clin Orthop; 186:112

Brinkman JM, et al (2008). Osteotomies arround the Knee: patient selection, stability of fixation and bone healing in high tibial osteotomies. J. Bone Joint Surg; 90-B:1548-57

Brown TD, et al (2006). Post-traumatic osteoarthritis. A first estímate of incidence, prevalence and burden of disease. J Orthop Trauma; 30:739-44

Brundtland GH (2007). The Bone and Joint Decade WHO Scientific Group meeting on burden musculoskeletal disease. Geneva.
    http://www.who.int/generaldirector/speeches/2000/english/...accessed

Callahan CM, Drake BG, Heck DA, Dittus RS (1994). Patients outcomes following tricompartimental total knee replacement. JAMA; 271:1349-57

Clark CR, Rorabech CH, MacDonald S, et al. (2001). Posterior-stabilized and cruciate-retaining total knee replacement: a randomized study. Clin Orthop; 392:208-12

Colizza WA, Insall JN & Scuderi GR (1995). The posterior stabilized total knee prosthesis. Assessment of polyethilene damage and osteolisis after a ten-year minimun follow-up. J Bone Joint Surg; 77-A:1713-20

Crockarell Jr. JR, and Guyton JL (2003). Arthroplasty of ankle and knee Chapter 6. Pp 245-313. In: Terry Canale S. Campell's Operative Orthopaedics Vol. One. Tenth Edition, Mosby, ISBN 0-323-01240-X. St. Louis

De Cárdenas OM, Álvarez RJ, Croas FA, et al (2008). Presentation of a protocol for Total Knee Arthroplasty. Rev Cubana Ortop Traumatol (on line), Vol 22 No. 2 pp. 0-0 ISSN 0864-215-X

De Cárdenas OM et al (2008). Revisión Knee replacement in an unusual case. Rev Cubana Ortop Traumatol (on line), Vol 22 No. 1 pp. 0-0 ISSN 0864-215-X

De Cárdenas OM (2010). Specials situations in Total Knee Arthroplasty. Proceeding of Cuban Orthopedic Congress ISBN 978-959-7158-95-0. Villa Clara, Sept.

De Cárdenas OM, Álvarez RJ, Croas FA, et al (2010). Kalisté Total Knee Arthroplasty System in patients with Rheumatoid Arthritis. Proceeding of Cuban Orthopedic Congress ISBN 978-959-7158-95-0. Villa Clara, Sept

Dennis DA, Kouistek RD, Strehl JB, et al (1998). Patients with PS-TKA demostrated greater flexion that patients with PCR-TKA when measured in weight bearing. J Arthroplasty; 13(7):748-52

Diduch DR et al (1977). Total Knee replacement in young active patients. J Bone Joint Surg; 79-A:571-82

Dorr LD (1993). Management of Bone Defects. Chapter 18, pp. 309-17. In: Rand JA. Total Knee Arthroplasty. Raven Press. New York. ISBN 0-88167-930-5

Dunbar MJ, Howard A, Bogoch EA, et al (2009). Orthopedics in 2020. Predictor of Musculoskeletal Need. An OAA-COA Symposium The Orthopaedic Forum. J Bone Joint Surg; 91:2276-86

El-Azab H, Halawa A, Anetzberger H, et al (2008). The effect of closed- and open- wedge high tibial osteotomy on the tibial slope: a retrospective radiological review of 120 cases. J Bone Joint Surg; 90-B:1193-7

Engh GA, & Parks NL (1994). The use a bone defect classification system in revisión Total Knee Arthroplasty. Orthop trans; 18:1138-9

Ensini A, Catani, Leardini A, et al (2007). Alignments and clinical results in conventional and navigated Total Knee Arthroplasty. Clin Orthop; 457:156-62

Ewald FC (1989). The Knee Society Total Knee Arthroplasty roentgenographic evaluation and Scoring system. Clin Orthop; 248:9-12

Giffin JR, Stabile K, Zantop T, et al (2007). Importancs of tibial slope for stability of the posterior cruciate ligament deficient Knee. Am J Sports Med; 35;1443-9

Hung CLW, Pan YW, Yuen CK, et al (2009). Interobserver and intraobserver error in distal femur transepicondylar axis measurement with computed tomography. J Arthroplasty; 26:96-100

Hungerford DS (1995). Malalignment, erosion and patella abscense. Chapter 11. Pp. 161- 75. In: Lotke PA. Master Technique in Orthopaedic Surgery Knee Arthroplasty. Lippincott Raven Publisher. Philadelphia. ISBN 0-7817-0032-9

Insall JN, Dorr LD, Scott RD, Scott WN (1989). Rationale of the Knee Society Clinical Rating System. Clin Orthop; 248:13-14

Jacobs WCH, Clement DJ, Wimenga AB (2008). Conservación del sacrificio del ligamento cruzado posterior en el reemplazo total de rodilla para el tratamiento de la Osteoartritis y la Artritis Reumatoide. (Revisión Cochrane traducida). Biblioteca Cochrane Plus; Número 2, Oxford, Update Software. Disponible en http://www.update-sofware.com. (Translated from the Cochrane Library, Issue. Chicester, UK, John Wiley & Sons. Ltd.

Dawson J., Fitzpatrick R, Murray D., Carr A (1998). Questionnaire on the perceptions of patients about total Knee replacement QPPTKR. J Bone Joint Surg; 80-B(1):63-69

Insall JN, Lachiewicz PF, Burnstein AH (1982). The posterior stabilized condylar prosthesis: A modification of the total condylar design. Two to four year clinical experience. J Bone Joint Surg; 64-A:1317-23

Johnson BP and Dorr LD (1999). Total Knee Arthroplasty after high tibial osteotomy. Chapter 12, pp. 178-92. In: Lotke PA. Master Technique in Orthopaedic Surgery Knee Arthroplasty. Lippincott-Raven Publisher. Philadelphia. ISBN 0-7817-0032- 9-1995

Katz MM et al (1987). Results of Total Knee Artroplasty after failed proximal tibial osteotomy for osteoarthritis; J Bone Joint Surg 69-A:225

Katz JN et al (2007). Association of hospital and surgeon procedure volumen with patient centered outcomes of total Knee replacement in a populatio-based cohort of patient age 65 years and older. Arthritis Rheum; 56:568-74

Leunox D, Hungerford D. & Krackow K (1987). Total Knee Arthroplasty following patellectomy. Clin Orthop; 223:220

Lingard EA, Berven S, Katz JN (2000). Management and care of patients undergoing Total Knee Arthroplasy: variations across different health care settings. Arthritis Care Res; 13:129-36

Lombardi Jr. AV, Mallory T, Fade RA, et al (2001). An algorithm for posterior cruciate ligament in Total Knee Arthroplasty. Clin Orthop; 392:75-87

Lombardi AV, Nett MP, Scott WN, et al (2009). Primary Total Knee Artrhoplasty. J Bone Joint Surg; 91 Suppl 5:52-5

Lotke PA (1999). Master Technique in Orthopaedic Surgery Knee Arthroplasty. Lippincott-Raven Publisher Philadelphia. ISBN 0-7817-0032-9-1995

Minns CJ, Baker KL, Dewey M, et al (2007). Effectiveness of phisiotherapy exercise after Knee Arthroplasty for Osteoarthritis: Systematic review and meta-analysis of randomised conrolled trials. BMJ; 335:812-5

Paletta GA & Laskin RS (1995). Total Knee Arthroplasty after a previus patellectomy. J Bone Joint Surg; 77-A:1708-12

Parvizi J. et al (2006). Management of stiffness following Total Knee Arthroplasty. J Bone Joint Surg *Am;* 88:175-181

Ranawat CS, Aglietti P, Shine J. (1976). A comparison of four model of Total Knee replacement prostheses. J Bone Joint Surg; 58-A:754-65

Ranawat CS, Padgett DE, Osashi Y (1989). Total Knee Arthroplasty for patients younger than 55 years. Clin Ortop; 248:27

Ranawat CS and Flynn Jr. WF (1999). Stiff Knee. Ankylosis and flexion. Chapter 10 pp. 141-59. In: Lotke PA. Master Technique in Orthopaedic Surgery. Knee Arthroplasty. Lippincott-Raven Publiser. Philadelphia. ISBN 0-7817-0032-9-1995

Ranawat ChS, Ranawat AS, Metha A (2003). Total Knee Arthroplasty rehabilitation protocol. What makes the difference? J. Arthroplasty; 18:27-30

Rand JA, Trousdale RT, Ilstrup DM et al (2009. Factors affecting the durability of Primary Total Knee Prosthesis. J Bone Joint Surg; 85-A:259-65

Rakin EA, Alarcon GS, Chang RW, et al (2004). NIH Consensus Statements on Total Knee Replacement. J. Bone Joint Surg; 86(6):1328-35

Robertsson O, Knutson K, Lewold S, et al (1997). Knee Arthroplasty in rheumatoid arthritis: a report from the Swedish Knee arthroplasty register on 4,381 primary operation 1985-1995. Acta Orthop Scand; 68:545-53

Rodríguez JA, Saddler S, Edelman S & Ranawat CH (1996). Long term results of Total Knee Arthroplasty in class 3 and 4 rheumatoid arthritis. J Arthroplasty; 11:141-15

Rubino LJ, Schoderhek RJ, Raymond Golish S et al (2008). The effect of plate position and size on tibial slope in high tibial osteotomy: a cadaveric study. J Knee Surg; 21:75-9

Shakespeare D., Kinsel V (2005). Rehabilitation after Total Knee Replacement. Time to go home? Knee; 12:185-9

Stuard MJ and Rand JA (1988). Total Knee Arthroplasty in young adults who have rheumatoid arthritis. J Bone Joint Surg; 70-A:84-7

Scott WN, Booth RE, Dalury DF et al (2009). Efficiency and economics in Joint Arthroplasty. J Bone Joint Surg; 91 Suppl 5:36-3

Scuderi GR, Insall JN (1989). The posterior stabilized Knee Prosthesis. Orthop Clin North Am; 20(1):71-8

Scuderi GR and Insall JN (1999). Varus and valgus fixed deformities. Chapter 8 pp. 111- 127 In: Lotke PA. Master Technique in Orthopaedic Surgery Knee Arthroplasty. Lippincott-Raven Publisher Philadelphia. ISBN 0-7817-0032-9-1995

Sculco TP (1999). Bone graft. Chapter 9, pp. 132-40 In: Lotke PA. Master Technique in Orthopaedic Surgery. Knee Arthroplasty. Lippincott-Raven Publisher. Philadelphia. ISBN 0-7817-0032-9.-1995

Stern S (2002). Cost considerations. An historical perspective. In: Scuderi GR & Tria Jr. AJ. Eds Surgical techniques in Total Knee Artroplasty. Springer-Verlag. New York

Whiteside, LA and Ohl MD (1990). Tibial tubercle osteotomy for exposure of the difficult Total Knee Arthroplasty. Clin Orthop; 260:6-9

Windsor RE, Insall JN, & Vincent KG (1988). Technical consideations of Total Knee Arthroplasty after proximal tibial osteotomy. J Bone Joint Surg; 70-A:547-555

Yan WP, Leung A, Lin KG, et al(2007). Interobserver and intraobserver errors in obtaining visually selected anatomical landmarks during registration process in non- image-based navigation assisted total Knee. J. Arthroplasty; 22:1050-61

9

Fixation of Periprosthetic Supracondylar Femur Fractures Above Total Knee Arthroplasty – The Indirect Reduction Technique with the Condylar Blade Plate and the Minimally Invasive Technique with the LISS

K. Kolb[1], P.A. Grützner[2], F. Marx[3] and W. Kolb[4]

[1]*Department of Trauma Surgery Klinikum am Steinenberg, Reutlingen*
[2]*Department of Trauma Surgery Unfallklinik Ludwigshafen*
[3]*Department of Trauma Surgery, Friedrich-Schiller-University, Jena*
[4]*Department of Trauma and Orthopaedic Surgery, Bethesda Hospital, Stuttgart*
Germany

1. Introduction

Supracondylar fractures of the femur after total knee arthroplasty are an uncommon but highly challenging injury (Streubel et al., 2010). The management of distal femoral fractures following a total knee replacement can be complex and requires the equipment, perioperative support and surgical skills of both trauma and revision arthroplasty services (Johnston et al., 2011, Nauth et al., 2011). The incidence of periprosthetic supracondylar femur fractures after total knee arthroplasties ranges from 0.3% to 2.5%. A patient with revision total knee arthroplasty has a significantly higher risk of supracondylar fracture above the prosthesis (2-4%) (Merkel & Johnson, 1986; Berry, 1999). Interprosthetic femoral fractures tend to occur more frequently in the supracondylar region above total knee arthroplasty components (Mamczak et al., 2010). Predisposing factors are female gender, poor bone stock, rotationally constrained implants, stress risers such as screw holes around the knee, malalignment of the prosthesis, endosteal ischaemia (bone cement, spongiosa preparation), anterior femoral notching, arthrofibrosis, chronic steroid use, rheumatoid arthritis, revision total knee arthroplasties, poliomyelitis and Parkinson's disease (Table 1, Aaron & Scott, 1987; Ayers, 1997; Berry, 1999; Bogoch et al., 1987; Cain et al., 1986; Cordeiro et al., 1990; Culp et al., 1987; Diehl et al., 2006; DiGioa et al., 1991; Figgie et al., 1990; Haddad et al., 1999; Hirsh et al., 1981; Lesh et al., 2000; Merkel et al., 1986; Moran et al., 1996; Ritter et al., 1988; Roscoe et al., 1989; Shawen et al., 2003; Short et al., 1981; Sisto et al., 1985; Wick et al., 2004; Zehntner & Ganz, 1993). A biomechanical study has shown that notching of the anterior cortex significantly lessens the load to failure by decreasing the bending strength by 18% and the torsional strength by approximately 40% (Lesh et al., 2000). In a retrospective study, the clinical results of 1089 consecutive total knee replacements demonstrated no difference in knees managed with or without anterior femoral notching (Ritter et al., 2005). This finding emphasises the potential for osseous remodelling to decrease the risk of fracture should an anterior notch occur (Dennis, 2001). Additionally, should an anterior notch of the distal part of the femur occur, the surgeon should consider implantation of a femoral component with an attached diaphysis-engaging stem to support the weakened distal part of the femur (Dennis, 2001).

Motions of stiff knees under anaesthesia have a high risk of periprosthetic supracondylar femur fractures (Diehl et al., 2006).

General	Femur
Patient depending factors	
Osteoporosis	Female gender
Bone disease (M. Paget)	
Rheumatoid arthritis	Arthrofibrosis
Steroid abuse	
Neurologic abnormalities	
Malalignment	
Infections	
Surgery dependant factors	
Revision total knee arthroplasty	Malalignment of the prosthesis
Removal of cement	Implantation error
Screw holes around the knee	Anterior femoral notching
Osteolysis due to wear	
Stress shielding	
Motion under anaesthesia	Endosteal ischemia
Prosthesis dependant factors	
	Intramedullary stems
	Constrained prosthesis

Table 1. Risk factors for periprosthetic supracondylar femur fractures above total knee arthroplasty modified according to (Diehl et al., 2006 ; Nauth et al., 2011)

Most periprosthetic femur fractures occur between two and four years after a total knee arthroplasty (Ehrhardt & Kuster, 2010). The number of these cases may rise quickly, given the projection that, by the year 2030, the implantation of total knee arthroplasties will increase to 3.48 million in the United States, an increase of 673% compared with 2005. The most frequent mechanism of injury is a low-velocity fall onto the knee in combination with torsion or axial compression, with a smaller proportion resulting from high-energy trauma (e.g., motor vehicle accidents) (Su et al., 2004)

The complication rate of these fractures is between 25% and 75%. Conservative treatment of displaced fractures with casting results in malalignment (25-100%), non-union (20-35%), loss of motion of the knee, and inability to maintain reduction of the fracture (Kolb et al., 2009). Surgical treatment provides the best restoration of mechanical alignment to the limb, permits early mobilisation to avoid the complications of prolonged bed rest, and may maximise healing potential in a region where blood supply is already compromised by providing stable fixation (Rorabeck & Taylor, 1999). In 1970, the AO (Arbeitsgemeinschaft für Osteosynthesefragen) published the first results of 112 supracondylar femoral fractures treated according to their principles using a condylar plate, a fixed angle device, with 74% good or excellent results (Wenzl et al., 1970).

The reported complications of operative treatment included deep infection (3%), fixation failure (4%), non-union (9%), and revision surgery (13%) (Herrera et al., 2008). The treatment of periprosthetic fractures around the knee can be challenging for a number of reasons (Healy et al., 1993; Kim et al., 2006; Rhinelander, 1972): (1) these fractures occur in patients with poor bone stock that can compromise potential fixation; (2) the majority of these patients are elderly and, because of their age may have retarded fracture healing; (3) the epiphyseal and frequently the intramedullary blood supplies of the distal femur are interrupted after total knee arthroplasty; (4) after a fracture of the distal part of the femur immediate reduction of total bone blood flow by nearly 50% through the physiological vasoconstriction in both the periosteal and intramedullary vessels further impairs blood supply; (5) the attachment of the ligamentous structures to the fracture fragment may predispose these knees to potential instability, necessitating the use of a constrained prosthesis with all their potential problems. The wide metaphyseal and diaphyseal spaces, osteopenia, and distal extension of the fracture often associated with these elderly patients can result in suboptimal internal fixation (Ricci et al., 2006). Fractures with stable prostheses are best treated with some meeans of internal fixation and without stem revision (Dennis, 2001).

Ideally, the treatment of a supracondylar femoral fracture above a total knee arthroplasty would be characterised as follows (Kregor et al., 2001):
-    The ability of the patient to return to pre-accident function,
-    A surgical technique that is minimally invasive,
-    Capability of immediate motion,
-    No need for bone-grafting,
-    Low risk of infection, and
-    Adaptability to various total knee designs.

In practice, flexible intramedullary nails, rigid retrograde IM nails, angled blade plates, cobra plates, dynamic condylar screws and Ilizarov external fixators have been used (Althausen et al., 2003; Beris et al., 2010; Chettiar et al., 2009; Gliatis et al., 2005; Maniar et al., 1996; McLaren et al., 1994; Rorabeck & Taylor, 1999; Zehntner & Ganz, 1993).

Fixation with conventional compression plates, though for the most part successful, has its limitations (Kubiak et al., 2006). Conventional plate osteosynthesis (CPO) with rigid fixation has shown a high complication rate that includes delayed or non-union, infection, hardware failure and re-fracture after plate removal (Bostman, 1983; Claes et al., 1999, Finsen & Benum, 1986; Hidaka & Gustilo, 1984; Kenwright & Goodship, 1989; Kessler et al., 1992; Mulier et al., 1997; Noorda & Wuisman, 2002; Riemer et al., 1992; Stoffel et al., 2003).

(Mast et al., 1989) pioneered the indirect reduction technique without disturbance of the soft tissue envelope around the fracture itself.

The concept of the indirect reduction technique is to provide reduction of the fracture through traction across the intact soft tissues and decreased surgical dissection of the fracture site (Mast et al., 1989). Minimally invasive plate osteosynthesis (MIPO) have been introduced to go one step further (Krettek et al., 1997). Locked plate fixators improved the stability of plate osteosynthesis significantly (Streubel et al., 2010; Kolb et al., 2010). The combination of locked plate fixators and the MIPO technique allows for plate osteosynthesis without bone grafts (Streubel et al., 2010; Kolb et al., 2010).

The aim of this report is to describe new planning methods and new techniques of internal fixation for supracondylar femur fractures above total knee arthroplasty.

2. Preoperative assessment

Preoperative clinical evaluation involves questions related to general factors that include smoking, peripheral vascular and neurological status, nutritional status, comorbidities such as diabetes, alignment of the injured leg, pre-injury range of motion of the knee, knee extensor mechanism, signs of loosening of the prosthesis (weight dependant pain, knee instability, reduced walking distance), infection and activity level. Radiographic assessment includes anterior posterior (a.p.), lateral and oblique radiographs of the knee and femur including the hip and former radiographs if available (Diehl et al. 2006; Ehrhardt & Kuster, 2010). Specifically, the lateral radiograph is used to assess (Kregor et al., 2001) the following: 1. the integrity of the femoral component-bone interface to assess potential loosening, 2. the bone block attached to the femoral component, and 3. the position of the cement mantle and flange for the femoral component. Modern CT scans provide more information concerning the integrity of the femoral-bone interface to assess potential loosening of the prosthesis (Kregor et al., 2001; Ehrhardt & Kuster, 2010). Both the type and classification of fractures and the type of prosthesis should be known preoperatively because this information is very important for choosing the right treatment option (Ehrhardt & Kuster 2010). The operative report should be available whenever possible (Ehrhardt & Kuster, 2010).

2.1 Classification

The classification system that is the most valuable to management was created by Rorabeck & Young (Fig. 1, Rorabeck & Taylor, 1999; Dennis, 2001). Their classification system takes

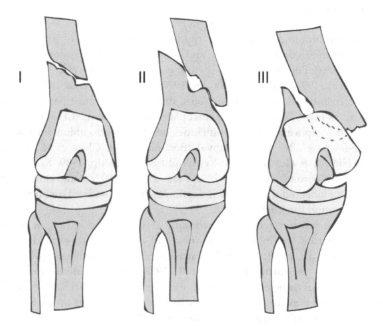

Fig. 1. The Classification system of supracondylar femoral fractures above total knee arthroplasties created by (Rorabeck & Young, 1999)

into account both the status of the prosthesis (that is, whether it is intact or failing) and the displacement of the fracture (Dennis, 2001).

(Su et al., 2004) developed their classification system because patients are increasingly being treated operatively and the bone stock of the distal segment continues to be considered a key limiting factor to obtaining adequate fixation (Herrera et al., 2008). Their classification system takes into account the height of the fractures (Table 2, Su et al., 2004).

Fracture Type	Fracture Height
I	Fracture above the femoral component
II	Fracture above the femoral component, fracture reaching the tip of the femoral component
III	Fractures below the tip of the femoral component

Table 2. Classification system of supracondylar femoral fractures above total knee arthroplasties created by (Su et al., 2004)

3. Treatment options

The goals of treating supracondylar femoral fractures above total knee arthroplasties are to obtain and maintain good postfracture alignment and stability to allow an early range of motion and bone healing (Culp et al., 1987; Rorabeck & Taylor, 1999; Dennis, 1998; Ehrhardt & Kuster, 2010). Acceptable alignments exhibit translations that are less than 5 mm, angulations that are less than 5°-10°, minimal rotations, less than 1 cm of femoral shortening, and proper tibiofemoral prosthetic joint alignments (DiGioia & Rubash, 1991). High malunion rates are common in association with varus, flexion, and internal rotation deformities typically seen as a result of forces exerted by the adductor and gastrocnemius muscle groups (Figgie et al., 1990; Dennis, 2001).

3.1 Non-operative treatment

The non-operative options include skeletal traction, application of a cast, pins and plaster, and cast bracing (Dennis et al., 2001). Traction has a high complication rate and is no longer an option. According to Rorabeck & Young, only fracture type I can be treated conservatively, 4-6 weeks with a cast and 6 weeks of mobilisation with a brace (Chen et al., 1994). However, this treatment may be associated with difficulty in maintaining the reduction, a prolonged period of immobilisation, reduced knee functions, malunion and non-union (McGraw, P.; & Kumar, A., 2010). Conservative treatment was followed by non-union in 20% and mal-union in 23% of the cases evaluated (Culp et al., 1987). Casting resulted in an average loss of motion of 26° (Culp et al., 1987). Of these fractures, 29% eventually required operative care (Harlow & Hofmann, 1994; Dennis, 2001).

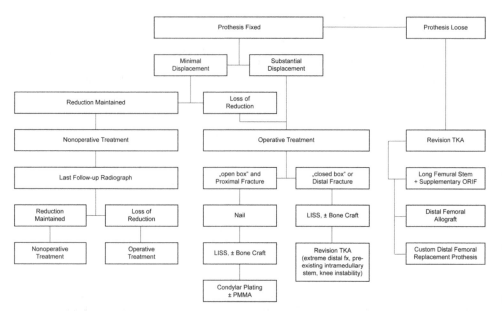

Fig. 2. Schematic of treatment options for supracondylar femoral fractures above total knee arthroplasties. TKA=total knee arthroplasty, PMMA=polymethylmethacrylate

3.2 Operative treatment

Several options are available to provide secure internal fixation of supracondylar fractures of the distal femur (Fig. 2, Ayers, 1997; Kolb et al., 2009). Many factors must be considered in choosing the most appropriate management method for these fractures including the patients general health, prefracture ambulatory status, fracture pattern, location, displacement, and type of implant (Su et al., 2004). Periprosthetic fractures above total knee arthroplasties have particular risks for failure, including wide metaphyseal and diaphyseal spaces, osteoporosis, small distal femoral fragments, and prosthetic anchorage pegs reducing the sites for fixation (Kolb et al., 2010). Surgical options include intramedullary devices, condylar buttress plates and, - more recently, – locking plates (internal fixators) that are typically placed in a submuscular manner (Herrera et al., 2008).

3.3 Coventional plate osteosynthesis

The two basic types of fixed angle devices are the condylar screw plate and the 95° condylar blade plate. They work best for more proximal fractures and when there is minimal comminution of the distal fragments (Ayers, 1997; Su et al., 2004). The advantages of the 95° condylar plate are that no bone has to be removed from the distal fragment when this device is inserted and that the blade is relatively thin (Healy et al., 1993). The blade can therefore, be placed closed to the lugs of the femoral component and close to the anterior femoral flange (Healy et al., 1993). Usually, the entry site for the blade chisel is at a height of 2.5-3 cm above the prosthetic joint line, depending on the configuration of the fracture and the prosthetic design (Moran et al., 1996). However, the angled 95° condylar blade plates do not provide sufficient stability in osteoporotic bone and might interfere with the fixation lugs of the femoral component, and the polymethylmethacrylate (Zehntner & Ganz 1993, Chen et al. 1994). Of the total numbers of conventional plate osteosynthese an average of 32% (range, 0-75%) primary bone grafts were used. A mean of 10% (range, 0-50%) of those with conventional plate osteosynthesis (CPO) had an implant failure and developed a non-union (Table 3, Kolb et al., 2009).

Authors, year of publication	Bone graft (n, % early/later)	Infection	Implant failure	Non-union (n, %)	Results of fixation
Sisto et al., 1985	0	0	0	0	Valgus 3° 1 (33%) Valgus 5° 2 (66%)
Merkel et al., 1986	2 (40%)	1 (20%)	0	0	Normal alignment
Figgie et al., 1990	4 (40%)	0	5 (50%)	5 (50%)	Varus 7° 5 (23%)?
Healy et al., 1993	15/3 (75%/15%)	0	0	0	Normal alignment
Zehntner et al., 1993	2 (30%)	0	0	0	Valgus 5° (range, 0-10°)
Moran et al., 1996	6/2 (40%/13%)	0	3 (20%)	3 (20%)	Shortening 2 cm 3 (20%) Valgus 17° 1 (7%) Varus 2° 1 (7%)
Ochsner et al., 1999	0	0	0	0	Varus

Table 3. Complications of conventional plate osteosynthesis (CPO) of fractures above fixed total knee arthroplasties (from Kolb et al., 2009).

The indirect reduction technique allows for the use of longer plates with less pullout force acting on the screws due to improvement of the working leverage and significant stress reduction in the plate (50%-85%) (Kolb et al., 2009; Gautier & Sommer, 2003; Stoffel et al., 2003). Various methods have been used to enhance fixation using internal fixation (McGraw, P.; & Kumar, A., 2010). In severely osteoporotic bone, polymethylmethacrylate can be used to enhance screw fixation (Zehentner & Ganz, 1993). An intramedullary autograft is another option to help restore bone stock and achieve quadric-cortical fixation of the screws (Tani et al., 1998). However, this technique has not been widely used because of donor-site morbidity, particularly in elderly patients (McGraw, P.; & Kumar, A., 2010).

Combining medial strut allografts with compression plates allows for fixation of severe osteoporotic fractures and failures of initial open reduction and internal fixation (Wang & Wang, 2002). Three patients with very low and comminuted fractures exhibited good results using intramedullary fibular strut allografts without donor-site morbidities(Kumar et al., 2008).

The epiphyseal and frequently the intramedullary blood supplies of the distal femur are interrupted after total knee arthroplasty (Healy et al., 1993). Immediate reduction of total bone blood flow after a fracture of the distal part of the femur through physiological vasoconstriction in both the periosteal and intramedullary vessels by nearly 50% further impairs blood supply (Rhinelander, 1972). Fractures above total knee arthroplasties may have greater tendencies to non-unions than do distal femoral fractures not associated with arthoplasties (Moran et al., 1996). Microangiographic studies have demonstrated that much of the vascular supply to the callus area derives from the surrounding soft tissue (Rhinelander, 1972). Conventional plate osteosynthesis produces compression between the implant and the bone and probably further impairs the blood supply (Fig 3 Healy et al., 1993; Wagner, 2003). Plates interfere significantly with the periosteal blood supply, resulting in bone necrosis (Perren et al., 1988). Direct manipulation of bone fragments in conventional plate osteosynthesis is a major cause of devitalisation of the bone fragments (Leunig et al., 2000). Medial dissection of soft tissue can disrupt this important blood supply and is, thus, to be avoided (Mast et al., 1989).

The extreme difference in healing time between conservative treatment (3 months) and compression fixation (15 months) indicates that the circumstances can be improved (Perren, 2003). Bone union depends on respecting the capacity of the soft tissues to maintain vascular supply to the bone, on the reduction of the fracture, and on applying the technique that best provides the necessary stability for union to occur (Wagner & Frigg, 2006). Surgical treatment should take biological, biomechanical and surgical aspects into account (Table 4, Korner et al., 2003).

AO principles THEN (Müller et al., 1970)	Influences through clinical experiences and experimental investigations	AO principles NOW (Wagner & Frigg, 2006)
1. Anatomical precise reduction	Applied science concerning: - bone healings, - blood supply through soft tissues and bone, - biological shortcommings of ORIF in multifragmentary shaft fractures lead to a new way of thinking. As a consequence, indirect reduction techniques were developed	Fracture reduction and fixation to restore anatomical relationships. Reductions need not be anatomical but only axially aligned in the diaphysis and the metaphysis. Anatomical reduction is required for intra-articular reductions. The principles of articular fracture care: - atraumatic anatomical reduction of the articular surfaces, stable fixation of the articular fragments, and - metaphyseal reconstruction with bone grafting and buttressing apply as they did at the beginning

2. Rigid fixation, absolute stability	The most notable change in the treatment of diaphysael fractures has been the shift from the mechanical to the biological aspects of internal fixation. The preservation of the viability and integrity of the soft tissue envelope of the metaphysis has been recognized as the key to success. Today the dominant theme in the fixation of fractures of the diaphysis is the biology of bone and the preservation of the blood supply to bony fragments, and no longer the quest for absolute stability. Major changes have occurred in the timing of the different steps of metaphyseal reconstruction, as well as in the fixation methods and techniques. The comprehensive classification of long bones has helped predict treatment and outcome.	Stabilisation with different grades of stability, from high (absolute stability) to low (relative stability). Appropriate construct stability. Stability by compression or splinting, as the fracture pattern and the injury require. The joint surfaces require anatomical reduction with absolute stability. The majority of diaphyseal fractures are treated with relative stability methods (eg. intramedullary or extramedullary splinting).
3. Preserving blood supply	The present concept still emphasises that the blood supply through the soft tissues and bone is the most important aspect in fracture care. - atraumatic soft tissue technique through the appropriate surgical approaches, - atraumatic reduction and fixation techniques are mandatory, - implants with new bone-implant interface	Preservation of the blood supply to soft tissues and bone by careful handling and gentle reduction techniques and a newly designed bone-implant interface
4. Early protective motion for rehabilitation because pain was abolished and union assured		Early and safe mobilisation of the part and the patient. Early active motion can also be carried out because splint fixation is stable enough to allow postoperative functional care

Table 4. Comparison of AO principles from 1970 and 2006 (from Wagner and Frigg, 2006).

3.4 Plate osteosynthesis with the indirect reduction technique

The concept of biological internal fixation entails preserving the biologic reactivity of the tissue as much as possible (Rozbruch et al., 1998). This process includes careful tissue dissection, epiperiosteal bone dissection, and indirect reduction of the fracture to avoid the stripping and de-vascularisation of bone fragments (Rozbruch et al., 1998). (Mast et al., 1989) pioneered the indirect reduction of fractures without disturbance of the soft tissue envelope around the fracture and reduced blood loss. One example of an indirect reduction method is the distraction of fragments using a distractor, an external fixator, a plate or traction applied to a limb (Wagner & Frigg, 2006). The fragments are reduced using ligamentotaxis, minimising the extent to which they are manipulated and preserving their blood supply (Babst et al., 2001; Rüedi et al., 1998; Wagner & Frigg, 2006; Vidal et al., 1979). Primary grafting, which is often used in CPO is not necessary (Kolb et al., 2009; Ricci et al., 2005; Ricci et al., 2006). Minimally invasive techniques (i.e., MIPO) go one step further (Krettek et al., 1997). The bridging plate is one of the early developments of an internal fixator (Brunner & Weber, 1982). Recent developments are the Schuhli nut developed by Mast (Kolodziej et al., 1998), the Zespol plate (Ramotowski & Granowski, 1991), the point contact fixator (PC-Fix) (Tepic et al., 1997), the less invasive stabilisation system (LISS) (Frigg et al., 2001), and the locking compression plate (LCP) (Frigg, 2003). Healing has been accelerated with the PC-Fix, so that it removal is possible after only 3 months (Wagner & Frigg, 2006). Local infection resistance has been improved, such that 750 times more Staphylococcus aureus were required to produce the same incidence of infection with the PC-Fix as with the dynamic compression plate (Arens et al., 1999).

3.5 Minimally invasive osteosynthesis with internal fixators and retrograde nails

Internal fixators and retrograde nails have advantages in minimally invasive osteosynthesis (MIO) compared to the condylar plate (Ehrhardt & Kuster, 2010). Numerous studies (Chettiar et al., 2009; Gliatis et al., 2005; Henry, 1995; Mittlmeier et al., 2005; Murrell & Nunley, 1995; Platzer et al., 2010; Rolston et al., 1995; Smith et al., 1996) recommend nailing in the posterior cruciate ligament retaining femoral component with an open box. The supracondylar nail preserves the fracture haematoma, does not require extensive soft-tissue stripping, and provides fair stability to the fracture (Figgie et al., 1990; Gardner et al., 2004; Gliatis et al., 2005; Kolb et al., 2008; Mittlmeier & Beck 2005; Stedtfeld et al., 2004). Problems associated with the use of a retrograde nail include malalignment due to a poor starting point, flexion malalignment as a result of the knee flexion required for access to the joint during reaming and nail placement, and insufficient distal stability (Horwitz & Kubiak, 2010). The intercondylar distance must be at least 11mm or 12 mm to accommodate the nail, and the knee flexion must be at least 60° (Diehl et al., 2006; Kolb et al., 2010; Rolston et al., 1995). Small distal fragments should have enough space for at least two screws (Diehl et al., 2006, Kolb et al., 2010; Mittlmeier et al., 2005). Many systems include an interference screw that can be placed in the most distal screw hole to convert the nail to a fixed-angle device (Horwitz & Kubiak, 2010). However, these systems still fail because the osteoporotic cancellous bone is inadequate, and it is not uncommon for a distal femoral fracture to drift into valgus at the site of the nail fixation (Horwitz & Kubiak, 2010). Angular correction and additional stability can be achieved bx placing blocking screws in the distal fragment (Stedtfeld et al., 2004). In a retrospective study, 14 supracondylar periprosthetic fractures obtained good functional outcomes, a low complication rate and 100% fracture unions (Chettiar et al., 2009).

3.6 Minimally invasive osteosynthesis with the Less Invasive Stabilisation System (LISS)

The LISS has theoretical advantages for the treatment of supracondylar femoral fractures above well-fixed total knee arthroplasties (Kolb et al., 2010). Broadly, the advantages of the LISS fixator are attributable to three factors (Kregor et al., 2001):

1. The ability to place multiple fixed-angled locked screws, offering improved stability of the distal fragment,
2. the ability to place percutaneous screws in the proximal femur without dissection of the metaphyseal/diaphyseal component of the fracture,
3. the ability to place 3 or 4 screws even in small distal fragments.

The bridge-plating technique produces minimal biological damage with locked flexible fixation (Ehinger et al., 2011; Thielemann et al., 1988; Rozbruch et al., 1998; Perren, 2002; Gautier & Jakob, 2004). The minimally invasive plate-osteosynthesis technique leaves the blood supply largely intact and reduces blood loss compared with the conventional plate osteosynthesis using a standard approach (Mast et al., 1989; Krettek et al., 1997; Grützner et al., 1997; Farouk et al., 1998; Krettek et al., 2001; Althausen et al., 2003; Kolb et al., 2003). It avoids the need for precise reduction and exposure of the bone, thus reducing surgical trauma (Thielemann et al., 1988; Gerber et al., 1990; Ganz et al., 1991; Rozbruch et al., 1998; Perren, 2002). The locked plates provided significantly greater fixation stability than the standard plate, blade plate, condylar buttress plate, dynamic condylar screws, or the retrograde nail in biomechanical studies involving axial loading with mild to moderate osteoporotic femurs (Egol et al., 2004; Ganz et al., 1991; Koval et al., 1997; Marti et al., 2001; Salas et al., 2011; Zlowodzki et al., 2004). The probability of periprosthetic fracture of the locking plate compared to the retrograde IM nail (in a deterministic finite element model of each construct type) was higher under the applied loading conditions (locking plate 21.8% versus IM nail 0.019%) (Salas et al., 2011). By using an internal fixator with locked screw heads, the screw loading is primarily bending and not pullout (Gautier & Sommer, 2003; Wagner & Frigg, 2006). Locked screws provide improved anchorage and safety and they cannot be stripped during their insertion because they limit the torque applied to the screw thread (Perren, 2003, Fig 3a and 3b). The pull out resistance of the LISS is increased with convergent screws in the femoral condyle. These plates are particularly useful in the presence of a proximal femur implant as they allow unicortical screw fixation that overlap the distal part of the proximal implant, thereby avoiding a stress riser between the two implants (McGraw & Kumar, 2010). Blood supply to the bone is preserved, and no contact between the fixator and the bone required (Kolb et al., 2010).

3.7 Osteosynthesis with the locking compression plate (LCP) and polyaxial locking plates

In September 1998, Professor Michael Wagner (of the Wilhelminen Hospital in Vienna) questioned whether it was possible to make the LISS screw-head hole compatible with conventional bone screws (Frigg, 2003). As a result the locking compression plate (LCP) was developed. It has a combined plate hole, which allows for the use of conventional bone screws or locked screws. The possibility of using the LCP as a compression plate (> primary fracture healing), an internal fixator (> secondary fracture healing) or in a specific combination (hybrid fixation) allows for ideal plate anchorage that is adapted to the bone (Frigg, 2003; Wagner, 2003).

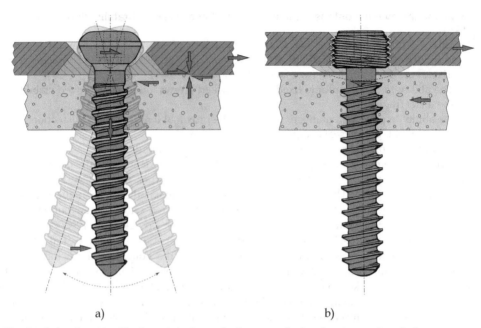

a)   b)

Fig. 3. a left – Longitudinal section through the screw hole of a conventional plate screw. The inclination of the screw is not locked. The screw is tightened with an axial traction of 2000 to 3000 N, the plate is compressed onto the bone producing friction which resists a tangential load of 1000 N (friction = 0.4 x 2500 = 1000 N). Fig. 3. b right – Longirudinal section through the locked screw of an internal fixator. Because of the steep conical surfaces ("Morse cone") the screw locks upon application of minimal torque. Therefore absence of compression between the plate and bone allows either point contact or no contact thus enabling reduction of the contact damage to the blood supply. This type of forece transmission does not depend on axial preloading of the screw (from Perren, 2002).

Polyaxial locking plates (POLYAX Locked Plating Systemt, DePuy, Warsaw, IN, USA), which allow screw angulation within a maximum 40-degree cone, are now available (Haydukewych et al., 2007). As the conical threaded head engages the bushing, the bushing expands, placing hoop stresses on the surrounding hole and effectively locking the screw (Haydukewych et al., 2007). Polyaxial locking plates offer more fixation versatility without an apparent increase in mechanical complications related to loss of reduction (Haydukewych et al., 2007). The non-contact bridging plate for distal femurs (NCB DF, Zimmer, Warsaw, IN, USA) combines conventional plating techniques with polyaxial screw placement and angular stability (Ehrhardt et al., 2008). Results of this combination technique show promise with regard to union and malunion rates in periprosthetic fractures in elderly and osteoporotic patients (Ehrhardt et al., 2008; El-Zayat et al., 2010). In a biomechanical study, the POLYAX supported smaller loads compared with the LISS and NCB while under axial loading (Otto et al., 2009). In addition, the mode of failure of the NCB plate, creating an intra-articular fracture propagating from the distal posterior screw hole, may be of some concern (Otto et al., 2009).

4. Preoperative planning

Indirect reduction and closed fixation techniques are technically much more demanding than an open procedure; thus, accurate preoperative planning is needed to choose the appropriate implant size and length, shape of the plate and the number, position and order of insertion of the screws (Mast et al., 1989). The common issues related to the use of locked supracondylar plates for extraarticular distal femoral fractures are appropriate plate length, malalignment, and interference with total knee arthroplasty pegs (Horwitz & Kubiak, 2010). Plate length is important in patients with osteoporosis, both for fixation of the condylar fragment and to avoid creation of stress risers in the femoral shaft (Horwitz & Kubiak, 2010). Use of a long plate, while leaving some screw holes without screws, provides better fixation with less chance of failure at the proximal part of the diaphysis due to either pullout of the screws or a fracture at the tip of the plate (Sanders et al., 2002). The newer techniques

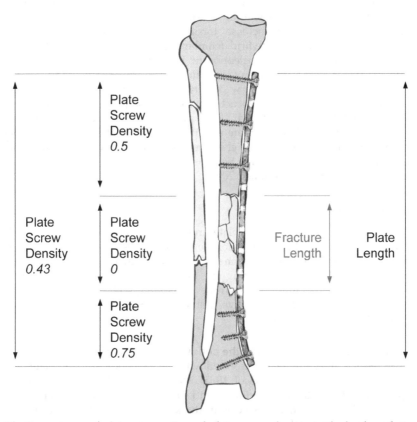

Fig. 4. The importance of plate-span ratio and plate-screw density in the bridge-plating technique. The schematic drawing shows a mechanically sound fixation of a comminuted diaphyseal fracture of the lower leg. The plate-span ratio is approximately 3, indicating that the plate is three times longer than the overall fracture area. The overall plate-screw density of the construct in this example is 0.43 & screws for a 14-hole plate (from Gautier and Sommer, 2003).

of indirect reduction and subcutaneous or submuscular implant insertion allow for increasing the plate length without additional soft tissue dissection (Gautier & Sommer, 2003). The plate length can be chosen according to the pure mechanical demands of the specific fracture that requires stabilisation (Gautier & Sommer, 2003). The working length has been shown to be the most important factor affecting axial stiffness and torsional rigidity (Stoffel et al., 2003). Increasing the working and plate lengths reduces considerably the von Mises stress in the LISS plate (Duda et al., 2002). In osteoporotic femurs, the use of self-tapping bicortical locking head screws with at least four or five screws in each fragment is recommended (Frigg & Wagner, 2006; Kregor et al., 2001).

As has been shown in total hip replacement, the LISS can be combined with periprosthetic screws, a locking attachment plate, or a cable system. The omission of one screw hole near the fracture site has been shown to significantly decrease, axial stiffness and torsional rigidity (by 64% and 36%, respectively (Stoffel et al., 2003).The number of screws has greater influence over shorter versus longer working lengths (Stoffel et al., 2003). Further more, more than three screws on either side of the fracture did little to increase axial stiffness; likewise, four screws did not increase torsional rigidity (Stoffel et al., 2003). In a biomechanical study locked and hybrid (combining of locked and unlocked) constructs demonstrated similar behaviour in osteoporotic bone; no differences between the locked and hybrid specimens were found at any cyclic interval (Gardner et al., 2006).

The plate-span ratio and the plate-screw density determine the ideal lengthof the internal fixator (Gautier & Sommer, 2003; Rozbruchet al., 1998). The plate-span ratio is the quotient of plate-length and fracture-length, while the plate-screw density is the quotient of the number of screws inserted into the plate and the number of plate holes (Rozbruch et al., 1998).The plate-span ratio should be higher than 2-3 in comminuted fractures and higher than 8-10 in simple fractures (Gautier & Sommer, 2003). The plate-screw densitiy should be below 0.5-0.4 (Fig. 4, Gautier & Sommer, 2003).

5. Surgical technique

The length of the 95° condylar blade plate and the LISS, positioning, and length of the screws are selected using the Association for Osteosynthesis/ASIF templates (Synthes Corporation). Leg length and axial alignment of the contralateral extremity are determined as described by (Kolb et al., 2009). Surgical procedures involved the tool preOp plan, developed by Siemens, to support osteosynthesis planning with regard to the 95° condylar blade plate and the LISS (Less Invasive Stabilisation System) (Synthes, West Chester, Pennsylvania) (Koudela et al., 2010).

5.1 Indirect reduction technique with the condylar blade plate

The indirect reduction technique is performed with the 95° condylar blade plate (Kolb et al., 2009; Müller et al., 1979; Ostrum & Geel, 1995). The surgical technique includes a standard lateral approach to the distal femur with the patient in a supine position. Hyperextension of the distal femoral fragment is corrected with the knee flexed to 60° over a supracondylar towel bump. After opening the fascia lata, the vastus lateralis muscle is elevated from the linea aspera, and the perforating vessels are preserved when possible. The lateral and anterior aspects of the femur are exposed. The posterior and medial soft tissues are not violated. The blade of the 95° condylar blade plate is inserted along the track previously made by the seating chisel parallel to a k-wire that marks the joint line. The window of the seating chisel is in the middle third of the anterior half of the distal femur, 2.5 cm above the prosthetic joint line and, if possible, anterior to the anchorage pegs of the prosthesis (Mast et al., 1989). Indirect reduction is obtained through manual traction or a compression-distraction device to obtain the appropriate axis, rotation and length of the femur. The plate is then attached to the proximal shaft with a Verbrugge clamp and fixed with screws. At least four divergent plate screws are used for proximal plate fixation. In three patients with severely osteoporotic bone, fractures were stabilised in combination with bone cement to enhance screw fixation. The screws are fully inserted into the cement while it is still soft after the plate is provisionally fixed to the femur, and the screws are tightened after the cement has set. Only one knee had a plate-bone interface failure after 4 weeks. Bone graft was required in only four patients with severely osteoporotic bone with comminution and in three in combination with bone cement.

5.1.1 Postoperative considerations
Postoperatively, patients are allowed toe-touch weight bearing for 6-8 weeks, except for one patient who has an associated tibial fracture. Two patients are mobilised with a glider cane. After removal of the suction drains on the second postoperative day, continuous passive motion is initiated.

6. Minimally invasive technique with the LISS

The standard anterolateral approach to the distal femur is performed on a radiolucent table with the patient in a supine position (Kolb et al., 2010). Hyperextension of the distal femoral fragment is corrected with the knee flexed over a supracondylar towel bump. Closed indirect reduction through manual traction with control of the axis, rotation and length, and temporary retention of the articular block on the shaft are attained. A 4 cm to 5 cm lateral incision is made over the distal femur. After sharp dissection through the skin and subcutaneous tissue, the iliotibial band is divided in line with its fibres. Atraumatic entry into the area between the vastus lateralis and the lateral femoral condyle (without visualising the metaphyseal part of the fracture) is performed. The perforating vessels are kept intact. The plate is placed slightly more distally than the recommended 1.0-1.5 cm, often directly adjacent to the femoral component to achieve maximal screw purchase (Kregor et al., 2001). The plate is used as an internal fixator and not as a reduction aid. The LISS was temporarily fixated using the aiming device with two 2.0 mm Kirschner wires (Fig. 5). At least four self-drilling monocortical locked screws are used for the articular block, and at least four self-tapping bicortical locked screws are used for the shaft. When interference occurs with an intercondylar box of the femoral component (in four patients), we use shorter self-tapping or periprosthetic screws. In two patients with interference from total hip replacements, periprosthetic locked screws were used in the proximal femoral fragment when the LISS overlapped a hip prosthesis. After a proximal screw pull-out due to malpositioning of the fixator, we obtain a true lateral view of the proximal shaft to ensure that the plate is centred on the bone in the lateral view before inserting the proximal screws, and we perform a mini-open approach over the proximal three holes of the fixator, facilitating the exact positioning of the fixator.

We require no intraoperative blood transfusion and no bone graft or soft tissue procedure.

6.1 Postoperative considerations
Active physiotherapy and continuous passive motion are initiated on day 2 after removal of the drains. Patients are allowed to partially bear weight (up to 20 kg) for 6 to 8 weeks.

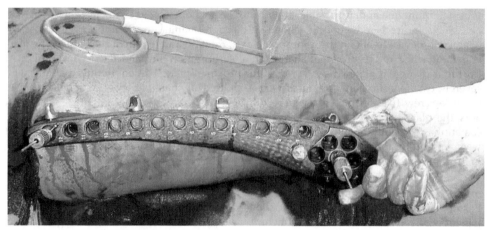

Fig. 5. Temporary fixation of the LISS with the aiming device with two 2.0 mm Kirschner wires.

7. Results and conclusions

The incidence of periprosthetic fractures is increasing as ageing populations throughout the world live longer (Kolb et al., 2010). Despite the increased risk of many of our patients all knees treated with the angled 95° condylar blade plate in indirect reduction technique healed without complications (Kolb et al., 2009). The angled 95° condylar plate in indirect reduction technique is still a good implant with good long-term results (Kolb et al., 2009). It works best in proximal fractures when there is minimal comminution of the distal fragment in the hands of a surgeon experienced with this device (Kolb et al., 2009). A minimally invasive, locked plating system permits stable fixation, early knee motion with good short- to mid-term results, and minimal complications (Kolb et al., 2010, Tables 5 and 6).

Authors Year of publication	Patients (n) for Follow-up (n, %)	Internal Fixation CPO/MIPO Nailing	Fracture Healing (weeks)	Mean Follow-up (years)	Good/Excellent Results (%) Scoring System
Sisto et al., 1985	3/3 (100%)	CPO (CP)	16 (12-20)	1.1	86 HSS knee score
Merkel et al., 1986	5/3 (60%)	CPO 4 (80%) Screws 1 (20%)	ND	3.0	76.3 KSS score
Cain et al., 1986	4/4	CPO 1 (25%) Rush pins 3 (75%)	Non-union 2 (50%)	2.5	25 Own rating system
Culp et al., 1987	30/22 (73%)	CPO (67%) Rush pins 2 (7%)	Non-union 1 (3%)	3.7	ND
Figgie et al., 1990	22/12	CPO 10 (45%) CP 5 (23%), Dual plating 2 (9%), CPB 2 (9%), Barr bolt and AO screws 1 (4%)	32 (16-64) Non-union 5 (23%)	ND	64 University knee score
Healy et al., 1993	20	CPO (CP/DCS 7/7, 35%, CBP 6, 30%)	16 (6-40)	2.2	84 KSS score

Zehntner et al., 1993	7/6 (86%)	CPO (CPB 6, 86%)	14 (12-16)	1.4	50 Cain rating system
McLaren et al., 1994	7/7 (100%)	Intramedullary supracondylar rod 7 (100%)	12	1.3	ND
Moran et al., 1996	15/15 (100%)	CPO (CP 9 60%, CBP 3 20% (2 with double plating)	12 (4-16), non-union 3 (20%)	2.5	KSS score
Ochsner et al., 1999	6/5 (83%)	CPO (Fork Plate) 6 (100%)	9	ND	ND
Wick et al., 2001)	6/6 (100%)	GSH nail 8 (100%)	12.4	1.4	69 Freeman score
Kregor et al., 2001	13	LISS 13/13 (100%)	ND	ND	ND
Althausen et al., 2003	11	LISS 5 (45%) Rush rod 4 (36%) CPO 2 (18%) Retrograde nail 1 (9%)	ND	ND	ND
Wick et al., 2004	18/18 (100%)	DFN (44%), GSH nail 1 (6%), LISS 9 (50%)		2.5	ND
Gliatis et al., 2005	10/10 (100%)	GSH 10 (100%)	12	2.9	59 WOMAC score
Ricci et al., 2006	24/22 (92%)	LCP 24 (100%)	12 (8-20), Non-union 3 (13%)	1.0	ND
O'Toole et al., 2006	14/11 (79%)	LISS 14 (100%)	ND	1.0	71 own score
Fulkerson et al., 2007	18	LISS 18	6.2 (3-19) months Delayed union 2 (11%) Non-union 3 (17%)	2.3	ND
Kolb et al., 2009	21/15 (71%)	CP	14 (12-16)	9 (712)	77 KSS score
Streubel et al., 2010	89/61 (69%) Group A (n=28), Group B (n=33)	Peri-Loc Distal Lateral Femur locking plate, Locking Condylar Plate, LISS	Delayed union 5 (18%), non-union 3 (11%) group A, delayed union 2 (6%), non-union 5 (15%) group B	Minimum follow-up 0.5	ND
Kolb et al., 2010	23/19 (83%)	LISS 23 (1005)	14 (9-21) Delayed union 2 (11%)	3.8 (2.2-5.6)	81 KSS score

Table 5. Results of surgically treated periprosthetic femur fractures above total knee arthroplasties

Authors Year	Malalignment	Bone graft (n, % early/late)	Infection (n, %)	Implant Failure	Scondary Surgical Procedure
Sisto et al., 1985	Valgus 3/5° ½ (33/66%)	0	0	0	0
Merkel et al., 1986	0	2 (40%), 1 (20%)	0	Intraoperative 1 Death	1 Above knee amputation
Cain et al., 1986	Valgus 10° 2 (25%)	0	0	0	0
Culp et al., 1987	3 (10%)	0	2 (7%)	0	2 Above knee amputations
Figgie et al., 1990	Varus 7° 5 (23%)	4 (18%)	0	5 (23%)	4 Revision osteosynthesis with bone grafting, 1 Revision TKA,
Healy et al., 1993	0	15/3 (75%)/(15%)	0	0	3 Revision osteosynthesis
Zehntner et al., 1993	Valgus 5° (0-10°)	2 (30%)	0	0	0
McLaren et al., 1994	0	0	0	0	1 Stress fracture at the proximal locking screw
Moran et al., 1996	Shortening 2 cm 3 (20%), Valgus 17° 1 (7%), Varus 2° 1 (7%)	6/2 (40%)/(13%)	0	3 (20%)	3 Revision osteosynthesis, 2 with bone graft
Ochsner et al., 1999	Varus 1 (17%)	0	0	0	1 Valgus osteotomy
Wick et al., 2001	Valgus 10° 1 (17%), Shortening 1 (17%)	0	0	0	0
Althausen et al., 2003	Rush rod valgus 13° 2 (50%), 10° 1 (25%),	0	0	0	ND

	Retrograde Nail varus 3° 1 (100%), Shortening >2 cm 1 (25%), CPO varus 4° 1 (50%)				
Kregor et al., 2001	0	0/1 (8%)	0	0	1 Revision osteosynthesis
Wick et al., 2004	Valgus 18° retrograde	0	1 (6%)	1 (6%) retrograde nail	1 Revision osteosynthesis 1 Hematoma
Gliatis et al., 2005	Valgus 35° 1 (11%)	0	0	0	ND
Ricci et al., 2006	Varus 6° 1 (4%), Valgus 7°/9°/13° 1/1/1 (4%)	0	2 (8%)	4 (17%) proximal screw failure	1 Above knee amputation 1 Debridement
O'Toole et al., 2006	0	0	0	0	0
Fulkerson et al., 2007	<5° Varus/Valgus angulation	0/1 (6%)	1 (6%)	1 (6%)	1 Revision to DCS and Dall-Miles cables, 2 Revision TKA, 1 Excision plasty
Kolb et al., 2009	Varus 5° 1 (5%)	4/1 (19%)/(5%)	0	1 (5%)	1 Revision osteosynthesis with bone graft and bone cement, 2 Hematomas
Streubel et al., 2010		2 (7%) Group A, 4 (12%) Group B	1 (4%) Group A, 1 (3%) Group B	0	8 Debridments, 6 Revision osteosynthesis
Kolb et al., 2010	Varus 7 1 (5%)	0	0	1 (5%)	1 Revision osteosynthesis

Table 6. Complications of surgically treated periprosthetic femur fractures above total knee arthroplasties

8. References

Aaron, R.K.; & Scott, R. (1987) Supracondylar fracture of the femur after total knee arthroplasty, Clin Orthop Relat Res, Vol.219, (June 1987), pp.136-139.

Althausen, P.L.; Lee, M.A.; Finkemeier, C.G.; Meehan, J.P.; & Rodrigo, J.J. (2003). Operative stabilization of supracondylar femur fractures above total knee arthroplasty: a comparison of four treatment methods, J Arthoplasty, Vol.18, No.7, (October 2003), pp.834-839.

Arens, S.; Eijer, H.; Schlegel, U.; Printzen, G.; Perren, S.M.; & Hansis, M. (1999). Influence of the design for fixation implants on local infection: experimental study of dynamic compression plates versus contact fixateurs in rabbits, J Orthop Trauma, Vol.13, No.7, (September-October 1999), pp.470-476.

Ayers, D.C. (1997). Supracondylar fracture of the distal femur proximal to a total knee replacement, Instruct Course Lect, Vol.46, pp.197-203.

Babst, R.; Hehli, M.; & Regazzoni, P. (2001). [LISS tractor. Combination of the "less invasive stabilization system" (LISS) with the AO distractor for the distal femur and proximal tibial fractures], Unfallchirurg, Vol.104, No.6, (June 2001), pp.530-535. German.

Beris AE, Lykissas MG, Sioros V, Mavrodonitis AN, Korompilias AV. (2010). Femoral periprosthetic fracture in osteoporotic bone after total knee replacement: treatment with external Ilizarov fixation, J Arthroplasty, Vol.25, No.7, (October 2010), pp.1168.e9-12.

Berry, D.J. (1999) Epidemiology: hip and knee, Orthop Clin North Am, Vol.30, No.2, (April 1999), pp.183-190. Review.

Böstman, O.M. (1983). Rotational refracture of the shaft of the adult tibia, Injury, Vol.15, No.2, (September 1983), pp.93-98.

Bogoch, E.; Hastings, D.; Gross, A.; & Gschwend, N. (1988). Supracondylar fractures of the femur adjacent to resurfacing and MacIntosh arthroplasties of the knee in patients with rheumatoid arthritis, Clin Orthop Relat Res, (April 1988), Vol.229, pp.213-220.

Brunner, C.; & Weber, B.G. (1982). Special Techniques in Internal Fixation, Springer, Berlin, Germany.

Cain, P.R.; Rubash, H.E.; Wissinger, H.A.; & McClain, E.J. (1986). Periprosthetic femoral fractures following total knee arthroplasty, Clin Orthop Relat Res, Vol.208, (July 1986), pp.205-214.

Chen, F.; Mont, M.A.; & Bachner, R.S. (1994). Management of ipsilateral supracondylar femur fractures following total knee arthroplasty, J Arthroplasty, Vol.9, No.5, (October 1994), pp.521-526.

Chettiar, K.; Jackson, M.P.; Brewin, J.; Dass, D.; & Butler-Manuel, P.A. (2009). Supracondylar periprosthetic femoral fractures following total knee arthroplasty: treatment with a retrograde intramedullary nail, Int Orthop, Vol.33, No.4, (August 2009), pp.981-985.

Claes, L.; Heitemeyer, U.; Krischak, G.; Braun, H.; & Hierholzer, G. (1999). Fixation technique influences osteogenesis of comminuted fractures, Clin Orthop Relat Res, Vol.365, (August 1999), pp.221-229.

Cordeiro, E.N.; Costa, R.C.; Carazzato, J.G.; & Silva Jdos, S. (1990). Periprosthetic fractures in patients with total knee arthroplasties, Clin Orthop Relat Res, Vol.252, (March 1990), pp.182-189.

Culp, R.W.; Schmidt, R.G.; Hanks, G.; Mak, A.; Esterhai, J.L.; & Heppenstall, R.B. (1987).
    Supracondylar fracture of the femur following prosthetic knee arthroplasty. Clin
    Orthop Relat Res, Vol.222, (September 1987), pp.212-222.
Dennis, D.A. (1998). Periprosthetic fractures following total knee arthroplasty: the good,
    bad, & ugly, Orthopedics, Vol.21, No.9, (September, 1998), pp.1048-1050. Review.
Dennis D.A. Periprosthetic fractures following total knee arthroplasty. (2001). J Bone Joint
    Surg Am, Vol.83, pp.120-130.
Diehl, P.; Burgkart, R.; Klier, T.; Glowalla, C.; & Gollwitzer, H. (2006) [Periprosthetic
    fractures after total knee arthroplasty, Orthopäde, Vol.35, No.9, (September 2006),
    pp.972-974. Review. German.
DiGioia, A.M.3rd.; & Rubash, H.E. (1991) Periprosthetic fractures of the femur after total knee
    arthroplasty. A literature review and treatment algorithm, Clin Orthop Relat Res,
    Vol.271, (October 1991), pp.135-142.
Duda, G.N.; Mandruzzato, F.; Heller, M.; Kassi, J.P.; Khodadadyan, C.; & Hass, N.P. (2002).
    Mechanical conditions in the internal stabilization of proximal tibial defects, Clin
    Biomech (Bristol, Avon), Vol.17, No.1, (January 2002), pp.64-72.
Egol, K.A.; Kubiak, E.N.; Fulkerson, E.; Kummer, F.J.; & Koval, K.J. (2004). Biomechanics of
    locked plates and screws, J Orthop Trauma, Vol.18, No.8, (September 2004), pp.488-
    493.
Ehinger, M.; Adam, P.; Abane, L.; Rahme, M.; Moor, B.K.; Arlettaz, Y.; & Bonnormet, F.
    (2011). Treatment of periprosthetic femoral fractures of the knee, Knee Surg Sports
    Traumatol Arthrosc, Mar 23. [Epub ahead of print].
Erhardt, J.B.; Grob, K.; Roderer, G.; Hoffmann, A.; Forster, T.N.; & Kuster, M.S. (2008).
    Treatment of periprosthetic femur fractures with the non-contact bridging plate: a
    new angular stable implant, Arch Orthop Trauma Surg, Vol.128, No.4, (April 2008),
    pp.409-416.
Erhardt JB, Kuster MS. (2010). [Periprosthetic fractures of the knee joint]. Orthopäde
    2010;39:97-108.
El-Zayat, B.F.; Zettl, R.; Efe, T.; Krüger, A.; Eisenberg, F.; & Ruchholtz, S. (2010) [Minimally
    invasive treatment of geriatric and osteoporotic femur fractures with polyaxial
    locking implants (NCB-DF).], Unfallchirurg, (November 18, 2010), [Epub ahead of
    print].
Farouk, O.; Krettek, C.; Miclau, T.; Schandelmaier, P.; & Tscherne, H. (1998) Effects of
    percutaneous and conventional plating techniques on the blood supply to the
    femur, Arch Orthop Trauma Surg, Vol.117, No.8, pp.438-441.
Figgie, M.P.; Goldberg, V.M.; Figgie, H.E. 3rd.; & Sobel, M. (1990) The results of treatment of
    supracondylar fracture above total knee arthroplasty, J Arthroplasty, Vol.5, No.3,
    (September 1990), pp.267-276.
Finsen, V.; & Benum, P. (1986). Refracture of the hip rare after removal of fixation device,
    Acta Orthop Scand, Vol.57, No.5, (October 1986), pp.434-435.
Frigg, R.; Appenzeller, A.; Christensen, R.; Frenk, A.; Gilbert, S.; & Schavan, R. (2001). The
    development of the distal femur Less Invasive Stabilization System (LISS), Injury,
    Vol.32, Suppl 3, (December 2001), pp.SC24-31. Review.
Frigg, R. (2003). Development of the Locking Compression Plate, Injury, Vo.34, Suppl 2,
    pp.B6-10. Review.

Fulkerson, E.; Tejwani, N.; Stuchin, S.; & Egol, K. (2007). Management of periprosthetic femur fractures with a first generation locking plate, Injury, Vol.38, No.8, (August 2007), pp.965-972.

Ganz, R.; Mast, J.; Weber, B.; & Perren, S.M. (1991). Clinical aspects of „bio-logical" plating, Injury, Vol.22, pp.4-5.

Gardner, M.J.; Helfet, D.L.; & Lorich D.G. (2004). Has locked plating completely replaced conventional plating, Am J Orthop, Vol.33, No. 9, (September 2004), pp.439-446. Review.

Gardner, M.J.; Griffith, M.H.; Demetrakopoulos, D.; Brophy, R.H.; Grose, A.; Helfet, D.L.; Lorich, D.G. (2006). Hybrid locked plating of osteoporotic fractures of the humerus, J Bone Joint Surg Am, Vol.88, No.9, (September 2006, pp.1962-1967.

Gautier, E.; & Sommer, C. (2003) Guidelines for the clinical application of the LCP, Injury, Vol.34, Suppl 2, pp.B63-76. Review.

Gautier, E.; & Jakob, R.P. (2004). Biomechanics of osteosynthesis by screwed plates. In Biomechanics and biomaterials in orthopedics, D.G. Poitout (Ed.), pp.330-350, Springer, New York, USA.

Gerber, C.; Mast, J.; & Ganz, R. (1990). Biological internal fixation of fractures. Arch Orthop Trauma Surg, Vol.109, No.6, pp.295-303.

Gliatis, J.; Megas, P.; Panagiotpoulos, E.; & Lambiris, E. (2005). Midterm results of treatment with a retrograde nail for supracondylar periprosthetic fractures ofm the femur following total knee arthroplasty, J Orthop Trauma, Vol.19, No.3, (March 2005), pp.164-170.

Grützner, P.; Winkler, H.; & Wentzensen, A. (1997). [New aspects and developments of plate osteosynthesis. Point Contact Fixateur-PC Fix-Indication-technology-experiences, OPJ, Vol.3, pp.332-338.

Haddad, F.S.; Masri, B.A.; Garbuz, D.S.; & Duncan, C.P. (1999). The prevention of periprosthetic fractures in total hip and knee arthroplasty, Orthop Clin North Am, Vol.30, No.2, (April 1999), pp.191-207. Review.

Haidukewych, G.; Sems, S.A.; Huebner, D.; Horwitz, D.; & Levy, B. (2007). Results of polyaxial locked-plate fixation of periarticular fractures of the knee, J Bone Joint Surg Am, Vol.89, No.3, (March 2007), pp.614-620.

Harlow, M.L.; & Hofmann, A.A. (1994). Periprosthetic fractures. In The knee, W.N. Scott (Ed.), pp.1405-1417, CV Mosby, St. Louis, USA.

Healy, W.L.; Siliski, J.M.; & Incavo, S.J. (1993). Operative treatment of distal femoral fractures proximal to total knee replacements, J Bone Joint Surg Am, Vol.75, No.1, pp.27-34.

Henry, S.L. (1995). Management of supracondylar fractures proximal to total knee arthroplasty with the GSH supracondylar nail, Contemp Orthop, Vol.31, No.4, (October 1995), pp.231-238.

Herrera, D.A.; Kregor, P.J.; Cole, P.A.; Levy, B.A.; Jönsson, A.; & Zlowodzki, M. (2008). Treatment of acute distal femur fractures above total knee arthroplasty: a systematic review of 415 cases (1981-2006), Acta Orthop, Vol.79, No.1, (February 2006), pp.22-27.

Hidaka, S.; & Gustilo, R.B. (1984). Refracture of bones of the forearm after plate removal, J Bone Joint Surg Am, Vol.66, No.8, (October 1984), pp.1241-1243.

Hirsh, D.M.; Bhalla, S.; & Roffman, M. (1981) Supracondylar fracture of the femur following total knee replacement. Report of four cases, J Bone Joint Surg Am, Vol.63, No.1, (January 1981), pp.162-163.

Horwitz, D.S. & Kubiak, E.N. (2010). Surgical treatment of osteoporotic fractures about the knee, Instr Course Lect, Vol.59, pp.511-523. Review.

Johnston, A.T.; Tsiridis, E.; Eyres, K.S.; & Toms, A.D. (2011). Periprosthetic fractures in the distal femur following total knee replacement: A review and guide to management, Knee, Jul 7. [Epub ahead of print].

Kenwright, J.; & Goodship, A.E. (1989). Controlled mechanical stimulation in the treatment of tibial fractures, Clin Orthop Relat Res, Vol.241, (April 1989), pp.36-47.

Kim, K.I.; Egol, K.A.; Hozak, W.J.; & Parvizi J. (2006). Periprosthetic fractures after total knee arthroplasties, Clin Orthop Relat Res, Vol.446, (May 2006), pp.167-175.

Kessler, S.B.; Deiler, S.; Schiffl.Deiler, M.; Uhthoff, H.K.; & Schweiberer, L. (1992). Refractures: a consequence of impaired local bone viability, Arch Orthop Trauma Surg, Vol.111, No.2, pp.96-101.

Kolb, K.; Koller, H.; Lorenz, I.; Holz, U.; Marx, F.; Grützner, P.; & Kolb, W. (2009). Operative treatment of distal femoral fractures above total knee arthroplasty with the indirect reduction technique: a long-term follow-up study, Injury, Vol.40, No.4, (April 2009), pp.433-439.

Kolb, K.; Grützner, P.; Koller, H.; Windisch, C.; Marx, F.; & Kolb, W. (2009). The condylar plate for treatment of distal femoral fractures: a long-term follow-up study, Injury, Vol.40, No.4, (April 2009), pp.440-448.

Kolb, W.; Guhlmann, H.; Friedel, R.; & Nestmann, H. (2003). [Fixation of periprosthetic femur fractures with the less invasive stabilization system (LISS)-a new minimally invasive treatment with locked fixed-angle screws], Zentralbl Chir, Vol.218, No.1, (January 2003), pp.53-59. German.

Kolb, W.; Guhlmann, H.; Windisch, C.; Marx, F.; kolb, K.; & Koller, H. (2008). Fixation of distal femoral fractures with the Less Invasive Stabilization Sytems: a minimally invasive treatment with locked fixed-angled screws, J Trauma, Vol.65, No.6, (December 2008), pp.1425-1434.

Kolb, W.; Guhlmann, H.; Windisch, C.; Marx, F.; Koller, H.; & Kolb, K. (2010). Fixation of periprosthetic femur fracture above total knee arthroplasty with the less invasive stabilization system: a midterm follow-up stady, J Trauma, Vol.69, No.3, (September 2010), pp.670-676.

Kolodziej, P.; Lee, F.S.; Patel, A.; Kassab, S.S.; Shen, K.L.; Yang, K.H.; & Mast, J.W. (1998). Biomechnical evaluation of the schuhli nut, Clin Orthop Relat Res, Vol.347, (February 1998), pp.79-85.

Korner, J.; Lill, H.; Müller, L.P.; Rommens, P.M.; Schneider, E. & Linke, B. (2003). The LCP-concept in the operative treatment of distal humerus fractures – biological, biomechanical and surgical aspects, Injury, Vol.34, Suppl 2, (November 2003), pp.B20-30. Review.

Koudela, K. Jr.; Koudelová, J.; Koudela, K. Sr.; Kunesova. M.; Kren, J.; & Pokorny, J. (2010). [Radiographic measurements in total knee arthroplasty and their role in clinical practice], Acta Chir Orthop Traumatol Cech, Vol.77, Vol.4, (August 2010), pp.304-311.

Koval, K.J.; Hoehl, J.J.; Kummer, F.J.; & Simon, J.A. (1997). Distal femoral fixation: a biomechanical comparison of the standard condylar buttress plate, a locked buttress plate, and the 95-degree blade plate, J Orthop Trauma, Vol.11, No.7, (October 1997), pp.521-524.

Kregor, P.J.; Hughes, J.L.; & Cole, P.A. (2001). Fixation of distal femoral fractures above total knee arthroplasty utilizing the Less Invasive Stabilizations System (L.I.S.S.), Injury, Vol.32, Suppl 3, pp.SC64-75:

Krettek, C.; Schandelmaier, P.; Miclau, T.; & Tscherne, H. (1997). Minimally invasive percutaneous plate osteosynthesis (MIPPO) using DCS in proximal and distal femoral fractures, Injury, Vol.28, (Suppl 1), pp.S-A20-30.

Krettek, C.; Müller, M.; & Miclau, T. (2001). Evolution of minimally invasive plate osteosynthesis (MIPO) in the femur, Injury, Vol.32, Suppl 3, pp.S-C14-S-C23.

Kubiak, E.N.; Fulkerson, E.; Strauss, E.; & Egol. K.A. (2006). The evolution of locked plates, J Bone Joint Surg Am, Vol.88, Suppl 4, (December 2006), pp.189-200. Review.

Kumar, A.; & Chambers, I. (2008). Management of periprosthetic fracture above total knee arthroplasty using intramedullary fibular allograft and plate fixation, J Arthroplasty, Vol.23, No.4, (June 2008), pp.554-558.

Lesh, M.L.; Schneider, D.J.; Deol, G.; Davis, B.; Jacobs, C.R.; & Pellegrini, V.D. Jr. (2000). The consequence of anterior femoral notching in total knee arthroplasty. A biomechanical study, J Bone Joint Surg Am, Vol.82, No.8, (August 2000), pp.1096-1101.

Leunig, M.; Hertel, R.; Siebenrock, K.A.; Ballmer, F.T.; Mast, J.W.; & Ganz, R. (2000). The evolution of indirect reduction techniques for the treatment of fractures, Clin Orthop Relat Res, Vol.375; (June 2000), pp.7-14. Review.

Mamczak, C.N.; Gardner, M.J.; Bolhofner, B.; Borelli, J. Jr.; Streubel, P.N.; & Ricci, W.M. (2010). Interprosthetic femoral fractures, J Orthop Trauma, Vol.24, No.12, (December 2010), pp.740-744.

Maniar, R.N.; Umlas, M.E.; Rodriguez, J.A.; & Ranawat, C.S. (1996). Supracondylar femoral fracture above a PFC posterior cruciate-substituting total knee arthroplasty treated with supracondylar nailing. A unique technical problem, J Arthroplasty, Vol.11, No.5, (August 1996), pp.637-639.

Marti, A.; Fankhauser, C.; Frenk, A.; Cordey, J.; & Gasser, B. (2001). Biomechanical evalutation evaluation of the less invasive stabilization system for the internal fixation of distal femur fractures, J Orthop Trauma, Vol.15, No.7, (September-October 2001), pp.482-487.

Mast, J.; Jacob, R.; & Ganz, R. (1989). Planning and reduction techniques in fracture surgery, Springer, New York, USA. .

http://www.medical.siemens.com/webapp/wcs/stores/servlet/ProductDisplay~q_catalo gId~e_-3~a_catTree~e_100010,1007665,12760,1032265~a_langId~e_-3~a_productId~e_202741~a_storeId~e_10001.htm

McGraw, P.; & Kumar, A. (2010). Periprosthetic fractures of the femur after total knee arthroplasty, J Orthop Traumatol, Vol.11, No.3, (September 2010), pp.135-141. Review.

McLaren, A.C.; Dupont, J.A.; & Schroeber, D.C. (1994). Open reduction internal fixation of supracondylar fractures above total knee arthroplasties using the intramedullary rod, Clin Orthop Relat Res, Vol.302, (May 1994), pp.194-198.

Merkel, K.D.; & Johnson E.W.jr. (1986). Supracondylar fracture of the femur after total knee
    arthtoplasty, J Bone Joint Surg Am, Vol.68, No.1, (January 1986), pp.29-43.
Stedtfeld, H.W.; Mittlmeier, T.; Landgraf, P.; & Ewert, A. (2004). The logic and clinical
    applications of blocking screws, J Bone Joint Surg Am, Vol.86, Suppl 2, pp.17-25.
Mittlmeier, T.; Stöckle, U.; Perka, C.; & Schaser, K.D. (2005). [Periprosthetic fractures after
    total knee joint arthroplasty, Unfallchirurg, Vol.108, No.6, (June 2005), pp.481-495;
    quiz 496. Review. German.
Mittlmeier, T.; & Beck, M. (2005). [Retrograde medullary locking in periprosthetic distal
    femoral fracture after condylar knee joint replacement], Unfallchirurg, Vol.108,
    No.6, (June 2005), pp.497-501. Review. German.
Moran, M.C.; Brick, G.W.; Sledge, C.B.; Dysart, S.H.; & Chien, E.P. (1996). Supracondylra
    femoral fracture following total knee arthroplasty, Clin Orthop Relat Res, Vol.324,
    (March 1996), pp.196-209.
Mulier, T.; Seligson, D.; Sioen, W.; van den Bergh, J.; & Reynaert, P. (1997). Operative
    treatment of humeral shaft fractures, Acta Orthop Belg, Vol.63, No.3, pp.170-177.
Müller, M.E.; Allgöwer, M.; & Willenegger, H. (1970). Manual of Internal Fixation, first ed.,
    Springer, New York, USA.
Müller, M.E.; Allgöwer, M.; Schneider, R.; & Willenegger, H. (1979). Manual of Internal
    Fixation, 2nd ed., Springer, New York, USA.
Murrell, G.A.; & Nunley, J.A. (1995). Interlocked supracondylar intramedullary nails for
    supracondylar fractures after total knee arthroplasty. A new treatment method, J
    Arthoplasty, Vol.10, No.1, (February 1995), pp.37-42.
Nauth, A.; Ristevski, B.; Begué, T.; & Schemitsch, E.H. (2011). Periprosthetic distal femur
    fractures: current concepts, J Orthop Trauma, Vol.25, Suppl 1, (June 2011), pp.S82-
    85.
Noorda, R.J,; & Wuisman, P.I. (2002). Mennen plate fixation for the treatment of
    periprosthetic femoral fracture: a multicenter study of thirty-six fractures, J Bone
    Joint Surg Am, Vol.84, No.12, (December 2002), pp.2211-2215.
Ochsner, P.E.; & Pfister, A. (1999). Use of the fork plate for internal fixation of periprosthetic
    fractures and osteotomies in connection with total knee replacement, Orthopedics,
    Vol.22, No.5, (May 1999), pp.517-521.
Ostrum, R.F.; & Geel, C. (1995). Indirect reduction and internal fixation of supracondylar
    femur fractures without bone graft, J Orthop Trauma, Vol.9, No.4, pp.278-284.
O'Toole, R.V.; Gobezie, R.; Hwang, R.; Chandler, A.R.; Smith, R.M.; Estok, D.M.2nd.;
    &Vrahas, M.S. (2006). Low complication rate of LISS for femur fractures adjacent to
    stable hip or knee arthroplasty, Clin Orthop Relat Res, Vol.450, (September 2006),
    pp.203-210.
Otto, R.J.; Moed, B.R.; & Bledsoe, J.G. (2009). Biomechanical comparison of polyaxial locking
    plates and a fixed-angle locking plate for internal fixation of distal femurs, J Orthop
    Trauma, Vol.23, No.9, (October 2009), pp.645-652.
Perren, S.M.; Coredy, J.; Rahn, B.A.; Gautier, E.; & Schneider, E. (1988). Early temporary
    porosis of bone induced by internal fixation implants. A reaction to necrosis, not to
    stress protection? Clin Orthop Relat Res, Vol.232, (Juliy 1988), pp.139-151. Review.
Perren, S.M. (2002). Evolution of the internal fixation of long bone fractures, J Bone Joint
    Surg Br, Vol.84, No.8, (November 2002), pp.1093-1110. Review.

Perren, S.M. (2003) Backgrounds of the technology of internal fixators, Injury, Vol.34, Suppl 2, pp.B1-3.

Platzer, P.; Schuster, R.; Aldrian, S.; Prosquill, S.; Krumboeck, A.; Zehetgruber, I.; Kovar, F.; Schwarmeis, K.; & Vecsei, V. (2010). Management and outcome of periprosthetic fractures after total knee arthroplasty, J Trauma, Vol.68, No.6, (June 2010), pp.1464-1470.

Ramotowski, W.; & Granowski, R. (1991). Zespol. An original method of stable osteosynthesis, Clin Orthop Relat Res, Vol.272, (November 1991), pp.67-75.

Rhinelander, F.W. (1972). Circulation in bone. In: Bourne GH, editor. 2nd ed., The biochemistry and physiology of bone, vol 2, 2nd ed. New York: Academic Press, p. 1-77.

Ricci, W.M.; Bolhofner, B.R.; Loftus, T.; Cox, C.; Mitchell, S.; & Borelli, J. Jr. (2005). Indirect reduction and plate fixation, without grafting, for periprosthetic femoral shaft fractures about a stable intramedullary implant, J Bone Joint Surg Am, Vol.87, No.10, (October 2005), pp.2240-2245.

Ricci, W.M. ; Loftus, T.; Cox, C.; & Borelli, J. (2006). Locked plates with minimally invasive insertion techniques for the treatment of periprosthetic supracondylar femur fractures above total knee arthroplasty J Orthop Trauma, Vol.20, No.3, (March 2006), pp.190-196.

Ricci, W.M.; Bolnhofner, B.R.; Loftus, T.; Cox, C.; Mitchell, S.; & Borrelli, J. Jr. (2006). Indirect reduction and plate fixation without grafting, for periprosthetic femoral shaft fractures about a stable intramedullary implant. Surgical technique, J Bone Joint Surg Am, Vol.88, Suppl 1 Pt2, (September 2006), pp.275-282.

Riemer, B.L.; Butterfield, S.L.; Burke, C.J 3rd.; & Mathews, D. (1992). Immediate plate fixation of highly comminuted femoral diaphyseal fractures in blunt polytrauma patients, Orthopedics, Vol.15, No.8, (August 1992), pp.907-916.

Ritter, M.A.; Faris, P.M.; & Keating, E.M. (1988) Anterior femoral notching and ipsilateral supracondylar femur fracture in total knee arthroplasty, J Arthroplasty, Vol.3, No.2, pp.185-187.

Ritter, M.A.; Thong, A.E.; Keating, E.M.; Faris, P.M.; Meding, J.B.; Berend, M.E.; Pierson, J.L.; & Davis, K.E. (2005). The effect of femoral notching during total knee arthroplasty on the prevalence of postoperative femoral fractures and on clinical outcome, J Bone Joint Surg Am, Vol.87, No.11, (November 2005), pp.2411-2414.

Rolston, L.R.; Christ, D.J.; Halpern, A.; O'Connor, P.L.; Ryan, T.G.; & Uggen, W.M. (1995). Treatment of supracondylar fractures of the femur proximal to a total knee arthroplasty, J Bone Joint Surg Am, Vol.77, No.6, (June 1995), pp.924-931.

Rorabeck CH, Taylor JW. Periprosthetic fractures of the femur complicating total knee arthroplasty. Orthop Clin North Am 1999;30:265-277.

Roscoe, M.W.; Goodman, S.B.; & Schatzker, J. (1989) Supracondylar fracture of the femur after GUERPAR total knee arthroplasty, Clin Orthop Relat Res, Vol.241, (April 1989), pp.221-223.

Rozbruch, S.R.; Müller, U.; Gautier, E.; & Ganz, R. (1998). The evolution of femoral shaft plating technique, Clin Orthop Relat Res, Vol.354, (September 1998), pp.195-208.

Rüedi, T.P.; Sommer,C.; & Leutenegger, A. (1998). New techniques in indirect reduction of long bone fractures, Clin Orthop Relat Res, Vol.347, (February 1998), pp.27-34. Review.

Salas, C.; Mercer, D.; DeCoster, T.A.; & Reda Taha, M.M. (2011) Experimental and probahilistic analysis of distal femoral periprosthetic fracture: a comparison of locking plate and intramedullary nail fixation. Part A: experimental investigation, Comput Methods Biomech Biomed Engin, Vol.12, No.2, (February 2011), pp.157-164.

Sanders, R.; Haidukewych, G.J.; Milne, T.; Dennis, J.; & Latta, L.L. (2002). Minimal versus maximal plate fixation techniques of the ulna: the biomechanical effect of number of screws and plate length, J Orthop Trauma, Vol.16, No.3, (March 2002), pp.166-171.

Shawen, S.B.; Belmont, P.J.Jr.; Klemme, W.R.; Topoleski, L.D.; Xenos, J.S.; & Orchowski, J.R. (2003) Osteoporosis and anterior femoral notching in periprosthetic supracondylar femoral fractures: a biomechanical analysis, J Bone Joint Surg Am, Vol.85, No.1, (January 2003), pp.115-121.

Short, W.H.; Hootnick, D.R.; & Murray, D.G. (1981). Ipsilateral supracondylar femur fractures following knee arthroplasty, Clin Orthop Relar Res, Vol.158, (July-August 1981), pp.111-116.

Sisto, D.J.; Lachiewicz, P.F.; & Insall, J.N. (1985). Treatment of supracondylar fractures following prosthetic arthroplasty of the knee, Clin Orthop Relat Res, Vol.196, (June 1985), pp.265-272.

Smith, W.J.; Martin, S.L.; & Mabrey, J.D. (1996). Use of supracondylar nail for treatment of a supracondylar fracture of the femur following total knee arthroplasty, J Arthroplasty, Vol.11, No.2, (February 1996), pp.210-213.

Streubel, P.N.; Gardner, M.J.; Morshed, S.; Collinge, C.A.; Gallagher, B.; & Ricci, W.M. (2010). Are extreme distal periprosthetic supracondylar fractures of the femur too distal to fix using a lateral locked plate? J Bone Joint Surg Br, Vol.92, Vol.4, (April 2010), pp.527-534.

Stoffel, K.; Dieter, U.; Stachowiak, G.; Gächter, A.; & Kuster, M.S. (2003) Biomechanical testing of the LCP – how can stability in locked internal fixators be controlled? Injury, Vol.34, Suppl 2, pp.B11-19.

Su, E.T.; Dewal, H.; & Di Cesare, P.E. (2004) Perisprosthetic femoral fractures above total knee replacements, Am J Acad Orthop Surg, Vol.12, No.1, (January-February 2004), pp.12-20. Review.

Tani, Y.; Inoue, K.; Kanecko, H.; Nishioka, J.; & Hukuda, S. (1998) Intramedullary fibular graft for supracondylar fracture of the femur following total knee arthroplasty, Arch Orthop Trauma Surg, Vol.117, No.1-2, pp.103-104.

Tepic, S.; Remiger, A.R.; Morikawa, K.; Predieri, M.; & Perren, S.M. (1997). Strength recovery in fractured sheep tibia treated with a plate or an internal fixator: an experimental study with a two-year follow-up, J Orthop Trauma, Vol.11, No.1, (January 1997), pp.14-23.

Thielemann, F.W.; Blersch, E.; & Holz, U. (1988). [Plate osteosynthesis of femoral shaft fracture with reference to biological aspects], Unfallchirurg, Vol.91, No.9, (September 1988), pp.389-394. German.

Vidal, J.; Buscayret, C.; Fischbach, C.; Brahin, B.; Paran, M.; & Escare, P. (1977). [New method of treatment of comminuted fractures of the lower end of the radius: „ligamentary taxis"], Acta Orthop Belg, Vol.43, No.6, pp.781-789. French.

Wagner, M. (2003). General principles for the clinical use of the LCP, Injury, Vol.34, Suppl 2, (November 2003), pp.B31-42. Review.

Wagner, M. & Frigg, R. (2006). Manual of Fracture Management, Internal Fixators, Concepts and Cases using LCP and LISS, Thieme, New York, USA.

Wang, J.W.; & Wang, C.J. (2002). Supracobdylar fractures of the femur above total knee arthroplasties with cortical allograft struts, J Arthroplasty, Vo.17, No.3, (April 2002), pp.365-372.

Wenzl, H.; Casey, P.A.; Hérbert, P.; & Bellin, J. (1970). Die operative Behandlung der distalen Femurfraktur. AO Bulletin, Chur AO: Arbeitsgemeinschaft für Osteosynthesefragen.

Wick, M, Müller, E.J.; & Muhr, G. (2001). [Supracondylar femoral fractures in knee endoprosthesis. Stabilizing with retrograde interlocking nail], Unfallchirurg, Vol.104, No.5, (May 2001), pp.410-413. German.

Wick, M.; Müller, E.J.; Kutscha-Lissberg, F.; Hopf, F.; & Muhr, G. (2004). [Periprosthetic supracondylar femoral farctures: LISS or retrogarde intramedullary nailing? Problems with use of minimally invasive technique], Unfallchirurg, Vol.107, No.3, (March 2004), pp.181-188. German.

Zehntner, M.K.; & Ganz, R. (1993). Internal fixation of supracondylar fractures after condylar total knee arthroplasty. Clin Orthop Relat Res, Vol.293, (August 1993), pp.219-224.

Zlowodzki, M.; Williamson, S.; Cole, P.A.; Zardiackas, L.D.; & Kregor, P.J. (2004). Biomechanical evaluation of the less invasive stabilization system, angled blade plate, and retrograde intramedullary nail for the internal fixation of distal femur fractures, J Orthop Trauma, Vol.18, No.8, (September 2004), pp.494-502.

10

Patient-Specific Patellofemoral Arthroplasty

Domenick J. Sisto[1], Ronald P. Grelsamer[2] and Vineet K. Sarin[3]

[1]Los Angeles Orthopaedic Institute, Sherman Oaks, California
[2]Mount Sinai Medical Center, New York, New York
[3]Kinamed Incorporated, Camarillo, California
USA

1. Introduction

In this chapter we review the topic of patellofemoral arthroplasty from a historical, technical, and clinical perspective. Emphasis is placed on the design rationale, surgical technique, and clinical results of so-called "patient-matched" or "patient-specific" patellofemoral arthroplasty in which the trochlear implant is matched to the anatomy of the individual patient through the use of pre-operative computerized imaging scans (Fig 1).

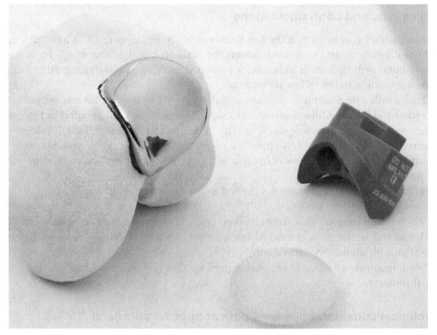

Fig. 1. Patient-specific patellofemoral implant mounted on patient-specific physical bone model, alongside a companion patient-specific drill guide & marking template and all-polyethylene patella button. Collectively these items constitute the patient-specific patellofemoral arthroplasty system described in this chapter.

The implants are inlayed into the articular cartilage without any intra-operative femoral bone resection. Clinical results involving patient-matched patellofemoral arthroplasty are presented with an average follow-up of 11 years. Case studies reviewing our collective experience with patient-matched trochlear implants in the setting of femoral trochlear dysplasia are also presented.

2. Historical perspective

The origins of patellofemoral arthroplasty (PFA or PFR) can be traced to 1955 with the introduction of the McKeever prosthesis (McKeever, 1955). This prosthesis consisted of a Vitallium® shell used to resurface only the patella. The procedure was eventually abandoned because of concerns regarding trochlear wear (Leadbetter et al, 2006). Blazina et al (1979) reported on the use of a patellofemoral prosthesis. In the decades that followed, a number of different patellofemoral prostheses were developed and studied (Lonner, 2004; Leadbetter et al, 2005; Lonner, 2007; Sisto & Sarin, 2008; Gupta et al, 2010). The clinical results with these designs have been highly variable, which has led to skepticism about the success of the procedure. A consensus view has emerged that appropriate patient selection and prosthesis design are the two most critical elements for achieving successful outcomes after patellofemoral arthroplasty (Arnbjornsson and Ryd, 1998; Kooijman et al, 2003; Lonner, 2004; Ackroyd et al, 2007; Lonner, 2007; Gupta et al, 2010).

3. Indications and contraindications

Previous authors (Grelsamer, 2006; Leadbetter et al, 2006; Lonner, 2007) have discussed in detail the indications and contraindications for patellofemoral arthroplasty. To summarize, patellofemoral arthroplasty is indicated for isolated patellofemoral degenerative arthritis of the knee, according to the following criteria:
- Degenerative or posttraumatic osteoarthritis limited to the patellofemoral joint, so that medial and lateral Ahlback scores (Ahlback, 1968) are less than or equal to 1 point;
- Severe symptoms affecting daily activity referable to patellofemoral joint degeneration unresponsive to lengthy non-operative treatment and conservative procedures;
- Patellofemoral malalignment/dysplasia induced degeneration with or without instability.

Contraindications include but are not limited to the following criteria:
- The lack of non-operative care;
- Pain referred from outside the patellofemoral compartment or even outside the knee;
- Medial and lateral tibiofemoral Ahlback scores (Ahlback, 1968) greater than 1 point;
- Systemic inflammatory arthropathy;
- Patellofemoral instability or malalignment that is uncorrectable at the time of arthroplasty.

4. Technical considerations for a patient-specific approach

4.1 Motivation

The shape and alignment of the human patellar trochlear groove is highly variable (Feinstein et al, 1996). Such variability presents a challenge for so-called "off-the-shelf" patellofemoral prostheses that feature a fixed geometry and a finite number of sizes. For patellofemoral compartments that deviate from an off-the-shelf implant's design paradigm, there exists an inherent tradeoff between fit and alignment that must be addressed intra-operatively. Many reported off-the-shelf implant failures are thought to be due to design deficiencies related to fit and alignment within the patellofemoral compartment (Lonner, 2004; Lonner, 2007; Gupta et al, 2010). The patient-specific approach to patellofemoral arthroplasty described in this chapter was conceived and developed in light of these challenges (Fig 2).

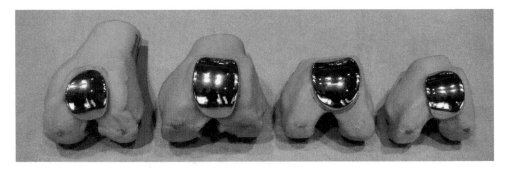

Fig. 2. Physical distal femur models from four patients treated with patient-specific patellofemoral arthroplasty (cartilage not shown). Note the substantial variation in trochlear groove geometry across this group, consistent with previously published findings. The patient-specific approach provides for a precise fit without bone resection or sculpting.

4.2 Design rationale
The design goal of patient-specific patellofemoral arthroplasty is to restore the mechanics of the patellofemoral compartment and maintain the native mechanics of the tibiofemoral compartments (Sisto & Sarin, 2006; Sisto & Sarin, 2008). Progression of arthritic disease into the medial and lateral knee compartments often contributes to the need for patellofemoral arthroplasty revision (Grelsamer, 2006). Poorly fitting off-the-shelf prostheses can detrimentally affect the mechanics of the knee joint (including the medial and lateral compartments), leading to disease progression into these compartments. Further, installing off-the-shelf prostheses can be a time-consuming process; and poorly fitting prostheses may require significant cement support. Patient-specific patellofemoral arthroplasty effectively addresses the design deficiencies and difficulties in surgical technique associated with off-the-shelf patellofemoral prostheses.

The patient-specific patellofemoral arthroplasty prosthesis described in this chapter is designed to custom-fit the bony anatomy; its bony contact surface is designed to conform to the bony anatomy of the patient's femoral trochlea using computed tomographic (CT) modeling (Fig 3). This approach allows for a precise fit of the implant to the trochlea without resection of subchondral femoral bone, as is necessary for so-called "onlay" off-the-shelf prostheses. Only removal of the overlying cartilage is necessary to obtain a precise fit with a patient-specific prosthesis. The trochlear prosthesis is designed to approximate normal patellofemoral kinematics by re-establishing a trochlear groove.

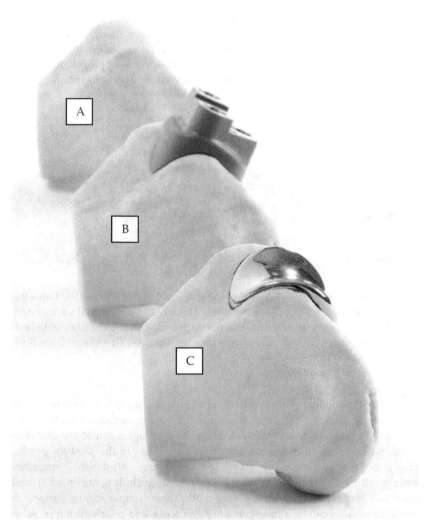

Fig. 3. Native patient-specific physical bone model (A), patient-specific bone model with companion patient-specific drill guide & marking template (B), and patient-specific bone model with companion patient-specific trochlear implant (C). Note the precise fit between patient-specific components and native unresected trochlear bone.

The distal margin of the patient-specific trochlear prosthesis is designed to rest 3 to 5 mm from the apex of the intercondylar notch. The prosthesis has a thickened lateral border to compensate for bone loss along the lateral edge of the trochlear groove and to provide congruency and tracking stability with the matching patellar implant. The thickened implant border does not anteriorize ("stuff") the patella relative to its pre-operative state because the anterior position of a given patella is defined by the thickness of the femoral implant's trochlear groove. The patient-specific femoral prosthesis may seem thick on lateral radiographs, but only because the radiograph is a 2-dimensional projection of a saddle-shaped structure.

The articular side of the patellofemoral implant has a radius of curvature matched to the curvature of a standard dome patellar implant. It is designed to constrain the patellar implant medially and laterally as it tracks along the trochlear groove. This design is, therefore, able to compensate for a deficient or dysplastic trochlear groove, which is often present in patellofemoral surgery candidates.

The bony-contact surface and the articulating surface of the patient-specific trochlear implant are "decoupled." The bony-contact surface is customized to fit the bony anatomy, while the articulating surface is designed to mate with a patella button prosthesis and provide medial-lateral constraint to the patella. The medial and lateral borders of the articular surface are thickened by a few millimeters to provide stability and congruency for the patella button.

The design rationale of patient-specific patellofemoral arthroplasty therefore eliminates the trade-off between fit and alignment that is inherent to off-the-shelf, particularly inlay, patellofemoral implants.

4.3 Stuffing

Overstuffing of the patellofemoral compartment has been cited (Lonner, 2007) as a concern over the use of patient-specific patellofemoral arthroplasty. Although this may be a theoretical concern, it has not been borne out by the clinical results. Moreover, the concept of patellofemoral overstuffing has been challenged. Merchant and colleagues (2008) state the following:

> The concept of overstuffing the patellofemoral joint has been simply and uncritically transferred from the femorotibial joint with no confirmatory studies. Because the capsule and inelastic ligaments secure the femorotibial joint, it is extremely important to balance these ligaments carefully during TKA and avoid a tibial insert that is too large. This will certainly overstuff this joint and lead to a poor result with decreased range of motion. The patellofemoral joint is a totally different articulation. Although the patellar ligament is inelastic, the quadriceps muscles are elastic and stretchable. This explains why the investigation by Bengs and Scott (2006) failed to support the claim of overstuffing by Conley et al (2007). More recently, Pierson et al (2007) reviewed 830 primary TKAs to determine the effects of so called overstuffing the patellofemoral joint. Their findings did "not support the widely held belief that stuffing of the patellofemoral joint results in adverse outcomes after total knee arthroplasty."

The trochlear prosthesis is designed to restore the anterior position of the non-degenerated patella. The thickness of normal articular cartilage is approximately 5 to 7 mm on the patella and 2 to 3 mm in the trochlea, yielding a combined total cartilage thickness of 7 to 10 mm (Grelsamer, 2000). The trochlear prosthesis typically is 2 to 5 mm thick along its center arc, the tracking arc of the patella. This thickness is a function of native trochlear groove depth (i.e., thinner implants are created for shallower grooves). The thinner implants are designed specifically to avoid overstuffing the more dysplastic trochleas. Coupled with an anatomic restoration of the patella, the extensor lever arm is intended to be unchanged or improved from the pre-operative condition (see Fig 6, described later in this chapter). If concerns about overstuffing still persist, accommodations can be made by resecting more bone on the patellar side or by selecting a thinner patellar implant.

5. Peri-operative technique

The peri-operative technique for patient-specific patellofemoral arthroplasty has been previously described (Sisto & Sarin, 2007; Sisto et al, 2010; Lombardi, 2011) and consists of pre-operative planning, intra-operative technique, and post-operative management.

5.1 Pre-operative planning

A CT scan of the patient's knee is obtained using the following settings as specified by the manufacturer of the prosthesis (Kinamed Incorporated, Camarillo, California, USA):

- Voltage: 120 to 140 kV;
- Amperage: 200 to 300 mA;
- Scan Region: 5mm distal to the femoral condyles to 10mm proximal to the patella.

Computer modeling is then used to create a 3-dimensional physical model of the patient's distal femoral bone, which is sent to the surgeon. The manufacturer identifies the perimeter of coverage of the trochlear implant on this model. If deemed necessary based on the presence of significant osteophytes or bony defects in or near the native trochlea, the surgeon may physically remove osteophytes from the model and communicate these changes by returning the model to the implant manufacturer. The final design for the trochlear implant is then created after surgeon approval.

If changes are made during the design review, during surgery the surgeon will modify the real trochlear groove in the same manner as was done on the physical model. For this reason, it is imperative that the physical model be available for visual examination in the operating theatre.

It must be noted that patellofemoral arthroplasty is not a substitute for a patellar realignment procedure. Patella tracking must be evaluated for instability and soft tissue imbalance (Lonner, 2004; Grelsamer, 2000). Malalignment of the patella is determined through physical examination and standard radiographic evaluation. Assessment of patellar tracking is important in pre-operative planning, as patellar instability is the most often reported cause of dysfunction after patellofemoral arthroplasty. Tightness of the lateral retinaculum is often associated with lateralization and patellar tilt, which may be determined upon physical examination. Examination of medial structures for deficiency should also be carried out, as well as assessment of the tibial tuberosity (Q angle). Axial and lateral radiographs are often sufficient to quantify measures of patellar malalignment, including patella alta or baja, medial-lateral displacement and patellar tilt. Treatments are generally customized to each patient, although it remains to be determined if there are one or more standard procedures that will be optimal for most patients (Grelsamer, 2000).

5.2 Intra-operative technique

A standard midline incision is made to expose the patellofemoral joint, and the patella is everted or tilted 90°. The length of the incision is typically two-thirds the length of a standard total knee incision because tibial exposure is not necessary. The margin of cartilage to be removed is determined by placing the patient-specific drill guide onto the trochlea. Because the cartilage remnants on the trochlea will initially not permit a proper fit of the patient-specific custom drill guide, the surgeon first approximates the proper position of the drill guide (using the CT-created physical bone model as a template). The surgeon outlines the drill guide with methylene blue and by way of a ring curette removes the cartilage inside that outline. Osteophytes are removed as necessary. The patient-specific drill guide is then placed on the subchondral bone of the trochlea and moved slightly back and forth until it seats in its intended position as determined by the CT scan. Two headless nails are then used to secure the drill guide and the three holes are drilled. The holes are then thoroughly irrigated to remove any debris that may be present.

The trochlear prosthesis is designed to be used in conjunction with a standard off-the-shelf all-polyethylene patellar button of onlay design with a 25 mm radius of curvature. The residual patellar thickness is the same as with total knee arthroplasty.

During trialing, particular attention is paid to potential subluxation or catching within the limitations of a patient under anesthesia (Lonner, 2004). If realignment is necessary, balancing is carried out in the same manner as a non-prosthetic or total knee arthroplasty. To correct patellar tilt or lateral displacement of the patella, a proximal realignment procedure such as a lateral retinacular release, medial plication, vastus medialis obliquus advancement, and/or medial patellofemoral ligament repair may be carried out (Grelsamer, 2000). In the presence of a high Q angle, a distal realignment procedure such as transfer of the tibial tuberosity may be carried out to correct alignment of the extensor mechanism (Grelsamer, 2000). Any realignment or soft-tissue balancing strategy should be oriented toward addressing specific identifiable pathology (Grelsamer, 2000).

Cementing is carried out in standard knee arthroplasty fashion. Particular care needs to be taken to avoid cement seepage into the notch or other compartments. The cartilage of the other compartments must be kept moist throughout the procedure to avoid deterioration. Patellofemoral tracking is again evaluated and soft tissue corrections are carried out as necessary to ensure optimal patellar tracking.

5.3 Post-operative management

The need for prophylaxis against deep venous thrombosis has not been shown for patellofemoral replacement surgery. Postoperative rehabilitation consists of range of motion exercises as with any knee arthroplasty. As a rule, though, progress will be much quicker than with total knee arthroplasty patients. Immediate full-weight bearing is allowed. Physical therapy to restore quadriceps strength is encouraged. Twisting activities are discouraged, but no additional specific activity modifications are recommended.

6. Clinical results

Previous investigators have reported on clinical results obtained with off-the-shelf and patient-specific patellofemoral arthroplasty.

6.1 Results with off-the-shelf implants

Published clinical results with off-the-shelf patellofemoral implants have been previously reviewed in detail (Lonner, 2007; Sisto & Sarin, 2008; Gupta et al, 2010; Charalambous et al, 2011). These references cover twenty one studies that each involved from 14 to 306 patients who received 8 different off-the-shelf designs, with follow-up ranging from 6 months to 21 years. These reports demonstrate that clinical results with off-the-shelf patellofemoral implant designs have been highly variable.

The Australian national joint replacement registry reports that the cumulative revision rate at five and seven years for off-the-shelf patellofemoral implants used in the setting of primary osteoarthritis is 15.2% and 22.4%, respectively (Australian Orthopaedic Association, 2010).

6.2 Results with patient-matched Implants
6.2.1 Prior investigation

In an earlier published investigation (Sisto and Sarin, 2006), 100% survivorship with excellent or good Knee Society scores was reported at a mean duration of follow-up of 73 (range, 32 to 119) months. The study was a retrospective review of a consecutive single-surgeon series of patient-specific patellofemoral arthroplasties performed between March 1995 and August 2002. There were 25 patellofemoral arthroplasties performed in 22 patients (three staged bilaterals), 16 of whom were female. Mean age at the time of index arthroplasty was 45 (range, 23 to 51) years.

Only patients whose medial and lateral compartments scored less than or equal to 1 point on the Ahlback scale were indicated for patellofemoral arthroplasty. The patellofemoral compartments for all knees scored at least 4 points. The mean pre-operative Knee Society functional score was 49 points, and the mean pre-operative Knee Society objective score was 52 points.

There were 18 excellent and 7 good results at 73 months of follow-up. The mean post-operative Knee Society objective score was 91 (range, 82 to 96) points, and the mean post-operative Knee Society functional score was 89 (range, 81 to 94) points. All patients exhibited good to excellent Knee Society Score status and no patient had required additional surgery or had component loosening.

6.2.2 Eleven year follow-up

The objective of the eleven year follow-up study was to evaluate the longer-term success of patient-specific patellofemoral arthroplasty in the original patient cohort. For assessment of

Question	Answer
Has your custom PFA been replaced?	No: 25 out of 25 Yes: 0
Does your PFA keep you from doing anything that you would like to do?	No: 23 out of 25 Yes: 2 out of 25
How satisfied are you with your PFA?	Very Dissatisfied: 0 out of 25 Somewhat Satisfied: 0 out of 25 Very Satisfied: 25 out of 25
Have you had additional surgery on this knee since your PFA?	No: 25 out of 25 Yes: 0
How often do you take pain medication because of pain in this knee?	Never: 25 out of 25 Sometimes (1-2x per week): 0 Often (>1 per day): 0
If you have pain, where is the pain coming from?	Inside of Knee: 3 out of 25 Kneecap area: 21 out of 25 Outside of Knee: 1 out of 25
Does this knee feel weak or unstable?	No: 25 out of 25 Yes: 0
Would you undergo PFA with this custom implant again?	No: 0 Yes: 25 out of 25

Table 1. The original cohort included 25 patellofemoral arthroplasties (PFAs) in 22 patients. Each patient from the original cohort answered via telephone the above-listed questions, which were selected and adapted from the validated "Total Knee Function Questionnaire" (Weiss et al, 2002). All patients were successfully contacted and no knees were lost. Average time from index patellofemoral arthroplasty to completion of the questionnaire was 11.3 years (range, 7.8 to 14.9 years).

longer-term follow-up, the validated "Total Knee Function Questionnaire" (Weiss et al, 2002) was adapted and administered via telephone to each patient from the above-mentioned prior study. The questions were designed to assess the status of each patient's patellofemoral arthroplasty as well as their degree of knee function.

The questionnaire was completed for all 25 knees (Table 1). No knees from the original study were lost to follow-up. At a mean duration of 11.3 years (range, 7.8 to 14.9 years) from the index arthroplasty, all 25 patellofemoral arthroplasties were still in place and all patients reported themselves as being very satisfied. There were no reports of weakness, instability, or additional surgery. Two patients reported that despite their patellofemoral arthroplasty, they were not participating in sports activities. All patients experienced some pain, but not enough to warrant medication. All 22 patients said they would undergo the procedure again.

This 11 year follow-up study demonstrates that patient-specific patellofemoral arthroplasty is a safe and effective treatment for patients with isolated patellofemoral arthritis of the knee. These results compare favorably with those involving off-the-shelf patellofemoral arthroplasties that have been reported on over the past 30 years (Leadbetter et al, 2005; Leadbetter et al, 2006; Lonner, 2007; Sisto and Sarin, 2008; Gupta et al, 2010).

6.3 Complications

Progression of arthritis into the tibiofemoral compartment is a recognized complication of patellofemoral replacement; when symptomatic, this scenario leads to conversion to a total knee arthroplasty. Progression is more likely to develop when the disease patellofemoral arthritis does not have a clear origin, such as idiopathic arthritis (Grelsamer, 2006). Despite attempts to balance the extensor mechanism, patellar maltracking after patellofemoral arthroplasty can occur, especially when the patient pre-operatively demonstrates high level malalignment and/or dysplasia.

7. Case studies

Our (DJS and RPG) collective experience with patient-specific patellofemoral arthroplasty dates back to 1995 and consists of 91 cases in 79 patients through May 2011. Patients in our cohort generally fall into one of two categories: those having a "normal" femoral trochlear sulcus angle, with or without patellar tilt; and those having a femoral sulcus angle greater than 145°, i.e. a shallow or even convex trochlea – dysplastic trochleas will exhibit a crossing sign on a true lateral radiograph (Bollier and Fulkerson, 2011). The following case studies serve as illustrative examples.

7.1 Normal trochlear anatomy

Patient J.O. is a 49 year old male who initially presented with severe anterior knee pain 14 years ago after sustaining a twisting injury to his knee that was treated with arthroscopic surgery followed by a soft tissue realignment procedure two years later. During this time, he developed progressive and disabling anterior knee pain. He could not walk up or down stairs without assistance and could not kneel, squat or climb without severe pain.

Physical examination revealed severe anterior knee tenderness with severe crepitus and grinding in the retro-patellar space. He had no ligament instability and no medial or lateral joint line tenderness. All provocative tests for meniscal and ligamentous injury were negative. The radiographs revealed severe patellofemoral arthritis and no medial or lateral joint line abnormalities (Fig 4).

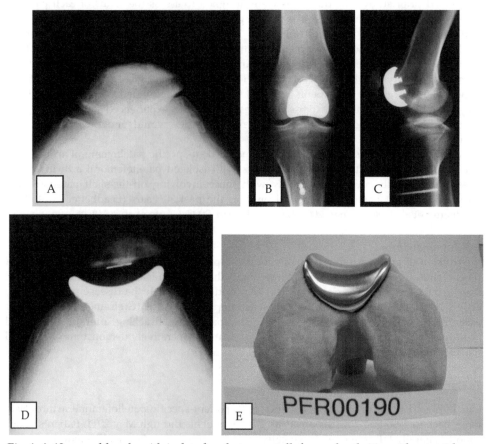

Fig. 4. A 49 year old male with isolated end-stage patellofemoral arthritis, without evidence of trochlear dysplasia as seen in pre-operative Merchant view (A), treated with a patient-matched patellofemoral prosthesis and all-polyethylene patella button. Post-operative anterior-posterior (B), lateral (C), and Merchant (D) views demonstrate proper orientation of patellofemoral prosthesis. Placement, fit, and alignment of the patient-specific trochlear implant was confirmed by the manufacturer using the patient-specific CT bone model prior to final polishing (E). See section 7.1 for additional case details.

The patient was initially treated with medications, heat, physical therapy and hyalgan injections without relief, and he remained symptomatic and disabled. In October 2009, he underwent a patient-matched custom patellofemoral arthroplasty of the right knee (Fig 4). Post-operatively, he has done remarkably well and has returned to his previous employment at the Los Angeles County Sheriff's Department. He currently has no pain and does not require any medications. He can ambulate up and down stairs without assistance and can kneel, squat and climb without pain.

7.2 Trochlear dysplasia

Patient D.B. is a 56 year old woman with anterior knee pain since her teenage years. Non-operative treatments had included activity modification, prescription and over-the-counter

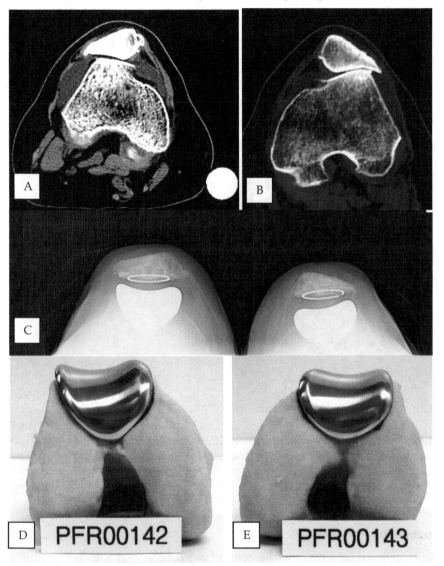

Fig. 5. A 56 year old female with bilateral isolated end-stage patellofemoral arthritis, with bilateral trochlear dysplasia (A, B), treated with patient-matched patellofemoral prostheses. Post-operative Merchant views (C) demonstrate proper orientation of patellofemoral implant components. Placement, fit, and alignment of both patient-specific trochlear implants were confirmed by the manufacturer using the patient-specific CT bone models prior to final polishing (D, E). See section 7.2 for additional case details.

pain medications, steroid and visco-supplementation injections, nutritional supplements, and physical therapy. Serum laboratory studies had not been suggestive of inflammatory arthritis.

Imaging studies demonstrated severe patellofemoral dysplasia and an absence of arthritis outside the patellofemoral compartment (Fig 5). She had undergone arthroscopies of both knees. She underwent patient-matched custom patellofemoral arthroplasty in September 2008 for her right knee and in December 2008 for her left knee.

Despite the chronically subluxed position of her patellae pre-operatively, an extensive intra-operative lateral release and medial plication have been sufficient to maintain her patellae centered within the patient-matched custom trochlear implant (Fig 5). She flexes easily to at least 120 degrees. The patient considers the procedure a success.

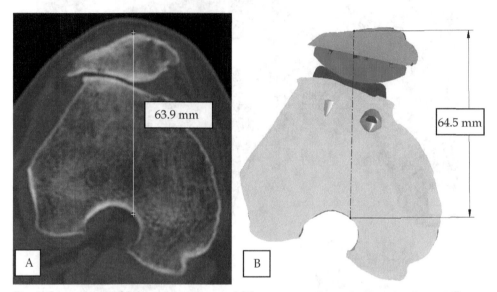

Fig. 6. Comparison of (A) pre-operative and (B) post-operative anterior-posterior patellar offset for the right knee described in Figure 5. Post-operative measurements were based on the known geometry of the patient-matched patellofemoral implant and the all-polyethylene patella selected at the time of surgery. In the presence of pronounced trochlear dysplasia (Figures 5A and 6A), treatment with a patient-specific patellofemoral arthroplasty prosthesis resulted in an insignificant net change in patellar offset (0.6 mm).

8. Conclusion

In this chapter we have reviewed the topic of patellofemoral arthroplasty from historical, technical, and clinical perspectives. The design rationale, peri-operative techniques, and 11 year clinical results of patient-matched patellofemoral arthroplasty have been reviewed and discussed. Experience with patient-matched trochlear implants in the setting of normal and dysplastic femoral trochleas have also been presented.

Patient-specific patellofemoral arthroplasty is a safe and effective treatment for patients with isolated patellofemoral arthritis. The results compare favorably with off-the-shelf patellofemoral arthroplasties that have been reported on over the past thirty years (Leadbetter et al, 2005; Leadbetter et al, 2006; Lonner, 2007; Sisto and Sarin, 2008; Gupta et al, 2010) and can be carried out more efficiently.

We believe the key elements that contribute to the success of patient-specific patellofemoral arthroplasty are as follows: (a) a strict inclusion criteria based on pre-operative radiographic evaluation; (b) a meticulous attention to soft-tissue balance and patellofemoral tracking at the time of arthroplasty; and (c) a patient-specific design and manufacturing methodology that ensures accurate and precise anatomic fit while simultaneously providing proper patellofemoral alignment and medial-lateral constraint.

9. References

Ackroyd CE, Newman JH, Evans R, Eldridge JD, Joslin CC (2007) The Avon patellofemoral arthroplasty: five-year survivorship and functional results. . *J Bone Joint Surg*, Vol. 89-B, pp. 310-5.

Ahlback S (1968) Osteoarthritis of the Knee. A Radiologic Investigation. *Acta Radiol Diagn (Stockh)*, Vol. 277, pp. 7-72.

Arnebjornsson AH and Ryd L (1998) The use of isolated patellar prostheses in Sweden 1977-1986. *Int Orthop*, Vol. 22, No. 3, pp. 141-4.

National Joint Replacement Registry of Australia, Annual Report (2010).

Bengs BC and Scott RD (2006) The effect of patellar thickness on intraoperative knee flexion and patellar tracking in total knee arthroplasty. *J Arthroplasty*, Vol. 21, pp. 650–655.

Blazina ME, Fox JM, Del Pizzo W (1979) Patellofemoral replacement. *Clin Orthop Rel Res*, Vol. 144, pp. 98–102.

Bollier M and Fulkerson JP (2011) The role of trochlear dysplasia in patellofemoral instability. *J Am Acad Orthop Surg*, Vol. 19, No. 1, pp. 8-16.

Charalambous CP, Abiddin Z, Mills SP, Rogers S, Sutton P, Parkinson R (2011) The low contact stress patellofemoral replacement: High early failure rate. *J Bone Joint Surg*, Vol. 93-B, pp. 484-9.

Conley S, Rosenberg A, Crowninshield R (2007) The female knee: anatomic variations. *J Am Acad Orthop Surg*, Vol. 15 (suppl 1), pp. S31–S36.

Feinstein WK, Noble PC, Kamaric E, Tullos HS (1996) Anatomic alignment of the patellar groove. *Clin Orthop Rel Res*, Vol. 331, pp. 64–73.

Fulkerson JP (2004) *Disorders of the Patellofemoral Joint*. 4th Edition. Philadelphia, PA. Lippincott Williams & Wilkins.

Grelsamer RP (2000) Current concepts review. Patellar malalignment. *J Bone Joint Surg*, Vol. 82-A, pp. 1639–1650.

Grelsamer RP (2006) Current concepts review. Patellofemoral Arthritis. *J Bone Joint Surg*, Vol. 88-A, pp. 1849–1860.

Gupta RR, Zywiel MG, Leadbetter WB, Bonutti P, Mont MA (2010) Scientific Evidence for the Use of Modern Patellofemoral Arthroplasty. *Expert Rev Med Devices*, Vol. 7, No. 1, pp. 51-66.

Kooijman HJ, Driessen AP, van Horn JR (2003) Long-term results of patellofemoral arthroplasty. A report of 56 arthroplasties with 17 years of follow-up. . *J Bone Joint Surg*, Vol. 85-B, pp. 836–40

Leadbetter WB, Ragland PS, Mont MA (2005) The appropriate use of patellofemoral arthroplasty. *Clin Orthop Rel Res*, Vol. 436, pp. 91–99.

Leadbetter WB, Seyler TM, Ragland PS (2006) Indications, Contraindications, and Pitfalls of Patellofemoral Arthroplasty. *J Bone Jt Surg*, Vol. 88-A(Suppl 4), pp. 122-137.

Lombardi AV (2011) Patellofemoral Arthroplasty: Custom Inlay Technique Offers a Patient Specific Approach. *Annual Meeting of the American Academy of Orthopaedic Surgeons*, pp. 142-144, San Diego, California, USA.

Lonner JH (2004) Patellofemoral Arthroplasty. Pros, Cons, and Design Considerations. *Clin Orthop Rel Res*, Vol. 428, pp. 158–165.

Lonner JH (2007) Patellofemoral Arthroplasty. *J Am Acad Orthop Surg*, Vol. 15, No. 8, pp. 495-506.

McKeever DC (1955) Patellar prosthesis. *J Bone Joint Surg*, Vol. 37-A, pp. 1074–1084.

Merchant AC, Arendt EA, Dye SF, Fredericson N, Grelsamer RP, Leadbetter WB, Post WR, Teitge RA (2008) The Female Knee. Anatomic Variations and the Female-Specific Total Knee Design. *Clin Orthop Rel Research*, Vol. 466, pp. 3059-3065.

Pierson JL, Ritter MA, Keating EM, Faris PM, Meding JB, Berend ME, Davis KE (2007) The effect of stuffing the patellofemoral compartment on the outcome of total knee arthroplasty. *J Bone Joint Surg*, Vol. 89-A, pp. 2195–2203.

Sisto DJ and Sarin VK (2006) Custom Patellofemoral Arthroplasty of the Knee. *J Bone Jt Surg*, Vol. 88-A, No. 7, pp. 1475-1480.

Sisto DJ and Sarin VK (2007) Custom Patellofemoral Arthroplasty of the Knee. Surgical Technique. *J Bone Jt Surg*, Vol. 89-A(Suppl 2), pp. 214-225.

Sisto DJ and Sarin VK (2008) Patellofemoral Arthroplasty with a Customized Trochlear Prosthesis. *Orthopedic Clinics of North America*, Vol. 39, No. 3, pp. 355-62.

Sisto DJ, Henry J, Sisto M, Sarin VK (2010) Patient-Specific Patellofemoral Arthroplasty. *Techniques in Knee Surgery*, Vol. 9, pp. 188-192.

Sisto DJ and Sarin VK (2011) Custom Patellofemoral Arthroplasty of the Knee: An Eleven Year Follow-Up. *Transactions of the Orthopaedic Research Society*, p. 1239, Long Beach, California, USA.

Weiss JM, Noble PC, Conditt MA, Kohl HW, Roberts S, Cook KF, Gordon MJ, Mathis KB (2002) What functional activities are important to patients with knee replacements? *Clin Orthop Rel Res*. Vol. 404. pp. 172-188.

11

Knee Arthrodesis with the Ilizarov External Fixator as Treatment for Septic Failure of Knee Arthroplasty

M. Spina[1], G. Gualdrini[2], M. Fosco[2] and A. Giunti[2]
[1]Department of Orthopaedics and Traumatology Surgery,
Ospedale Borgo Trento, Azienda Universitaria Integrata, Verona
[2]First Department of Orthopaedics and Traumatology Surgery,
Istituto Ortopedico Rizzoli, Bologna
Italy

1. Introduction

Femoral–tibial fusion remains one of the last treatment choices for recurrent septic failure of knee prostheses. It can be achieved by different surgical techniques, such as intramedullary nailing, mono/biaxial or circular external fixators, and fixation with long plates and screws.

In other studies, the rate of knee fusion following septic prosthetic loosening has been reported to range from 27% [1] up to 31-33% [2, 3] and even 41-42% [4, 5]. However, authors often do not report the way that fusion is achieved; others use an unspecified external fixation with a success rate ranging from 67 to 90% [6-9], and with a mean fusion time that ranges from 4.4 to 6 months.

More precisely, other authors report that fusion rates with the Ilizarov circular external fixator range from 64-75% [10, 11] to 83-93% [12, 13] and even up to 100% [14]. Mean fusion times range from 6.8 to 13 months.

Among our series of 58 septic knee prostheses treated in our ward from 1990 to 2007, 17 (29.3%) underwent femoral–tibial fusion. The fusions were attempted in all cases with the Ilizarov circular external fixator. The choice of fusion was dictated by bad local conditions of the knee (Fig. 1), the precarious general health status of the patient, and his determination to

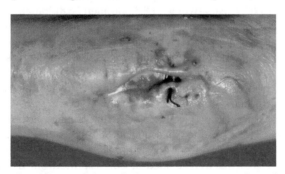

Fig. 1. Precarious local condition of the right knee in a septic prosthesis loosening

find a definitive solution to the problem. Another important factor was the number of failed prosthetic revision procedures due to septic loosening (Fig. 2).

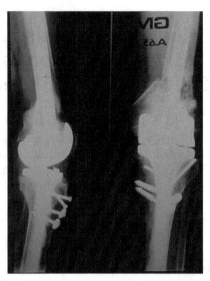

Fig. 2. A/P and L X-ray of a septic knee revision prosthesis loosening

The objective of our study was to evaluate the reliability of the Ilizarov circular external fixator as a surgical technique for knee arthrodesis, and to compare it to other fusion procedures.

2. Materials and methods

The data for this investigation were collected and analyzed in compliance with the procedures and policies set forth by the Helsinki Declaration, and all patients gave their informed consent. The study was authorized by the local ethical committee.

The series included 17 femoral–tibial fusions, representing 29.3% of all septic knee prosthetic loosenings (58) treated on the First Ward of the Rizzoli Orthopedic Institute from 1990 to 2007 (Table 1). Nine patients were women (53%) and eight were men (47%); the mean age at the time of fusion was 62.9 years (women 68.3 and men 56.8), ranging from 26 to 80 years. Eleven patients had a secreting fistula. The microbiological culture examination was positive for Staphylococcus epidermidis in eight cases, Staphylococcus aureus in four cases, Enterococcus in four cases, and other bacterial species to lesser degrees (Fig. 3). The culture examination was negative in four patients (23.5%), even when there were local conditions, and laboratory (ESR and CRP elevated) and radiological (locally increased uptake in total body scintigraphy with marked granulocytes) evaluations were positive for infection. Ten patients had previously been surgically treated for primary arthritis (58.8%), four for posttraumatic arthritis (23.5%), one for sequelae of tuberculous arthritis (5.9%), one for rheumatic arthropathy (5.9%), and one for arthropathy following pigmented villonodular synovitis (5.9%). Five patients were treated at our institute from the implantation of the primary prosthesis, whereas the remaining 12 patients were initially treated at other institutes. The Cierny–Mader classification was used for clinical and anatomopathological assessment [15], while the Engh classification was used to evaluate bone defects [16]. According to the Cierny–Mader system, ten patients (58.8%) belonged to group IV Bls, four patients (23.6%) to group IV Bs, and the remaining patients (17.6%) to group IV Bl.

A	B	C	D	E	F	G	H	I	L	M	N	O	P	Q
67	F	Rheumatoid Arthritis	SX	NO	Staphylococcus Aureous	YES	4B L-S	2	NO	3	Healed	8	None	-4 cm
57	F	Osteoarthritis	DX	YES (one revision TKA)	Staphylococcus Epidermidis and Aureous. Enterococcus	YES	4B L-S	2	NO	8	Healed	24	Small fistula (after 16 months)	-6 cm
51	M	Tubercular arthropathy	SX	YES (one revision TKA)	Staphylococcus Agalactiae, Epidermidis, Haemoliticus	NO	4B L-S	2	NO	8	Healed	6	Thrombo-phlebitis	-2 cm
80	F	Osteoarthritis	DX	YES (one revision TKA)	Pseudomonas Aeruginosa	NO	4B S	2	NO	3	Healed	50	None	-4 cm
55	M	Osteoarthritis	DX	NO	Not isolated	NO	4B S	2	NO	5	Not healed	6	Intolerance	/
70	F	Osteoarthritis	SX	NO	Staphylococcus Epidermidis	YES	4B L-S	3	YES	7	Not healed	†	Nonunion	/
64	F	Posttraumatic osteoarthritis	DX	NO	Staphylococcus Aureous	YES	4B L-S	2	NO	5	Healed	8	None	-4 cm
48	M	Posttraumatic osteoarthritis	SX	NO	Staphylococcus Epidermidis	YES	4B L	2	NO	8	Healed	28	None	-3 cm
70	F	Osteoarthritis	SX	YES (one revision TKA)	Not isolated	NO	4B S	2	NO	2	Not healed	6	Intolerance	/
74	M	Osteoarthritis	DX	NO	Not isolated	YES	4B L-S	3	YES	16	Healed	15	None	-3 cm
70	F	Osteoarthritis	DX	NO	Not isolated	YES	4B L-S	3	YES	6	Healed	66	None	-5 cm
65	M	Posttraumatic osteoarthritis	DX	NO	Staphylococcus Epidermidis, Pseudomonas Aeruginosa	YES	4B L-S	3	YES	14	Healed	101	None	-6 cm
64	F	Osteoarthritis	SX	NO	Enterococcus Fecalis	YES	4B L	3	YES	12	Healed	17	None	-6 cm
73	F	Osteoarthritis	DX	YES (two revisions TKA)	Streptococcus, Staphylococcus Epidermidis	YES	4B L-S	3	YES	20 (2 attempt)	Not healed	24	Nonunion	/
26	M	Posttraumatic osteoarthritis	SX	NO	Staphylococcus Epidermidis	NO	4B L	3	NO	18	Healed	32	None	0 cm
66	M	Osteoarthritis	SX	NO	Enterococcus, Pseudomonas Aeruginosa	NO	4B S	2	NO	4	Healed	8	None	-3 cm
70	M	Pigmented villonodular synovitis arthropathy	SX	NO	Staphylococcus Aureous, Epidermidis, Enterococcus	YES	4B L-S	2	NO	16	Healed	82	None	-4 cm

A Age at fusion, B Sex, C Initial diagnosis, D Side, E Revision, F Bacteria, G Fistula, H Cierny-Mader Classification, I Engh Classification, L Cement spacer, M Mean Time to Fusion (months), N Result, O Follow up (months), P Problems/Obstacles/Complications, Q Limb shortness (centimeters)

Table 1. Summary of the data on the patients included in this study

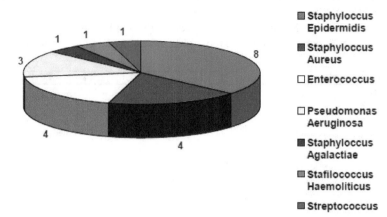

Fig. 3. Type and distribution of the isolated microbes

According to the Engh classification, ten patients (58.8%) were considered type II, and the remaining (41.2%) were considered type III. Different surgical treatments were performed depending on the Engh classification.

For type II Engh patients the treatment involved:

- Injection of the fistulous tract, when present, with methylene blue dye;
- Removal of prosthetic components and cement mantle, samples taken for microbiological culture testing, than surgical debridement and regularization of the femoral and tibial bone surfaces;
- Femoral–tibial stabilization under compression with the Ilizarov external fixator, applying 5–6 mm diameter percutaneous half-pins with a hydroxyapatite coating for femoral arches, a distal femoral ring, and a pair of tibial rings stabilized with Kirschner wires;
- Specific or wide-ranging antibiotic therapy for four/six weeks.

For Engh type III patients (except in one case) the treatment involved:

- Injection of the fistulous tract, when present, with methylene blue dye
- Removal of prosthetic components cement mantle, samples taken for microbiological
- culture testing, than surgical debridement and regularization of the femoral and tibial bone surfaces
- Application of antibiotic-loaded cement spacer stained with methylene blue (Fig. 4)
- Hinged brace and specific or wide-ranging antibiotic therapy for four/six weeks
- Assessment of infection indices and clinical condition, then further surgical debridement followed by femoral–tibial fusion with the external fixator
- Specific or wide-ranging antibiotic therapy for four/six weeks if the culture exam is positive at the time of fusion.

An additional surgical stage with the application of an antibiotic-loaded cement spacer is used for 4–6 weeks in patients belonging to Engh group III, because in our experience surgical debridement alone may not be sufficient to eradicate the infection in cases with large bone defects.

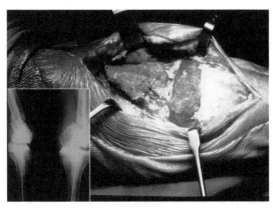

Fig. 4. a Antibiotic-loaded cement spacer stained with methylene blue following knee prosthesis removal. b A/P and L X-ray of a knee with cement spacer in situ

The type of antibiotic used in the spacer depended on the result of the microbiological test performed previously. In our series, in most cases we used vancomycin at a dose of 2–4 g of antibiotic per 40 g of cement.

In a 26-year-old patient with a final limb shortening of 11 cm, femoral and tibial lengthening were performed at same time as the fusion.

Patients who were considered healed showed a continuous cancellous trabecular pattern from femur to tibia at standard radiographs (Fig. 5) and no clinical and instrumental signs of an active infection. Stability at the fusion site was evaluated with the varus–valgus stress test. The femoral–tibial fusion was assessed both radiographically and clinically.

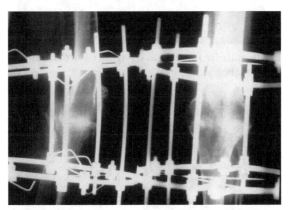

Fig. 5. A/P and L X-ray showing continuity of the trabecular–medullary pattern in a patient treated with Ilizarov's external fixator

3. Technical notes for assembling the external fixator

3.1 Femoral component
The fixator is anchored to the femoral diaphysis by three or four 5–6-mm percutaneous half-pins coated in hydroxyapatite and fixed to two Ilizarov arches of the same diameter but

different lengths (the distal one is longer). The arches are positioned perpendicular to the long axis of the femur. Four screws are recommended for patients over 60 kg in body weight. The distal arch is connected to a ring with a size proportional to the diameter of the knee and anchored to the distal femur by two Ilizarov wires.

3.2 Tibial component

The femoral distal ring is connected by three hinged rods to two rings of the same diameter that are anchored to the proximal tibial diaphysis by Ilizarov wires. For good fusion it is important that the fixator is connected to bone by Ilizarov wires on both sides of the subsequent fusion. In this setup the circular external fixator is bulky but effective. The hinged connection allows compression at the fusion site with deviations in flexion, external rotation and valgus of the tibia with respect to the femur. Proximal percutaneous screws and Ilizarov wires often cause local swelling of the skin. This is the most uncomfortable aspect for the patient (Figs. 6, 7).

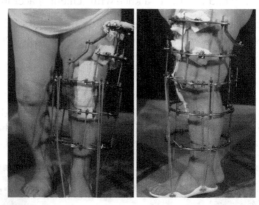

Fig. 6. Left knee in a patient treated by fusion using an Ilizarov circular external fixator. A splint is present to support the foot

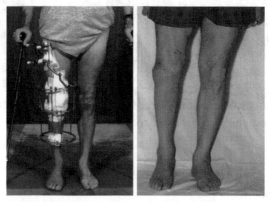

Fig. 7. Type IV Bls patient treated using an Ilizarov external fixator for left knee fusion. Functional stable limb bearing was achieved after 101 months

4. Results

Among the 17 patients, 13 fusions were achieved at the first surgical attempt in a mean time of 9.3 months (range 3–18 months) (Figs. 8, ,9) the mean follow-up was 30 months (range 6–101 months) (Table 1).

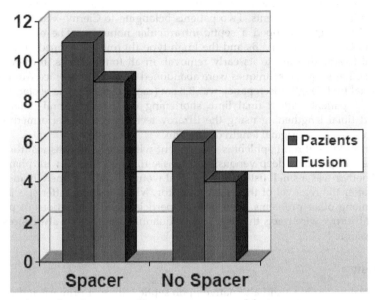

Fig. 8. Comparison of patients according to treatment and fusion rate

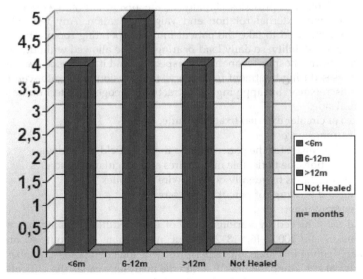

Fig. 9. Duration of treatment with Ilizarov fixator in healed patients

To assess difficulties that occur during treatment with the Ilizarov external fixator, Paley's classification was used [17] to distinguish problems, obstacles and complications. Problems represent difficulties that require no operative intervention to resolve, while obstacles represent difficulties that require an operative intervention. All intraoperative injuries and all problems that are not resolved before the end of treatment are considered true complications. In our cohort there were four complications (23.5%) that were responsible for treatment failure in four patients. Two patients belonging to Cierny–Mader IV Bls and the Engh type III group developed a septic intrarticular nonunion. The other two patients belonging to Cierny–Mader IV Bs and the Engh type II group developed an intolerance to the external fixator that led to its early removal. In all four patients, further attempts at fusion with other surgical techniques were abandoned and a hinged brace was applied. The mean residual limb length discrepancy was 3.8 cm (range 0–6 cm). One obstacle occurred in a 26-year-old patient with a final limb shortening of 11 cm; femoral–tibial fusion and femoral and tibial lengthening using the Ilizarov technique were performed at the same time, thus restoring the original length of the limb.

Problems included a thrombophlebitis in a patient with severe venous insufficiency of the lower limbs and previous deep venous thrombosis; this was treated with pharmacological therapy. Another was a small fistula at a surgical wound that developed in another patient 16 months after the removal of the external fixator, which resolved after specific antibiotic therapy. Among other problems, there were superficial wound infections of percutaneous screws and Ilizarov wire tracts that were never quantified but which always resolved with local disinfection.

5. Discussion

Femoral–tibial fusion is a valid alternative upon septic failure of primary and revision total knee arthroplasty, and is usually well tolerated by patients.

This treatment restores good limb loading, decreasing pain and eliminating infection.

Circular external fixation provides stability at the fusion site and correct femoral–tibial alignment in flexion, external rotation and valgus deviation. Any type of correction is possible without the need to take the patient into the operating room. The circular fixator provides very good stability, so daily load-bearing may be allowed without limitation. It is a low-cost option from a hospital economics perspective, and it ensures a low risk of infection. In particular cases during treatment for femoral–tibial fusion, the fixator can restore severe limb-length discrepancy by applying a distraction osteogenesis technique on the tibial and/or femoral side.

Disadvantages of circular external fixator include:

- A long learning curve
- Objective discomfort for the patient due to the wide field of the device
- Nonrigid fixation due to flexible metal wires and percutaneous screws
- Cutaneous infections frequently occur at wire entry sites
- Loosening and breakage of percutaneous screws
- Long treatment times.

Knee arthrodesis achieved by various types of intramedullary nailing has a success rate ranging from 67 to 100% [6, 18–24] in a mean time of about six months. Using intramedullary nailing in a knee with a periprosthetic infection poses a number of problems, such as the risk of spreading the infection into the medullary canal, the difficulty involved in treating infection recurrence, the possibility of nail migration or breakage, and the impossibility of performing a compression at the fusion site and clinically assessing its stability during treatment [23, 25].

The technique of femoral–tibial fusion with a monoaxial or biaxial external fixator has a success rate that ranges from 68 [26] to 89% [27] and up to 100% [28, 29]. These fixators, especially monoaxial ones, are fairly well tolerated by patients. However, they do not allow significant changes in the axis, and, due to their structural characteristics, they are rigid and not entirely reliable for complete load-bearing [30].

Finally, bone fusion with dual compression plates has a success rate ranging from 80 [31] to 100% [32]. The authors, however, report high rates of complications (18.2%) such as stress fractures and persistent infection. Healing in some cases was achieved after repeated surgical attempts. Bone fixation with plates and screws is rigid and enables axial

Author(s)	N° of Knees	Classification Used	Fusion rate	Mean Time to fusion (range) in months	Mean residual limb shortness	Complications	Mean FU in months
Johannsen HG et al (2005) [11]	8	none	75%	3,5 (3-4)	3,5 cm	12,5% (1 chronic osteomyelitis)	10
Manzotti A et al (2001) [12]	6	none	83%	6,8 (10,3-5,1)	-	None	34,2
Garberina MJ et al (2000) [10]	19	none	68%	4,6 (3-6,8)	-	26,3% (2 fractures, 2 valgus angulation, 1 wound infection)	32
Oostenbroek & van Roermund (2001) [13]	15	Mild/Moderate/Severe loss of bone	93%	12 (6-24,7)	4 cm	80% (2 femoral fractures 3 osteitis 3 frame instability 1 non-union 1 femoral angulation 1 heel decubitus 1 pneumonia infection)	52
David R et al (2001) [14]	13	none	100%	6,4 (4,6-8,4)	3,7 cm	7,7% (1 wound infection)	40,8
Spina M et al (2009)	17	Combined Engh/ Cierny-Mader	76,5%	9,3 (3-18)	3,8 cm	11,7% (1 Thrombophlebitis, 1 small fistula)	30

Table 2. Literature review of knee arthrodesis with an Ilizarov circular external fixator

compression [33]. It is, however, a complex procedure that is very invasive and at risk of infection. Nichols et al. [32] advise against this technique in the presence of widespread infection.

The existing literature on femoral–tibial fusion with an Ilizarov circular external fixator reports success rates that vary in different studies from 64 [10] to 100% [14] (Table 2). In our series, the rate of complete healing was 76.5% at the first surgical attempt in a mean time of 9.3 months. Failures consisted of four patients (23.5% of the entire group); two of these patients had bad general health conditions; one patient died a few months after removal of the external fixator; another did not heal despite a second attempt at fusion with an Ilizarov external fixator. The other two patients were affected by an anxious–depressive syndrome that contributed to severe intolerance to the external fixator, so its early removal was inevitable. This event accounted for 50% of the failures, so we believe in the importance of carefully assessing the patient's ability to cooperate before treatment.

Our selection of an Ilizarov circular external fixator was dictated by its low cost, versatility, stability under load, possibility to performing modifications during treatment, and low risk of septic dissemination. Nevertheless, in our opinion, careful patient selection is required, as old age and psychological intolerance are generally compromising factors. The treatment time is long and an experienced surgeon is needed to assemble the external fixator and manage it later.

6. References

[1] Husted H, Toftgaard Jensen T. Clinical outcome after treatment of infected primary total knee arthroplasty. Acta Orthop Belg. 2002;68(5):500–507. [PubMed]

[2] Blom AW, Brown J, Taylor AH, Pattison G, Whitehouse S, Bannister GC. Infection after total knee arthroplasty. J Bone Joint Surg Br. 2004;86(5):688–691. doi: 10.1302/0301-620X.86B5.14887. [PubMed] [Cross Ref]

[3] Weng X, Li L, Qui G, Li J, Tian Y, Hen J, Wang Y, Jin J, Ye Q, Zhao H. Treatment of infected total knee arthroplasty. Zhonghua Wai Ke Za Zhi. 2002;40(9):669–672. [PubMed]

[4] Bengston S, Knutson K, Lidgren L. Treatment of infected knee arthroplasty. Clin Orthop Relat Res. 1989;245:173–178. [PubMed]

[5] Hanssen AD, Trousdale RT, Osmon DR. Patient outcome with reinfection following reimplantation for the infected total knee arthroplasty. Clin Orthop Relat Res. 1995;321:55–67. [PubMed]

[6] Mabry TM, Jacofsky DJ, Haidukewych GJ, Hanssen AD. Comparison of intramedullary nailing and external fixation knee arthrodesis for the infected knee replacement. Clin Orthop Relat Res. 2007;464:11–15. [PubMed]

[7] Figgie HE, III, Brody GA, Inglis AE, Sculco TP, Goldberg VM, Figgie MP. Knee arthrodesis following total knee arthroplasty in rheumatoid arthritis. Clin Orthop. 1987;224:237–243. [PubMed]

[8] Klinger HM, Spahn G, Schultz W, Baums MH. Arthrodesis of the knee after failed infected total knee arthroplasty. Knee Surg Sports Traumatol Arthrosc. 2006;14(5):447–453. doi: 10.1007/s00167-005-0664-3. [PubMed] [Cross Ref]

[9] Rudolph F, Fengler F, Hein W. Arthrodesis as an alternative in infected knee arthroplasty. Beitr Orthop Traumatol. 1989;36(8):374–380. [PubMed]

[10]   Garberina MJ, Fitch RD, Hoffmann ED, Hardaker WT, Vail TP, Scully SP. Knee arthrodesis with circular external fixation. Clin Orthop. 2001;382:168-178. doi: 10.1097/00003086-200101000-00023. [PubMed] [Cross Ref]

[11]   Johannsen HG, Skov O, Weeth ER. Knee arthrodesis with external fixator after infected knee arthroplasty. Ugeskr Laeger. 2005;167(35):3295-3296. [PubMed]

[12]   Manzotti A, Pullen C, Deromedis B, Catagni MA. Knee arthrodesis after infected total knee arthroplasty using the Ilizarov method. Clin Orthop Relat Res. 2001;389:143-149. doi: 10.1097/00003086-200108000-00020. [PubMed] [Cross Ref]

[13]   Oostenbroek HJ, Roermund PM. Arthrodesis of the knee after an infected arthroplasty using the Ilizarov method. J Bone Joint Surg Br. 2001;83:50-54. doi: 10.1302/0301-620X.83B1.10572. [PubMed] [Cross Ref]

[14]   David R, Shtarker H, Horesh Z, Tsur A, Soudry M. Arthrodesis with Ilizarov device for failed knee arthroplasty. Orthopedics. 2001;24:33-36. [PubMed]

[15]   Cierny G, Mader JT, Penninck JJ (1985) A clinical staging system for adult osteomyelitis. Contemp Orthop 10(5)

[16]   Engh GA, Ammeen DJ. Bone loss with revision total knee arthroplasty: defect classification and alternatives for reconstruction. AAOS Instr Course Lect. 1999;48(22):167-175.

[17]   Paley D. Problems, obstacles, and complications of limb lengthening by the Ilizarov technique. Clin Orthop Relat Res. 1990;250:81-104. [PubMed]

[18]   Wilde AH, Stearns KL. Intramedullary fixation for arthrodesis of the knee after infected total knee arthroplasty. Clin Orthop Relat Res. 1989;248:87-92. [PubMed]

[19]   Bargiotas K, Wohlrab D, Sewecke JJ, Lavinge G, DeMeo PJ, Sotereanos GN. Arthrodesis of the knee with a long intramedullary nail following the failure of a total knee arthroplasty as the result of infection. Surgical technique. J Bone Joint Surg Am. 2006;89:103-110. doi: 10.2106/JBJS.F.01125. [PubMed] [Cross Ref]

[20]   Senior CJ, Assuncao RE, Barlow IW. Knee arthrodesis for limb salvage with an intramedullary couplet nail. Arch Orthop Trauma Surg. 2007;128:683-687. doi: 10.1007/s00402-007-0386-8. [PubMed] [Cross Ref]

[21]   Volpi R, Dehoux E, Touchard P, Mensa C, Segal P. Knee arthrodesis using a customized intramedullary nail: 14 cases. Rev Chir Orthop Reparatrice Appar Mot. 2004;90(1):58-64. [PubMed]

[22]   Lai KA, Shen WJ, Yang CY. Arthrodesis with a short Huckstep nail as a salvage procedure for failed total knee arthroplasty. J Bone Joint Surg. 1998;80(3):380-388. [PubMed]

[23]   Waldman BJ, Mont MA, Payman KR, Freiberg AA, Windsor RE, Sculco TP, Hungerford DS. Infected knee arthroplasty treated with arthrodesis using a modular nail. Clin Orthop Relat Res. 1999;367:230-237. doi: 10.1097/00003086-199910000-00029. [PubMed] [Cross Ref]

[24]   Jorgensen PS, Torholm C. Arthrodesis after infected knee arthroplasty using long arthrodesis nail. A report of five cases. Am J Knee Surg. 1995;8(3):110-113. [PubMed]

[25]   Donley BG, Matthews LS, Kaufer H. Arthrodesis of the knee with an intramedullary nail. J Bone Joint Surg Am. 1991;73(6):907-913. [PubMed]

[26]   Rand J, Bryan R, Chao E (1987) Failed total knee arthroplasty treated by arthrodesis of the knee using the Ace-Fisher apparatus. J Bone J Surg 69:39.

[27] Parratte S, Madougou S, Villaba M, Stein A, Rochwerger A, Curvale G. Knee arthrodesis with a double mono-bar external fixators to salvage infected knee arthroplasty: retrospective analysis of 18 knees with mean seven-year follow-up. Rev Chir Orthop Reparatrice Appar Mot. 2007;93(4):373–380. [PubMed]

[28] Fidler MW. Knee arthrodesis following prosthesis removal: use of the Wagner apparatus. J Bone Joint Surg. 1983;65B:29–31.

[29] Wade PJ, Denham RA. Arthrodesis of the knee after failed knee replacement. J Bone Joint Surg Br. 1984;66:362–366. [PubMed]

[30] Hak DJ, Lieberman JR, Finerman GA. Single plane and biplane external fixators for knee arthrodesis. Clin Orthop Relat Res. 1995;316:134–144. [PubMed]

[31] Munzinger U, Knessl J, Gschwend N. Arthrodesis following knee arthroplasty. Orthopade. 1987;16(4):301–309. [PubMed]

[32] Nichols SJ, Landon GC, Tullos HS. Arthrodesis with dual plates after failed total knee arthroplasty. J Bone Joint Surg Am. 1991;73(7):1020–1024. [PubMed]

[33] Christie MJ, Boer DK, McQueen DA, Cooke FW, et al. Salvage procedures for failed total knee arthroplasty. J Bone J Surg Am. 2003;85:S58–S62.

Part 3

Computer Assisted Total Knee Arthroplasty

12

Possibilities of Computer Application in Primary Knee Replacement

František Okál, Adel Safi, Martin Komzák and Radek Hart
Department of Orthopaedics & Traumatology
General Hospital Znojmo
Czech Republic

1. Introduction

Frequency of knee joint osteoarthritis has been growing over the last years. Range of degeneration involvement of the knee joint varies from unicompartmental to tricompartmental. The medial part of the knee is damaged most frequently. The solution of serious knee joint degeneration is a total replacement by endoprosthesis. It is indicated not only in the case of idiopathic gonarthrosis, but also in rheumatoid arthritis, osteonecrosis, post-traumatic arthritis or in different arthropathies. The fundamental condition for long term survival of a knee joint endoprosthesis (TKR) is the right position of femoral and tibial components with mechanical axis correction of a lower limb. Endoprosthesis implanted in wrong position can lead to acceleration of polyethylene wear and component release. Abnormal varus or valgus position have already been proved as a main cause of component failure. A malposition of femoral and tibial components has also a great influence on patella tracking during knee movement and on possible patellofemoral complications. That is why single bone resectiones must be performed with a great emphasis on the precision and in relation to the mechanical axis of the limb. Surgeons use a scale of different targeting equipments which serve preferably to the best possible matching of the bone cuts to the patient's geometry. The results show that even in cases of surgeon's great experience in TKR up to 30 % of operated cases have a four-degree and larger deviation of tibiofemoral angle from the ideal mechanical axis after bones resections. That is why computer navigation systems have been developed to eliminate the error of surgeon (Insall et al., 1985). The computer navigation systems were integrated into a routine orthopaedic practice more than thirteen years ago. After that the navigation became quickly a common tool at many working places for primary implantations of knee endoprosthesis. Instrumentation for mechanical targeting of resections described earlier have certain restrictions which cannot be exceeded. For example, it is a certain degree of freedom such as a rotation of a femoral and tibial components or impossibility to reach their perfectly accurate position with regard to the resected bones. It may be said that standard targeting deviced are constructed for the standard bone geometry.

The first study of navigation in orthopaedics reporting the use of infrared radiation was made by the group of Saragaglia (Grenoble, France) in years 1994 -1996 and in 1997 these surgeons implanted the first total endoprosthesis of a knee joint (Laskin, 1984; Bitter et al., 1994) under the assistance of the OrthoPilot navigation system (B.Braun-Aesculap,

Tuttlingen, Germany). In 1995 independently of the above mentioned group Krackow and Mihalko conducted a project of the development of a system for computer controlled TKR with the use of the Optitrack equipment (Northern Digital, Ontario, Canada). The first navigated implantation of TKR was made by this group in 1997 as well (Krackow, 1983). This project led to the creation of the Knee Track Module (Stryker Howmedica Osteonics, Allendale, NJ). Both systems - OrthoPilot and Knee Track Module represents first kinematic navigation systems.

We distinguish 4 basic types of navigation nowadays:

1. Kinematic navigation (imageless, CT-free) – is used for data registration through combination of physical palpation and kinematics. Data are transferred into a computer by means of infrared radiation. This type is the most often used way of navigation in orthopaedic surgery.
2. Fluoroscopy based navigation – it registers combined data obtained by physical palpation and kinematics but it uses C-arm at the beginning. Images are created by a computer on the basis of this information. Then surgeon operates on the radiologic replica of patient's anatomic area. The system is more frequently used in traumatology and in spine surgery.
3. CT-based navigation – it uses computer tomography for data collection. Today, it is used the mostly in a revision surgery and spine surgery.
4. MR-based navigation – it uses magnetic resonance for data collection. It is used mainly in neurosurgery.

The most simple and the most practical of these methods is the kinematic navigation. Anatomical structures are digitized by orientation palpation points with a portable "pointer". During bone resection computer shows surgeon the ideal position of instruments and optimal bone cuts. Computer equipped systems, which consist of standard resection patterns on the one hand and highly accurate navigation system on the other hand, are a natural consequence of current computer technology integration into surgery. Computer software reduces the risk of surgeon's error and enables fast and accurate placement of resection blocks (Hart & Janeček, 2003). It eliminates the use of intramedullary and extramedullary targeting devices and so reduces the risk of pulmonary embolism.

The aim of this chapter is to present the experience of authors with using of kinematic navigation systems and computer generally in the implantation of total and unicompartmental knee joint replacements. It points out to advantages and disadvantages of a navigation application during surgeries and to the importance of pre-operative planning by the help of digital images in connection with a surgical planning station. It also refers to special circumstances when the computer navigation technology can be the only one possibility of the implantation of the knee endoprosthesis.

2. Computer navigation in standard or minimally invasive total knee replacement

Authors of the article have been working with kinematic navigation systems routinely since the beginning of the year 2000. The study, which was published in the 2003 by the senior surgeon (Hart et al., 2003), was the third randomized study evaluating the use of navigation in a standard TKR surgery in world literature. Higher accuracy in case of the use of navigation in comparison with a standard instrumentarium in TKR has already been confirmed. Navigation system usually consists of five basic parts: 3D-camera with a control unit, infrared diodes, computer system, foot switch and mobile case with transformer (Fig. 1). A camera placed on a tracing bar localizes the position of diodes in an operative field. The camera is connected with the control unit and it enables to distinguish diode deviation already from the distance of tenths of one millimeter. Three diodes are needed at least during surgery. These are placed on nondeformable basis and they can be anchored by fastening mechanism on relevant bicortical screws, palpator or resection blocks. The computer system is formed by a computer itself and a keyboard with mouse. The computer gets information about diodes movement, it evaluates information and transfers it into a graphic form on a monitor. The foot switch has two pedals and it enables surgeon to control individual steps of the navigation system.

Before an operation we take standing weight bearing X-rays of the whole lower limb of a frontal plane and a standard X-rays of a sagittal plane. We evaluate relevant axis and angles, measure size of deformity and plan the size of endoprosthesis components in both planes in a way mentioned in the following subchapter by the help of PACS system with its application module. The patient's preparation before surgery does not differ from a standard procedure. The navigation system (camera) is being placed into the opposite side with regard to the surgeon into the distance of approximately 2 m.

Minimally invasive (MIS) or less invasive approach is an alternative to a common approach to the knee joint in TKR. Its use in connection with the navigation was published by the team of authors in 2006 (Hart et al., 2006). The procedure itself with the use of navigation does not differ from a standard parapatellar approach (Hart et al., 2005). In this case the navigation system serves as "the third eye" of the surgeon working in reducting operative field. The skin incision length is usually up to 12 cm. Subvastus approach does not disturb the extensor apparatus. M.vastus medialis is lifted and arthrotomy is made. It is followed by percutaneous insertion of original bicortical self drilling screw into the distal femur approximately 7 cm above the articular surface. We insert the second screw similarly into the proximal tibia about 10-12 cm below the articular surface. Then diodes are fastened on both screws. We fasten the third diode as a mobile one on a palpator (pointer).

Further step is to determine the real anatomy of a lower limb. A mechanical axis is determined by three points – by the center of hip, knee and ankle joints. First, we enter the information about the center of knee joint into the computer by a palpator with the fixed diode. Next, we determine the center of a hip joint. Movement of the femur in all planes has one fixed point which is the center of the femoral head. We determine the center of a hip joint by circular movements in a slight flexion. As the third, we localize the center of the ankle joint. We fasten an elastic tape on the area of tarsus during the surgery and the mobile diode on it. Then we enter data into the soft-ware by the movement in the ankle joint to the maximum extent of flexion and extension. Last we precisely determine the center of a knee joint. One of the possibilities how to determine the center of the knee is palpation of one anatomic point on each side of a joint. The second possibility is to use the same kinematic procedure as in the ankle joint: first is done of the determination rotation axis by tibial rotation round its longitudinal axis in flexion of $90°$ and second is to get the second transverse axis by movements of flexion – extension.

Then follows is the collection and saving of information relating to orientation points in the knee area which is necessary to do for an accurate placement of resection blocks and for the accurate size of the femoral component. A palpator with a fixed mobile diode is used for it.

The size of a femoral component is given by the distance of a dorsal condylar line and anterior femoral corticalis. We palpate medial and lateral epicondyles as well to determine the exact rotation of the femoral component. Next, we check orientation points in the area of the ankle joint. A malleolar line serves to an additional confirmation of the ankle joint center.

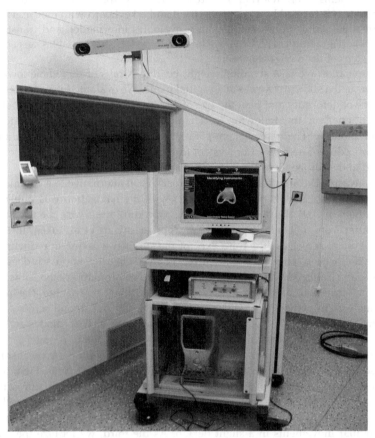

Fig. 1. Kinematic navigation system

After setting of all orientation points, an axis reconstruction of a lower limb appears on the monitor, both in a sagittal and frontal plane. Numeric data appear on the monitor as well besides the graphic illustration. In the frontal plane we get the information about the deformity in the sense of varus – valgus. The program will illustrate the degree of flexion contracture too. In this moment, it is necessary to compare computer specified values with preoperative measured values on X-ray photographs. If we find out (exceptionally) a difference greater than 5° in both planes, it is necessary to recheck fixation quality of both diodes and to repeat the whole procedure. First of all the proximal tibia is resected. A mobile diode is fasten to a resection block and we follow on the monitor the accuracy of its placement on proximal tibia. Both, the block orientation in a sagittal plane and frontal plane and the height of resection, are illustrated. We fix the block to the bone first by one pin to secure the zero deviation from the ideal position in a sagittal plane and the requested level of resection. Then, the resection block position in a frontal plane is corrected and after reaching the zero deviation in the frontal plane, the resection block is fixated by the second pin.

After the proximal tibia resection the balancement of collateral ligaments is being found out. After balancing of the collateral ligaments, it is being approached to balancing of extension and flexion gaps. After that the femoral resection follows. First, we reach zero position (90° to the femoral mechanical axis) in a sagittal and then in a frontal plane. The block is fixed to the femur by two pins and articular surface is resected.

After the application of a relevant trying components including an polyethylene insert of suitable height, the collateral ligaments balance is checked again. Graphic and numeric expression of the real limb mechanical axis is being watched on a monitor and values shown are compared with actual clinical findings. If the result is satisfactory, original components are implanted. The mechanical axis of the limb is being checked again during hardening of the bone cement.

A prospective study has been accomplished in author's institution (Hart et al., 2006) in which results of knee joint replacements in 40 patients implanted by MIS approach were compared with 40 endoprosthesis implanted through a standard approach. Arthritis of 3rd and 4th degree was indication for all these surgeries. Less pain and faster rehabilitation was found early after surgery in MIS group. This difference was only found until 10th day after surgery. This difference was not obvious after 6 and 12 weeks after the surgery. TKR implantation accuracy was preserved with the use of the computer navigation system in cases with MIS approach in comparison with the standard approach.

3. Comparison of preoperative digital planning with computer navigation in TKR

The knowledge of mechanical and anatomical axis construction of lower limb and basic angles is necessary for a correct planning and also for a post-operative evaluation of obtained component position. The connecting line between the centre of the femoral head and the centre of the knee joint is called the mechanical axis of the femur, the connecting line between the centre of the knee and the ankle joint is called the mechanical axis of the tibia. The line between the femoral head centre and the ankle joint centre (the Mikulicz's line) constitutes the mechanical axis of the lower limb. If it runs through the centre of the knee joint, femoral and tibial mechanical axes are parallel. In case of a varus knee deformity the mechanical axis of lower limb runs medially from its centre and the medial angle between femoral and tibial mechanical axes is smaller than 180°. In case of a valgus deformity the mechanical axis of a lower limb runs laterally from the knee joint centre and the medial angle between femoral and tibial mechanical axes is greater than 180°.

The right position of a lower limb during of X–ray examination is important for an accurate preoperative planning. The AP X-ray is performed under the load in standing patient in such a position so that the patella aims forward. The rotation of the lower limb within 10° does not influence the result of axis measurement significantly (Whietside & Arima, 1995). Greater external rotation of the limb simulates a varus deformity, the internal rotation simulates a valgus deviation. Severe gonarthrosis is usually connected with a flexional contracture which causes a possible mistake of measurement during the preoperative planning. The lateral X-ray of the knee is also taken in the standing patient with his knee in extension. Weight–bearing radiographs of the whole lower limb are necessary for an accurate determination of axial relations.

PACS (Picture Archiving and Communication System) system serves to the X-ray photographs storing. It is a storing and communication system of image data which supports both photos distribution and their description and arrangement. It serves to acceptance, storing, distribution and picture display. It is becoming an essential part of orthopaedic surgeon's everyday practice in connection with an orthopaedic planning station. Orthopaedic planning tools enable more accurate preoperative templating of TKRs than former standard templating (Fig. 2.).

It is possible to measure angles on the femoral and the tibial and the relation of femoral and tibial axis by means of a planning station on digitalized X-rays. It is possible to plan height of needed proximal tibial and distal femoral resection and to template femoral and tibial component sizes and polyethylene inlay height and their positions. Accuracy of TKR can be checked postoperatively in the same way. There was compared a lower limb axis deviation measured by PACS before and after a surgery with values gained by kinematic computer navigation preoperatively in the authors´ institution (Hart et al., 2010). There was also compared the size of components measured during the pre-operative planning by PACS, with sizes measured by the navigation during the surgery. There were 311 total knee endoprosthesis evaluated from January 2009 till September 2010 (21 months). All surgeries were done by experienced surgeons. Primary gonarthrosis was an indication for knee replacement in 278 cases. After proximal tibial osteotomy or fractures of the knee 33 TKR were done. Surgical technique was the same in all patients. In 253 cases was used the replacement with preservation of posterior cruciate ligament, in 58 cases with its resection. In all cases both components were fixated by bone cement.

Before and after surgery X-ray weight-bearing images of the whole lower limb were taken. By the help of PACS with the application of the orthopaedic planning station there was measured a lower limb axis before surgery (the angle between the mechanical femoral axis and the mechanical tibial axis) and components sizes and these values were compared with values measured by computer navigation during the surgery. The value of the deformity of lower limb axis measured by computer navigation before and after implantation was recorded during the surgery. The load during the surgery was imitated by axial pressure on a heel in the axis of operated lower limb. Postoperative radiological control was carried out on the seventh postoperative day with the full weight bearing. Agreement between components sizes planned by the orthopaedic planning station in PACS and really implanted components with the use of computer navigation was 73 % (in 227 endoprostheses) in the femoral component, 91 % (in 283 endoprostheses) in a tibial component and 48 % (in 149 endoprostheses) in polyethylene inserts.

In the majority of cases of disagreements smaller femoral (92 %) or tibial (90 %) component was implanted than which had been planned preoperativelly, in case of polyethylene inlay it was mostly necessary to use higher sizes (86 %). The cause of disagreement on the femoral component size in 84 total endoprostheses (27 %) was greater difference between a flexion and extension gap than 3 mm according to navigation. This is not possible to be found out

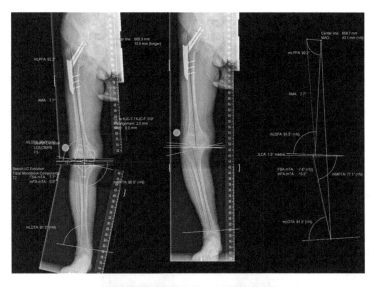

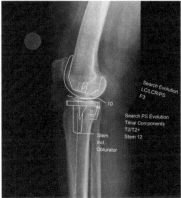

Fig. 2. The X-rays with preoperative templating by the orthopaedic planning station in PACS.

by the preoperative planning on X-ray photographs. Also a tibial component implantation of another size planned by PACS (9 %) had its cause in the size change of an implanted femoral component (the difference between both components would be larger than two sizes). In cases of 77 total replacements (92 %) there was the necessity to implant smaller femoral component by one size to balance tighter flexion gap. It was less frequent that the flexion gap was larger than extension one. This imbalance was solved by larger femoral component (8 %). Preoperative planning of the tibial component size by the help of PACS is relatively accurate because its size is determined only by AP and mediolateral dimensions of the tibial plate are and it is not influenced by flexional or extension gaps. The greatest disagreement was registered in polyethylene inlay planning - in 162 total endoprostheses (52 %). In 116 cases (72 %) there was implanted higher polyethylene insert by 2 mm than what had been planned preoperatively by PACS system. In 23 replacements (14 %) there was implanted higher polyethylene insert by 4 mm and in 23 cases (14 %) lower insert by 2 mm. The cause of this disagreement is usually knee joint balancing done by releasing of soft tissues on medial side in cases of varus deformity or on lateral side in cases of a valgus deformity.

These results show that the preoperative planning by digital templating estimates femoral component and polyethylene insert sizes only approximately, while tibial component sizes quite precisely. The computer navigation has its main significance in determination of the femoral component size depending on collected data accuracy and on flexional and extension gap balancing. The height of polyethylene inlay is determined by resection sizes of a proximal tibia and distal femur, by balancing of gaps and by knee joint stability during testing of trial inserts after cementing of original components.

The average mechanical axis measured preoperatively by PACS was 5.3° of varus (range 20.5° valgus to 16.9° varus). The mechanical axis measured by the navigation before endoprosthesis implantation was on the average 1.8° of varus (the range 13° valgus to 11° varus). Agreement in both measurements (with the difference less than 3°) was achieved only in 171 total replacements (55 %). The Table 1 shows an absolute value distribution of a lower limb mechanical axis deviation measured by PACS before surgery and by navigation at the beginning of the surgery.

In 190 patients (61 %), where the mechanical axis deviation measured by PACS was smaller than 10°, was an agreement with values measured by the navigation in 87 % of cases (165 endoprostheses). In 121 patients with the deviation of the mechanical axis preoperatively more than 10° (39 %) the agreement with values measured by the navigation was only in 5 % of cases (6 replacements). The reason for this difference is the relation between the force acting on the knee joint and the amount of lower limb deformity. In X-ray examination of the whole lower limb under the load the axial deformity of knee joint gets worse due to body weight. This deformity in ligaments is emphasized with a bigger axial deviation. The measurement of the mechanical axis deviation preoperatively by the navigation takes place only in a lying position with exclusion of the weight of the body. That is why the value is always smaller than the value measured during the preoperative planning. The bigger is the axis deviation measured by PACS, the bigger is the difference between values. Pressure on the heel in the axis of a lower limb during the navigation simulates the limb load insufficiently.

deviation (mFA - mTA)	number and % of the patients (MediCAD®2.06)	number and % of the patients (OrthoPilot)
0° - 5.0°	34 (11 %)	47 (15 %)
5.1° - 10.0°	156 (50 %)	255 (82 %)
> 10.0°	121 (39 %)	9 (3 %)

Table 1. The deviation of the axis of lower limb measured by orthopaedic planning system in PACS and by kinematic navigation system preoperatively.

The average mechanical axis measured by the navigation after the total endoprosthesis implantation was 0.4° varus (range, 3.0° valgus to 2.0° varus). The mechanical axis measured by PACS after the surgery was on average 0.5° varus (range, 3.5° valgus to 4.2° varus).

Agreement in both measurements (with the difference less than 3°) was achieved in 90 % of cases (280 endoprostheses). These results show the importance of navigation in total endoprosthesis implantations - the axis deviation within the range of 0° – 2.0° was measured post-operatively in 280 patients (90 %) by to the navigation and in 274 patients (88 %) by PACS. The axial deviation over 4° was not recorded by the navigation and only in 3 patients (1 %) by PACS. The Table 2 shows an absolute value distribution of the lower limb axis after endoprosthesis implantation measured by the navigation and PACS.

deviation (mFA - mTA)	number and % of the patients (MediCAD®2.06)	number and % of the patients (OrthoPilot)
0° - 2.0°	274 (88 %)	280 (90 %)
2.1° - 4.0°	34 (11 %)	31 (10 %)
> 4.0°	3 (1 %)	0

Table 2. The deviation of the axis of lower limb measured by orthopaedic planning system in PACS and by kinematic navigation system postoperatively

4. Computer navigation of valgus knee kinematics before TKR

Computer navigation technique can be used for a surgical approach choice in TKR implantation. Valgus deformity was analysed in the author's institutions in 50 patients. At the beginning of a surgery there were fixated navigation markers to the tibia and femur in these valgus limbs and data were collected for the navigation just before surgical approach was chosen. After data registration (software for correcting osteotomy) changes in values of a lower limb axis deformity in various of knee joint flexion (0°, 30°, 60°, 90°, 120°) were observed. In case of persistance of axis valgus deformity throughout the whole range of a knee movement it is called "right" valgus, in case of gradual transition of valgus deformity into varus during flexion it is called "false" valgus. In a „right" valgus knee there is a mismatch between both condyles in both the vertical and anteroposterior dimensions, the lateral condyle is generally smaller. (Šváb et al., 2010). In a „false" valgus knee there is no mismatch between anteroposterior dimensions of both condyles, the knee axis changes from valgus into varus with increased degree of flexion and lateral soft tissue structures are that's why not so contracted as in „true" valgus knee deformity, where the knee stays in valgus deviation during the whole range of motion.

In case of the "right" valgus deformity the lateral parapatellar approach according to Keblish is preferred because of an easier release of tight lateral structures. In case of the false deformities a standard medial parapatellar approach can be used. Valgus deformity of a lower limb was measured preoperatively by the navigation within the range from 4° to 13° (on average 7.8°). The right valgus deformity was observed during the knee joint passive flexion in 34 patients (68 %). The average value of the valgus knee joint deformity in extension in the group with the right valgus was 7.9° (range, 4° to 13°). Deviation value in this group decreased gradually during flexion in all cases. The difference in the degree of axis deviation between 0° and 120° of flexion in this group was on average 5.5° (range, 1° to 10°). Changes of the axial deviation depending on the degree of the knee joint flexion are illustrated in figure 3.

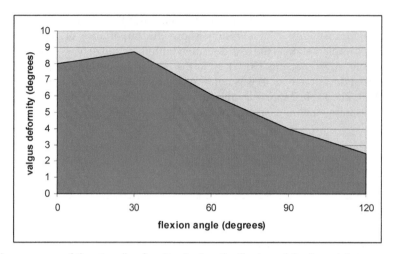

Fig. 3. The progress of the „true" valgosity during the flexion of the knee joint

The false valgus deformity of a knee joint was registered in 16 patients (32 %). In this group the average value of the valgus deformity was 7.5° (range, 6° to 9°). The varus deviation of the mechanical axis was already observed in 60° or 90° of flexion. The difference in the degree of the axis deviation of the limb between 0° and 120° of flexion in this group was on average 12.0° (range, 10° to 14°). Changes of the axial deviation depending on the degree of knee joint flexion with pseudovalgus are illustrated in figure 4.

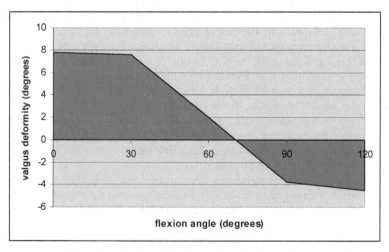

Fig. 4. The progress of the „false" valgosity during the flexion of the knee joint.

Because of the analysis of the knee joint valgus deformity by the computer navigation at the beginning of the surgery the operative time extended on average by 6 minutes (range, 4 to 11 minutes). The navigation was used consequently after the switch on the TKR a module for total endoprosthesis implantation.

5. Kinematic navigation in TKR with distal femoral disturbances

Kinematic navigation system is usually used to precise the knee endoprosthesis implantation. In cases of distal femoral deformity or in the presence of metal material in the distal femur is the navigation the best way how to solve this problem (Fig. 5).

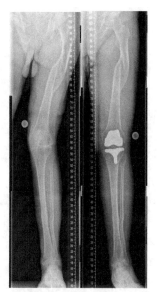

Fig. 5. The X-rays show the deformity of the femur, before and after implantation of TKR

The deformity can be caused by an injury or chronic osteopathy. Some metal material can be present after fracture osteosynthesis or after a revision implantation of hip joint total endoprosthesis. In these cases it is not possible to use standard intramedullary targeting devices and the kinematic navigation system is the best possibility how to implant the femoral component of the knee joint replacement correctly. 13 patients with the femoral deformity or presence of some metal material in the area of the distal femur have been operated in the authors´ institution. It was the condition after the distal femoral metaphyseal fracture with left plate in 4 patients. In 5 patients it was the condition after femoral diaphyseal fracture treated by an intramedullary nail (in one case the nail was broken). In 1 patient the femoral fracture was healed with an extended fragment malposition ad latus. In 3 patients the long stem femoral component of a hip replacement was present. In all these patients a standard implantation of a knee joint replacement was done with use of the computer navigation technique. The record lower limb axis has been restored in all these patients.

6. Kinematic navigation system for prevention of the hypocorrection or hypercorrection of the mechanical axis in UKA

The importance of kinematic navigation during the implantation of unicompartmental replacements is high. It can be used for knee surfaces resection but first of all for a simple control of the axial limb deviation during the implantation of the UKA. At the beginning of the surgery it is necessary to fix navigation markers percutaneuosly at the femur and tibia, to collect data (software for correction osteotomy) and to display the measured lower limb axis (Fig. 6).

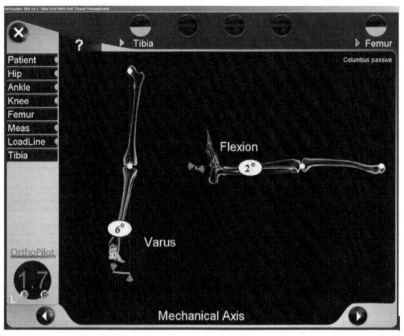

Fig. 6. The axis of the lower limb shown on the display of kinematic navigation system before UCA implantation

Then we implant the knee joint unicopartmental replacement throught a standard medial parapatellar approach and standard surgical technique. After the fixation of tibial and femoral components by bone cement the navigation is used for the right choice of polyethylene insert height with regard to its stability and especially the limb axis. The right size of the polyethylene insert is chosen so that the lower limb mechanical axis would be straight. There were implanted 67 unicompartmental replacements in the authors´ institution from April 2008 till September 2010 (30 months) (Fig. 7).

In 32 patients the replacement was made in a standard way without navigation, in 35 patients with the kinematic navigation. There were 20 men of average age 69.5 years (range, 54 to 82 years) and 47 women of average age 69.2 years (range, 49 to 85 years). In 29 cases a right knee was operated and in 38 cases a left knee. The medial compartmental replacement was done in all patients. All surgeries were made by experienced surgeons. In the group of patients operated without the use of navigation the average lower limb axial deviation was measured before the surgery was 5.1° varus (range, 1.0° to 12.6°). The average axial deviation measured radiologically in the long weight bearing X-rays after surgery was 2.1° of valgus (range, 8.5° valgus to 5.2° varus). The overcorrection of the lower limb mechanical axis into valgus without the use of navigation happened in 20 patients (63 %). The hypercorrection of axis into valgus > 2.0° happened in 12 patients (38 %). Varus deformity > 2.0° after surgery was recorded in 6 patients (18 %). The Table 3 shows the distribution of an absolute value of a lower limb mechanical axis after the unicompartmental endoprosthesis implantation measured by the planning station PACS.

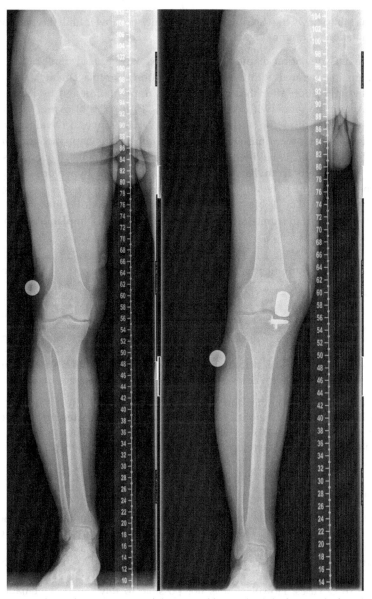

Fig. 7. The X-rays show the correction of the axis of lower limb before and after the surgery

valgus deformity	number of patients	varus deformity	number of patients
0.1° - 2.0°	8 (25 %)	0° - 2.0°	6 (19 %)
2.1° - 4.0°	8 (25 %)	2.1° - 4.0°	3 (9 %)
> 4.0°	4 (13 %)	> 4.0°	3 (9 %)

Table 3. This table shows the distribution of deformity of a lower limb mechanical axis after UCA implantation without navigation system

The average axis deviation of the lower limb was 4.1° varus (range, 1.0° to 9.0°) in the group of patients operated with the use of navigation (35 replacements). Axial deviations measured by navigation after the endoprosthesis implantation and by PACS 7 day after the surgery were the same (with the difference $\leq$ 2°) in 92 % of cases. The average axial deviation measured after the surgery was 0.5° varus (range, 5.1° valgus to 6.5°). The overcorrection of the lower limb mechanical axis into valgus happened only in 6 patients (17 %) with the use of the navigation. In these cases the hypercorrection was due to the prevention of mobile polyethylene core dislocation. The axis hypercorrection into valgus $\geq$ 2.0° happened in one patient (3 %). Varus deformity > 2.0° after the surgery was found in 4 patients (12 %). The Table 4 shows absolute value distribution of the lower limb mechanical axis after the unicompartmental endoprosthesis implantation measured by planning station PACS.

valgus deformity	number of patients	varus deformity	number of patients
0.1° - 2.0°	5 (14 %)	0° - 2.0°	25 (71 %)
2.1° - 4.0°	1 (3 %)	2.1° - 4.0°	3 (9 %)
4.0° <	0	4.0° <	1 (3 %)

Table 4. The table shows the distribution of deformity of a lower limb mechanical axis after UCA implantation with navigation system

The kinematic computer navigation represents significant help for the right choice of mobile polyethylene inlay height. An implant failure is threatening in cases of varus deformity reversing. In cases of more frequently observed hypercorrection into valgus lateral gonarthrosis usually develops. Both situations must be later solved by a conversion on TKR.

7. Conclusion

The importance of the kinematic computer navigation of knee endoprosthesis lies above all in the reduction of out-layers. This fact is important especially for beginning orthopaedic surgeons. The kinematic navigation should prevent from wrong resection of distal femur or proximal tibia. Navigation succeeds in 88 % cases (Hart et al, 2003) to reach the deviation from an ideal axial position of a lower limb less than 2°. Without the navigation it is observed in 70 % cases. However, it is not possible to rely on the kinematic navigation absolutely (as it is only auxiliary method). The key factor of the navigation system successful use during the whole surgical procedure is to keep an unchanged position of femoral and tibial diodes. Change of their position can influence dramatically the result of the whole navigation process. It is possible to avoid this complication in osteoporotic skeleton by an accessory Kirschner wire which prevents from the screw rotation. The time waste during the surgery, which represents time less than 10 minutes in hands of experienced surgeons, is not significant with regard to the above mentioned navigation system advantages.

Another substantial benefit of the computer navigation in a total knee joint endoprosthesis implantation is incases after fractures of the femur, where osteosynthesis material is left or after bone healing in a malposition which makes impossible to carry out the distal femoral resection with the use of an intramedullary targeting device. The navigation helps routinely also at the beginning of the surgery to distinguish the right valgus deformity from the false one. According to it we choose the suitable surgical approach. In unicompartmental knee joint replacements it is possible to choose the right polyethylene inlay height by the help of the navigation so that the lower limb mechanical axis is restored as accurately as possible. In this way we avoid axis overcorrection into valgus in most cases and subsequent decompensation of the lateral compartment and later necessity of conversion on TKR.

8. References

Hart, R., Janeček, M., Chaker, A. & Bucek, P. (2003). Total knee arthroplasty implanted with and without kinematic navigation. *International orthopaedics*, 27, 6, 366-369, DOI: 10.1007/s00264-003-0501-6

Hart, R. & Janeček, M. (2003). *Osové postavení dolní končetiny a poloha komponent kolenní endoprotézy s přihlédnutím ke kinematické počítačové navigace*, Neptun, , ISBN 80-902896-5-7, Praque, Czech Republic

Hart, R., Krejzla, J., Janeček, M. & Mahel, P. (2005). Minimally invasive total knee replacement surgery with use of the kinematic navigation. El Mochel Movie.

Hart, R., Janeček, M., Čižmář, I., Štipčák, V., Kučera, B. & Filan, P. (2006). Minimal-invasive und navigierte implantation von knietotalendoprothesen, radiologische analyse und frühe klinische ergebnisse. *Der Orthopäde*, 35, 5, 552-557, ISSN: 0085-4530

Hart, R., Janeček, M., Safi, A. & Okál, F. (2010). Digital temlating compared with kinematic navigation in TKR, *Proceedings of 10th Annual Meeting of CAOS-International*, Paris, France, June 2010

Insall, J.N., Binazzi, R., Soudry, M. & Mestriner, L.A. (1985). Total knee arthroplasty. *Clinical orthopaedics*, 192, 13-22, ISSN 1528-1132

Krackow, K.A. (1983). Approaches to planning lower extremity alignment for total knee arthoplasty and osteotomy about the knee. *Advances in operative orthopaedics*, 7, 69-88

Laskin, R. S. (1984). Alignment of total knee components. *Orthopedics*, 7, 62-72

Ritter, A.M., Faris, M.P., Keating, E.M. & Meding, J.B. (1994). Postoperative alignment of total knee replacement, its effect on survival. *Clinical orthopaedics*, 299, 153-156 ISSN 1528-1132

Šváb, P., Hart, R., Bárta, R. & Šmíd, P. (2010). Computer navigation of valgus knee kinematice before TKR, *Proceedings of 14th National Conference of Orthopaedy*, Praque, Czech Republic, May 2010

Whietside, L.A & Arima, J. (1995). The Anteroposterior axis for femoral rotational alignment in valgus total knee arthroplasty. *Clinical orthopaedics*, 321, 168-172.

13

Strategies to Improve the Function, Kinematic and Implants' Positioning of a TKA with Minimally Invasive Computer-Assisted Navigation

Nicola Biasca[1] and Matthias Bungartz[2]
[1]Orthopedic Clinic Luzern AG, Hirslanden Clinic St. Anna, Luzern
[2]Klinik für Orthopädie und Unfallchirurgie, Lehrstuhl für Orthopädie der
Friedrich-Schiller-Universität Jena, Waldkrankenhaus
„Rudolf Elle" Eisenberg
[1]Switzerland
[2]Germany

1. Introduction

Total Knee Arthroplasty (TKA) is a well established, highly successful procedure, with numerous long-term follow-up studies reporting clinical success rates of 72-100% at 10-20 years in terms of pain reduction, functional improvement and overall patient satisfaction [1-5]. Although TKA is generally successful, and despite the advances in surgical techniques, instrumentation and implant designs, between 5 to 8% of all patients still develop complications such as anterior knee pain, loosening, instability, malpositioning, infection or fractures [6-8]. Imperfection in the coronar, sagittal and axial alignments of the femoral and/ or of tibial components, improper ligament balancing and incorrect joint line restoration can lead to soft tissue imbalance and inability to re-establish optimal kinematics and the overall biomechanics of the joint, with persistent anterior knee pain, patellar maltracking, instability or limitation of movement [9-14, 15].

Several investigators have demonstrated on the basis of conventional radiography and computer-tomography that TKA, implanted with computer-assisted navigation and conventional approach, has more accurate component alignment than TKA implanted conventionally [9, 15-29].

The introduction of minimally invasive surgery (MIS) has gained in importance in orthopedics and especially in TKA. Patient`s demand for high activity level after TKA, concerns about postoperative pain, fast rehabilitation process, possible reduction in duration of hospitalization and costs in connection with the necessity of health care savings have led to the rapid advancement of less invasive surgical approaches and techniques as well as the development of new instrumentation by the orthopedic implant industry.

Regardless of the numerous advantages of minimal-invasive TKA, concern is driven about loss of accuracy for implant placement and increased complications related to skin slough and infection when a minimally invasive approach is used [30, 31]. Furthermore reduced operative visualization, a steep learning curve, an increased risk of complications, excessive skin trauma and compromised implant fixation and alignment are topic of objection. In addition few surgeons have expressed concern about minimally invasive surgery and its relevance to TKA as well as the safety of operations performed "through a keyhole" and are convinced that at present there is no credible evidence that smaller incisions significantly benefit the patient receiving MIS TKA. By contrast, proponents of MIS TKA report that MIS patients, compared to patients undergoing conventional TKA, Experience shortened hospital stay, less pain-control medications, faster recovery of knee range of motion and decreased blood loss all without compromise of accuracy or short-term outcome [32-34].

2. Computer-assisted navigated orthopedic surgery

The principle of computer-assisted surgery in orthopedics is based on the creation of a digital map for the different steps during operation. Using this map, the surgeon is guided through the operating process. The development of the digital image is based on three different basic ideas.

One system uses anatomical information which is achieved from pre-operatively performed CT- or MRI-scans, the second system is "peri-operatively-imaged" in which anatomical imaging occurs in the operating suite at the time of surgery. This requires a specially modified fluoroscopy unit, which entails the presence of a relatively bulky and expensive apparatus during surgery. These two systems display the "image-based systems". The third group on the contrary is "image-free" and relies on information acquired during surgery. This "image-free" navigation allows the surgeon to quantify data, receive real-time dynamic intra-operative maneuvering feedback and to obtain more reproducible results.

A very important feature of this navigation system is its ability to provide instant feedback regarding *in vivo* kinematics of the joint at different stages of the operation. Alignment and ligament stability can be assessed with the trials in place to ensure proper function. Furthermore, this system allows the surgeon to measure the coronal, sagittal and axial deformities, the alignments and the stability of the joint before, during and after the implantation of a TKA. These characteristics of the navigation system provide the unique opportunity to assess *in vivo* the kinematics of the knee during surgery and implement beneficial changes of the components or alteration in components selection.

We were using at the Orthopedic Clinic at the Hospital Oberengadin in Samedan an "image-free" navigation system (Stryker® Leibinger Knee Navigation System, Stryker® Leibinger, precisioN Knee Navigation Software V 4.0). This system is available in an active wireless PC-based guidance system, which is based on an image-free navigation method, and thus does not require pre-operative computer tomography or intra-operative fluoroscopy. It comprises a module for analyzing the alignment of the leg, the alignment of the resection planes and thus of the prosthetic components. The system also allows the surgeon to quantify the kinematics of the knee and the balancing of the soft tissue (Further details on the Stryker® Knee Navigation System are available on http://www.europe.stryker.com/).

2.1.1 Surgical procedure

The patient is placed supine on a standard operating table. A tourniquet is applied after exsanguination of the limb, and standard skin preparation and draping are undertaken. To obtain best exposition of all structures during the procedure, two distally positioned leg holders are fixed on the operating table to allow full flexion and extension of the leg. Flexing the knee thereby exposes the posterior structures whereas extension facilitates access to the anterior anatomy of the knee.

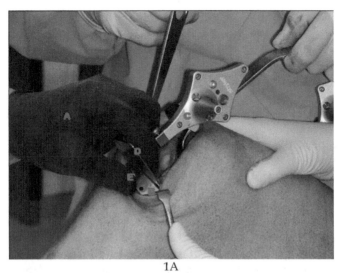

1A

Fig. 1A. The proximal tibial resection requires the surgeon to position the MIS Cutting Guide in relation to the three axes of freedom controlling the varus/ valgus, the depth and the posterior slope, with a freehand technique (A). The cutting guide block/ tracker construct (B-C-D) is then hold by the surgeon with a "tripod grip" (A). The universal tracker (C) is attached to the resection plane probe (D), which in turn is placed into the captured slot of the cutting guide block (B). The cutting guide block (B) is pinned into place with three pins (E).

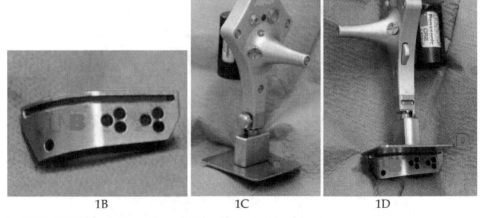

1B   1C   1D

Fig. 1B-D. MIS TKA must be performed with accurate instruments:
Fig. 1B. The cutting guide block (B).
Fig. 1C. The universal tracker (C) is attached to the resection plane probe (D).
Fig. 1D. The universal tracker (C) is attached to the resection plane probe (D), which in turn is placed into the captured slot of the cutting guide block (B).

Fig. 1A-D. Proximal tibial resection

As standard approach we used a mid-vastus approach [35-38]. To enable a better exposure and visibility of the lateral compartment the patella was osteotomized freehand to 12-14 mm bone thickness for later resurfacing in order to reconstruct preoperative thickness. All interventions were performed by a single surgeon (NB), who is a high volume arthroplasty surgeon and uses computer-navigation routinely for over six years.

Two pin trackers need to be fixed rigidly at the beginning of the operation on the lateral distal femur and on the ventral proximal tibia, both within the surgical access zone (For further details information's please see the references 24 and 25).

The digitizing pointer is now used to mark the key anatomical landmarks. After that procedure the surgeon is able to reproduce the correct joint kinematics at any time of the operation in any position of the leg with the Knee Navigation System software. After analyzing the kinematics curves and axis, bone cuts are performed using the information obtained from the navigation system.

We usually prefer starting with tibial cut first. The proximal tibial cut is made in a one-step procedure, controlling the desired posterior slope, varus/ valgus and depth. The degree of posterior slope of the tibial cut is aimed to match the original posterior slope of the tibial plateau as measured in the pre-operative lateral x-ray [16]. Using freehand technique, the position of the probe is adjusted according to the image and data shown on the computer. MIS TKA must be performed with accurate instruments that are coordinated with the procedure. The guide is held with a "tripod grip" technique (Figures 1A-D), and the visual movements of the guide can be monitored in real time on the screen (Figure 2).

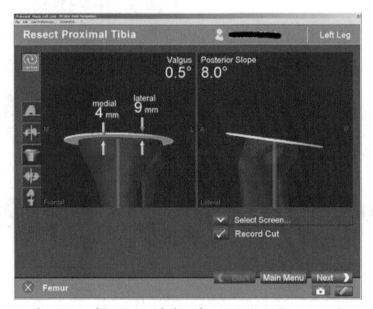

Fig. 2. The virtual position of cutting guide/ tracker construct is now an active tool, which can be monitored (i.e. the varus/ valgus angle, the slope angel and the depth) on the computer navigation screen.

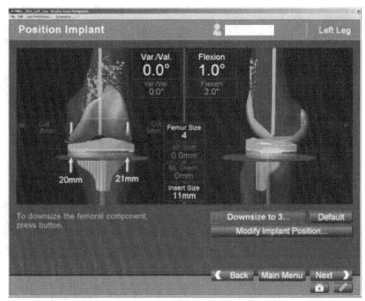

3A

Fig. 3A. "Implant Position": The system allows the surgeon to check the position of the implant.

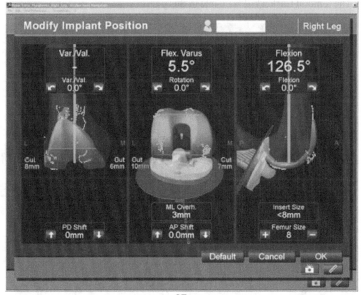

3B

Fig. 3B. "Modify Implant Position": This system allows the surgeon to modify the flexion/ extension, varus/ valgus, internal/ external rotation, anterior/ posterior shift, proximal/ distal shift of the femoral implant and to adjust its implant size relative to femur.

Fig. 3A. and 3B. Implant Position and Modify Implant Position:

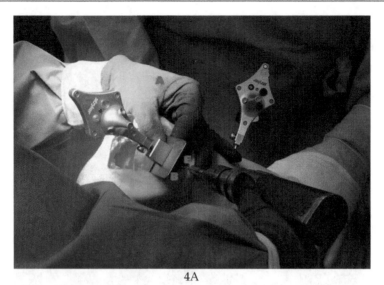

4A

Fig. 4A. With the freehand technique (A) the same cutting guide block (B) is used with the universal tracker (C) and with the resection plane probe (D) in the captured slot (E) and placed on the external border of the medial distal femur condyle (F). Similar to tibial cutting, a freehand technique with the cutting guide block (B-C-D) is used for the distal femoral resection. The block is pinned into place with three pins (E). The femoral tracker (G) is visible in this picture.

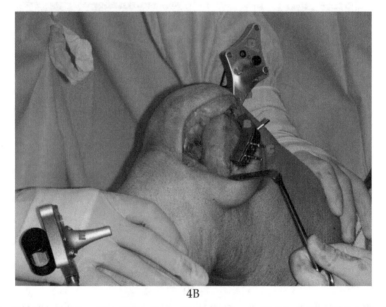

4B

Fig. 4B. The distal femoral resection (A) is done with the cutting guide block (B), which is fixed with three pins (C) and the surgeon can now use a saw blade to cut the desired distal femoral (A) resection. The femoral tracker (D) and tibial trackers (E) are visible in this picture. Now the distal femoral bone resection can be done with the saw through the cutting guide block.

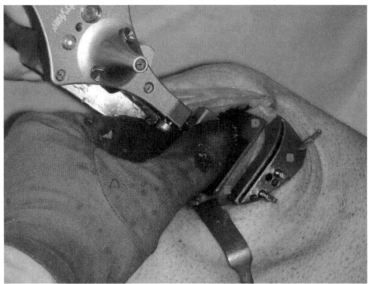

4C

Fig. 4C. Control of the corrected resection of the distal femoral bone with the freehand technique (A):
After resection with the cutting guide block (B), the universal tracker (C) in connection with the
resection plane probe (D) can verify the accuracy of the cut of the distal femoral bone surface (E), re-
correct the resection if it is necessary and finally record the distal femoral cut on the screen. In this
picture the resection plane probe (D) is hold on the distal femoral bone cut surface (E) to record the
resection result.

Fig. 4A-C. Distal femoral resection

Afterwards, the surgeon has the possibility to continue with the bone resection of the
distal femur. In a two-step process, using two femoral cutting blocks, the cutting guide
and the femoral alignment guide and the resection plane probe, the cuts are performed.
Distal femoral resection requires control of the flexion/extension, varus/ valgus and
depth of bone resection, based on our decision of the implant positioning and sizing
(Figures 4A-C).
The rotational alignment is subsequently established with the femoral alignment guide and
resection plane probe. The femoral component rotation is aimed to be 0° in relation to the
special algorithm of surgical transepicondylar axis and the Whiteside line as provided by
the computer software. Care is taken to avoid notching the ventral femoral cortex. We
finally finish the femur preparation with the femoral resection guide and the femoral
trochlea with the corresponding resection guide. Hereby care is taken to release any flexion
contracture and to remove all the posterior femoral osteophytes. The femoral component is
then inserted and, once correctly seated, the fixation lugholes are drilled.
Subsequently the tibial bone resection is finalized: The appropriately sized tibial baseplate
is inserted and its rotation is determined through self-adjustment by flexing and
extending the knee with the trial femoral and inlay components implanted. The tibial
component rotation is marked, and later the component is implanted with the desired
rotation [39, 40].

2.1.2 Trial component insertion

Before the insertion of the trial components, the tibial and femoral bone cuts are again verified with a small resection plane probe, which is directly applied on the resection planes of the affected bone. Every cut is recorded and stored by the system, and can be used for post-operative evaluation and quality control. After completion and digital check of the tibial, femoral and soft tissue preparation, the trial components are inserted and once again the correct position of the trial components is checked with a small resection plane probe for position. Subsequently, the patella preparation is finished and patellar tracking is checked with the implant trials in place.

2.1.3 Trial components soft tissue assessment

After the insertion of the trial components, limb alignment and soft tissue balancing are assessed with the intra-operative kinematics by moving the limb from extension to full flexion under neutral, varus and valgus stress, manually applied through the heel of the foot, carefully keeping the same rotation. Using this information, the surgeon can simulate changes of polyethylene insert and soft tissue release by repeating the assessment. In this way one can obtain a constant dynamic feedback in the process of balancing the knee (Figures 5A and B).

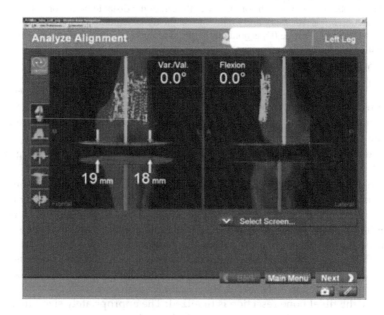

5A

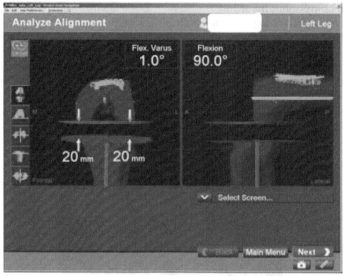

5B

Fig. 5A. and B. The Gap monitoring enables the surgeon to analyze varus/valgus, extension/flexion as well as the gap in extension (A) and flexion (B) upon performance of all cuts with a mechanical tensioner to ensure equal medial and lateral tension in both flexion and extension. This maneuver can also be done through the all ROM under neutral, varus and valgus stress.

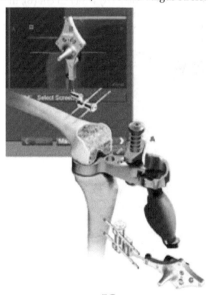

5C

Fig. 5C. Schematic view of the gap monitoring in flexion with a mechanical tensioner (A). The femoral tracker (B), the tibial tracker (C) and the screen (D) are visible in this picture.

Fig. 5A-C. Gap monitoring

2.1.4 Definite component insertion

All our patients received a posterior-stabilized "Scorpio" total knee prosthesis (Stryker® Howmedica Osteonics, Freiburg, Germany). After jet-lavage (approx. 3 L of Ringer Solution) of the resection planes the femoral and tibial components are cemented with the Stryker® Compact Vacuum Cement Mixing System. It is still possible to control the position of the tibial and femoral components with the resection plane probe and, if necessary, improve (Figures 6A and B). Then again the definitive position is documented with the navigation system.

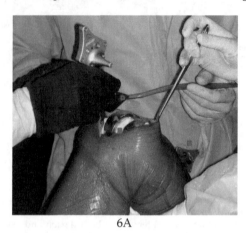

6A

Fig. 6A. After insertion of the femoral component (A) with cement (B), the surgeon has the possibility to check the position of the femoral component with the universal tracker (C) and the resection plane probe (D) and if necessary to improve its position before the cement is fully polymerized. The femoral tracker (E) is visible in this picture.

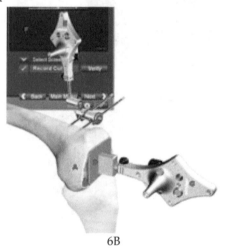

6B

Fig. 6B. Schematic view to check the position of the femoral component with the universal tracker (C) and the resection plane probe (D). In this schematic view, without a Prosthetic component, the distal femoral condyle (A), the distal femoral cut surface (B), the femoral tracker (E) and the screen (F) are visible.

Fig. 6A. and B. Final control of the position the femoral component

Any excessive cement is removed under direct vision. In the same way the femoral component is cemented, a polyethylene inlay trial is then inserted and thereafter the patellar component is embedded with cement. After the cement is fully polymerized, the tourniquet is released and subtle hemostasis performed. Before the final choice of the inlay size is made, it is still possible to assess the joint and soft tissue balance using different size of polyethylene inlay trials and to show the resulting kinematics analysis on screen.

2.1.5 Wound closure

The joint is accurately irrigated and an intraarticular drain is inserted. The arthrotomy is closed with interrupted absorbable sutures (Vicryl 2.0) with the knee at 90º of flexion. After putting a second, subcutaneous drain, the subcutaneous layer is closed with Vicryl 2.0, and the skin is closed with Ethycrin 4.0.

Subsequently the final outcome and the kinematics are documented, recorded and compared to the initial data to assess the success of any correction (Figures 7A and 7B).

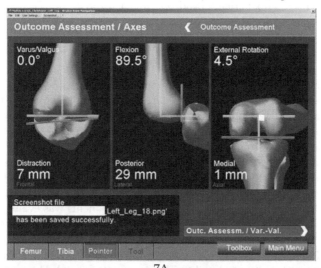

7A

Actual	min					+96°	max
+ Flexion - Hyperextension	-0.5°	+0.0°	+30.0°	+45.0°	+60.0°	+90.0°	+129.0°
+ Valgus - Varus	-1.5°	-1.0°	+0.5°	+0.5°	+1.0°	+0.0°	-0.5°
+ Internal - External	-8.0°	-8.0°	-5.0°	-5.0°	-5.0°	-3.0°	+4.0°
+ Compression - Distraction	-10	-10	-13	-11	-7	+0	+12
+ Medial - Lateral	+6	+6	+5	+5	+6	+7	+8
+ Anterior - Posterior	+10	+10	-8	-15	-22	-30	-38

7B

Fig. 7A. and B. The final outcome of the 3-dimensional axis (A) is documented on the screen as a value with a chart (B).

2.2 Postoperative treatment

For post-operative pain control, our patients first receive a "one-off sciatic nerve block (SB)" and then a continuous femoral nerve block (FB) [41, 42], combined with oral analgesics for both groups. Physical therapy is started as early as 4 to 6 hours post-operatively (continuous passive motion) and consequently intensified under supervision of an experienced physiotherapist (i.e. continuous passive motion 3 times a day, early ambulation, walking exercises, active bending and extending exercises, active knee stretching exercises, walking up and down stairs, leg press, ergometer-bike riding, coordination exercises, getting up from a seated position, strengthen exercises, etc.). Patients are allowed to full weight bearing as tolerated. Patients are discharged from the hospital once they are able to flex the knee joint to 120°, to perform an unassisted straight-leg raise, to walk independently with or without crutches, to rise from a chair to standing and sit from standing without support, and to ascend and descend a full flight of stairs. All patients receive Low Molecular Weight Heparin (LMWH, i.e. Fraxiparine®, Nadroparin) or a direct oral Factor Xa inhibitor (i.e. Xarelto®, Rivaroxaban) for deep venous thrombosis prophylaxis for 6 weeks. Outpatient physical therapy is started immediately after discharge. The Patients are evaluated clinically and radiographically in the office at 6 weeks, 3 months and 6 months.

2.3 Radiographic follow-up

All patients received full-length standing antero-posterior radiographs pre-operatively, at 6 weeks as well as 6 and 12 months post-operatively ("Philips® Multidiagnost 3"). Pre- and post-operative mechanical axes (i.e. the coronal mechanical axis of the limb, the Hip-Knee-Angle) were determined from radiographs. A mechanical axis of more than 3° varus/ valgus was determined as outlier as defined previously [17, 18]. Conventional radiographic assessment involved short-leg-length weight-bearing antero-posterior (AP) radiographs, as well as non-rotated short-leg-length lateral radiographs at 30° of knee flexion and patella axial radiographs. The alignment of the prosthetic components was evaluated on the short-length standard radiographs. Radiographic parameters, including the coronal femoral component angle, the sagittal femoral component angle, the coronal tibial component angle and the sagittal tibial component angle (i.e. tibial slope angle) were evaluated to determine the correct position of the femoral and tibial components [43, 44]. The coronal alignment of the femoral component was measured in relation to the anatomical femoral axis (ideal value = 96°) and of the tibial component in relation to the anatomical tibial axis (ideal value = 90°). To determine the sagittal angle of the femoral and tibial components, a perpendicular line, drawn from the midline of the femoral respectively tibial components, was compared with the midline of the distal segment of the femur and of the proximal segment of the tibia using the Knee Score reference lines [45]. Although little consensus on the ideal reference for defining the slope of the tibia on the lateral radiograph is reached, we used the technique described by Catani et al. and Yoo et al., measuring the slope of the tibial component on conventional short-length sagittal view radiographs with reference to the proximal anatomic axis [16, 46]. Pre- and post-operative sagittal tibial component angles (i.e. tibial slope angle) were compared on conventional short-length lateral radiographs in 30° of knee flexion. All patients also received standardized CT-scans of both knees 6 weeks postoperatively to evaluate rotational alignment of the components according to the technique described by Berger et al. for our follow-up study [47].

3. Results and discussion

3.1 CN TKA versus MIS CN TKA

In a previous study we compared two groups of patients either with a standard medial parapatellar approach (CN-TKA group) or with a minimal invasive mid-vastus approach (MIS CN-TKA group) [For further detailed information please see the references 48]. No inaccuracies of the Knee Navigation System (i.e. dirty reflectors, camera or rounding errors), or of the references pin itself (i.e. loosening of the reference pin intraoperatively and consequent inaccuracies in reference readings) were found. No switch to the conventional implantation method was necessary. Postoperative recovery of the patients was uneventful, there were no infections or wound healing disorders in both groups. No patients were lost to follow-up.

3.1.1 Clinical outcome

The mean postoperative range of motion (ROM) after 3 months was significantly higher in MIS CN-TKA (125° MIS CN-TKA group vs. 118° CN-TKA group) (p = 0.037). However, 6 months after operation there was no statistical relevant difference in range of motion between the two groups (125° vs. 122°) to be found. The Knee Society Clinical Rating Score (i.e. the knee and function scores) had improved in both groups to almost identical values 6 months after the operation. The mean length of hospital stay was significantly reduced in the MIS CN-TKA group (p < 0.0005) resulting in a total duration of 8 days (range 6 - 9 days) versus 17 days (range: 8 - 31 days) in the CN-TKA group. We found no statistically difference between operation time and blood loss in the computer-assisted MIS TKA compared to the conventional CN-TKA group [For further detailed information please see the reference 48].

3.1.2 Radiological outcome

The radiographic coronal mechanical axis of the limb (i.e. the Hip-Knee-Angle) improved to an orthograde level in both groups (CN TKA 0.5° versus MIS CN-TKA 0.7 °). We found no outliers in both groups regarding alignment .

The tibial slope was significantly reconstructed to match the preoperative value not only in the conventional CN-TKA group (CN-TKA: mean value 1.6°) but also in the minimally invasive CN-TKA group (MIS CN-TKA: mean value 1.4°). The same accuracy was found for the implantation of the tibial component in the coronal alignment with no statistically significant difference between the conventional CN-TKA group (CN-TKA: mean value 91.3°) and the minimally invasive CN-TKA group (MIS CN-TKA: mean value 91.4°).

With regard to the accuracy of the coronal alignment of the femoral component we found a correct implantation of the femoral component in all cases and there was no statistically significant difference between both groups (CN-TKA (96.2°) vs. MIS CN-TK (95.2°)). The post-operative radiological analysis of the sagittal alignment of the femoral component in relation to the anatomical femoral axis revealed slight more flexion of the femoral components in both groups than planned pre-operatively (CN-TKA: mean value 6.9° versus MIS CN-TKA: mean value 7.8°). However, the intra-operative alignment of the sagittal femoral cut showed an accurate value closed to 1° of flexion not only in the conventional CN-TKA group (CN-TKA Group: mean value of 0.58°, standard deviation

0.44°, Range 0.00 - 1.50), but also in minimally invasive CN-TKA group (MIS CN-TKA Group: mean value of 1.03°, standard deviation 0.40°, Range 0.50 - 2.00). Moreover, the anterior flange of the femoral component was parallel to the dorsal femoral cortex in every patient of both groups.

3.1.3 Computed tomography outcome

The Analysis of the postoperative CT scans revealed a statistically significant reconstruction of the desired rotational alignment of the femoral component parallel to the transepicondylar axis not only in the conventional CN-TKA group (CN-TKA: mean value 0.7°) but also in the minimally invasive CN-TKA group (MIS CN-TKA: mean value 1.3°) (p = 0.018). No outliers in the rotational alignment of the femoral prosthesis could be documented [For further detailed information please see the reference 48].

3.2 Discussion

It is well known by now that malposition of TKA affects implant fixation and leads to an increased risk of loosening, instability and decreased survival of the prosthesis. Computer-assisted navigation systems have been designed to increase the precision of implantation of TKA allowing the surgeon to reproduce the mechanical axes measured on full-length standing radiographs of the lower limb and reduces the number of outliers in the alignment of the limb compared to traditional mechanical instrumented TKA [9, 15-19, 21, 22, 48-54]. Two recent meta-analysis comparing alignment outcomes for computer-assisted navigated versus conventional TKA indicate a significant improvement in component orientation and mechanical axis, when computer-assisted navigation is used [55, 56]. Our analysis demonstrated that it is possible to achieve straight mechanical axes not only in the conventional but also in the minimally invasive approaches by using a computer-assisted navigation. Additionally intra-operative alignment of the femoral and tibial bone resection was accurate in all three planes not only in the conventional but also in the minimally invasive computer navigated TKA group. Similar intra-operative results have been published and our results showed the same accuracy of the intra-operative bone resections with the navigation system as the above mentioned [9, 16-18, 22].

However, the solely measurement of mechanical axis alone appears too basic as an indicator of correct limb alignment and long-term outcome. Accurate angles of the individual components in the coronal and sagittal planes, correct axial alignment and proper ligament and soft tissue balancing contribute to the success of knee replacement surgery and should be taken in consideration as well. The results of these data were also accurate in both groups using the computer-assisted navigation technique.

Different studies have compared computer-assisted systems with traditional implantation for improvement of component orientation. Most authors showed that the coronal alignment (i.e. the varus/ valgus alignment) of the femoral component was improved with the use of navigation [9, 16-18, 57-59]. Only few studies did not report an improvement in component alignment between patients in who navigation was used [60, 61]. Despite the fact that in these studies the senior authors have more experience with conventional than navigated TKA, the reduction of outliers was greater in the navigation group. However, all these studies investigated TKA implanted using conventional approach.

We were also able to demonstrate that, by using a computer-assisted navigation system, it is possible to implant the femoral and tibial components in the desired coronal and sagittal planes not only with the conventional but also with a minimally invasive approach. The post-operative radiographic analyses of the coronal alignment of the femoral and tibial components showed reliable results in both groups without any outliers in either group [For further detailed information please see the references 48].

Few further studies found the same accurate reconstruction of the sagittal alignment of the femoral component by using the navigation system, however with a standard conventional approach [9, 16, 19, 24, 25, 49, 57, 58, 62].

Literature documents that the influence of computer-assisted navigation on the alignment of the tibial component remains unclear. Several authors confirmed that the coronal alignment of the tibial component (i.e. the varus/ valgus alignment) is improved with the use of navigation [9, 24, 62], whereas other authors did not find evidence for improvement in coronal alignment [19, 49]. We found the same preciseness for the implantation of the tibial component in the coronal plane in the conventional as well as in the minimally invasive approach. Furthermore, we could demonstrate that the sagittal tibial component angle (i.e. the tibial slope angle) can be accurately and reproducibly reconstructed to match the original value of the tibial plateau in both computer-assisted approaches. Although some studies disagree that the alignment in the sagittal plane of the tibial component can be improved with navigation, our result confirmed, as it has been reported by other authors, that the surgeon can use, in practical terms, computer-assisted navigation to accurately restore the tibial slope during TKA using minimally invasive approaches as well [19, 24, 25, 28, 48, 49, 58, 63-68].

Even small abnormalities of rotational alignment of the components have a considerable influence on patellar tracking, varus/ valgus stability and on the overall biomechanics of the joint. The accuracy to adjust the rotational alignment of the femoral component is a prerequisite to avoid malfunctioning TKAs. Debate still exists whether a navigation system does improve the rotational alignment of the femoral component or not [67]. Several reference axes have been proposed to establish proper rotational alignment of the femoral components [63]. Of these axes, the transepicondylar axis approximates the flexion-extension axis of the knee. Furthermore, although there is no consensus about the best landmarks to gauge femoral rotation, alignment according to the surgical epicondylar axis seems to come closest to allowing physiological biomechanics [7, 8, 10, 67]. Debate continues with regard to how accurately and easily the transepicondylar axis can be located intra-operatively. Siston et al. found high variability in rotational alignment of the femoral component in a cadaver study [63]. This variability may be explained by the higher or lower ability of the surgeon to identify intra-operatively the medial epicondyle with its bone ridge and sulcus and the attachment of the deep and superficial fibers of the medial ligament, by the learning curve of the surgeon associated with the use of navigation and finally by the individual surgeon's skills. The algorithm of the Knee Navigation Software to establish the proper femoral rotational alignment by averaging the angle subtended by the Whiteside's line and the transepicondylar axis, gives the surgeon the possibility to improve the accuracy of the femoral rotational alignment without excessively increasing operative time. The analysis of our post-operative rotational alignment of the femoral component by CT-scans revealed a statistically significant reconstruction of the desired rotational alignment of the prosthesis parallel to the transepicondylar axis not only in the conventional but also in the minimally invasive computer-assisted navigated approaches. These results are in agreement with other studies using standard approaches, computer-assisted navigation and an improved computer tomography protocol [16, 17, 24, 68].

Although it has been reported that the rotational mismatch between the femoral and tibial components is decreased with navigation, controversy still exists as to whether navigation systems do improve the rotational alignment of the tibial component in the axial plane [24, 68, 69]. We used the technique describe by Dalury and Eckhoff et al., whereby the orientation of the tibial tray was determined by allowing it to float into position with respect to the femoral component while the knee was placed through a full arc of flexion and extension [39, 40]. We were able to document an accurate alignment of the tibial component in the CT scan postoperatively in both computer-assisted navigated groups as well. However, we do believe that a navigation system that relies only on digitization of landmarks to establish the rotational alignment of the tibial component is not reliable enough. Further research is therefore necessary.

In addition to component malpositioning, tibiofemoral instability is another very important factor that might lead to implant failure and chronic pain. Some studies point out that 30% to 35% of the revision TKA were due to an uncorrected joint stability [20-21]. Tibiofemoral instability often represents a failure to correct the soft tissues balancing throughout the full range of motion and to adjust the flexion and extension gaps at the time of the primary arthroplasty. Furthermore, it is important to take the different behavior of involved ligaments on the medial and lateral aspects into consideration as well. This instability can be in extension, midflexion and/ or in flexion. Stability and function of TKA are strictly related to the interplay among the prosthetic component alignment, the articular surface geometry (flat or congruent polyethylene insert), the type and designs of prosthesis (cruciate-retaining versus cruciate-substituting prosthesis), as well as the balancing of the soft tissue and muscle action. Of all these factors, implant component alignments, joint line restoration and soft tissue balancing "can and must be" assessed and restored by the surgeon during the intervention. Calculation of the joint line height both at the femur and tibia is usually performed by measurements on pre- and post-operative radiographs using standard anatomical indices, which are very inaccurate and not reproducible. The computer assisted navigation system allows the surgeon to measure and restore accurately the alignments of the prosthetic components in all three geometrical planes, femoral joint height and the tibial joint line, as well as the desired soft tissue balancing [54].

An established concept is the preparation of a rectangular joint gap in TKA. With a posterior stabilized TKA, flexion and extension gaps can be different. This has been regarded as an important goal achieving good joint function. However, the lateral tibiofemoral joint is physiologically lax, and as consequence the flexion gap may not be rectangular. Van Damme et al. reported in a cadaveric study on normal non-arthritic knee joint an increased laxity lateral compared to medial in full extension, and an increased lateral laxity from 0° to 90° flexion [70]. Because of technical difficulties, only few data are available on the physiological laxity of the joint. Such analysis can only be performed if the flexed knee is imaged three-dimensionally both in neutral position and under a varus/ valgus stress. Tokuhara et al. analyzed quantitatively the stability of the medial and lateral tibiofemoral joint for normal knees in an open MRI [71]. Their results indicate that the flexion gap in a normal knee is not rectangular and that the lateral joint gap is significantly lax. Recent biomechanical studies have further shown that flexion of the knee is associated with a significant medial-pivot internal rotation of the tibia [72-75]. Thus, in rotation the medial condyle is immobile and the lateral condyle is mobile on the tibial surface.

Since 1977, several studies have investigated the relationship between soft tissue release and the resulting changes in the tibiofemoral gaps in TKA using optical encoders, pressure-sensitive film, fluoroscopy or knee analysis system [76-79]. Computer-assisted surgical technology enables the surgeon to measure and assess knee behavior during operation, allowing real-time monitoring of knee's behavior from extension to flexion and soft tissue balance. In a previous study, we measured the mechanical axis and the varus/ valgus stability of the joint at different time points with the computer-assisted navigation and we documented a similar increased lateral joint laxity before and after implantation of the components at 45° and 90° of knee flexion. We even found that the overall laxity was decreasing beyond 45°/ 60° of flexion to maximal flexion [80]. Therefore, knee navigation allows the surgeon to objectively quantify and monitor kinematics and stability of the TKA through the full ROM pre-, intra- and post-operatively. Leaving the knee too lax after TKA may theoretically lead to tibiofemoral instability and excessive tightness of the joint in different position may cause stiffness. However, differently from TKA alignment, no data are available to define what is a well-balanced knee intra- and/or post-operatively. We suggested as ideal laxity for TKA a varus/ valgus laxity of an approximately total joint-line opening between 1.5° to 2° to be achieved from maximal extension to 45°/ 60° flexion and decreasing to 0.5° to 1.0° by further increasing flexion [80]. These findings serve as a benchmark for future soft tissue laxity measurements and additional work should be performed to validate these proposed values. The computer navigation will help to correlate the collected data and clinical outcomes more objectively than in the past and enable the setting of more accurate limits for soft tissue management.

Despite some motivating factors, including a potential reduction in duration of hospitalization and costs, one should not discount that the patient-driven desires include their concerns about postoperative pain, prolonged rehabilitation, and less than- ideal functional outcomes associated with conventional TKA. Various authors have also reported superior clinical results and decreased cost using minimally invasive techniques for TKA [24, 32, 43, 51. 52]. Obtaining these results with standard approaches and conventional instruments seem to cause much more soft tissue damages leading to an arduous recovery period for the patients. Although the length of the skin incision is shorter in the MIS approach, MIS knee surgery should not be defined by the size of the skin incision, but rather by the method of soft tissue handling once the skin is incised. Therefore, we should better substitute the misnomer "minimally invasive surgery" (MIS) for "soft-tissue sparing" surgery. We believe that minimal trauma of the soft tissue and bone results in better post-operative function and accelerated rehabilitation.

In a previous study, we were able to demonstrate that minimally invasive computer-assisted navigated TKA is able to achieve these objectives. With the minimally invasive approach patients were mobilized more aggressively reaching full weight bearing and profit by earlier discharge. Postoperative ROM after 3 months was significantly higher in MIS CN-TKA, but after 6 months differences were minimal. Clinical scores were identical for both groups six months after surgery. However, these clinical scores have turned out not to be ideal for the evaluation of patient satisfaction immediately after a computer-assisted navigated TKA with a conventional or MIS approach [81-83]. It would have been more appropriate to use patients' self-reported measures of outcome, such as the WOMAC and the SF-36 score systems. In addition, a recent prospective randomized controlled study demonstrated a positive correlation between accurate mechanical alignment after TKA and functional and quality-of-life patients' outcomes [84]. At all post-operative follow-up intervals from 6 weeks to 12 months the total IKSS score were significantly better in patients with a mechanical axis within 3o of neutral compared to those greater than 3o. Moreover, the SF-12 physical scores at all intervals from 3 months were also significantly better for patients with a mechanical axis within 3o of neutral, and at 12 months these patients demonstrated better SF-12 mental-scores as well. Furthermore, another recent study showed, that TKA with good alignment lead to better function with quicker rehabilitation and earlier hospital discharge as well [85]. Therefore, the use of a computer-assisted navigation not only leads to reproducible accuracy of implant positioning in all three planes, but also to better functional outcomes with quicker rehabilitation and earlier hospital discharge due to the advantages of minimally invasive techniques.

3.3 Conclusion
Modern computerized knee navigation systems, appropriately used, aid surgeons to accurately optimize mechanical and axial alignments of the components in all three planes to avoid any malrotation and/ or any errors in coronal, sagittal and axial alignments. These advantages can be achieved not only in the conventional but also in minimally invasive approach without loss of accuracy. There is an increasing statistical evidence of a positive correlation between accurate mechanical alignment after TKA and a better functional as well as quality-of-life patient outcomes. Nevertheless the surgeon has to keep potential pitfalls in association with the computer-assisted procedures in mind. If used correctly, the system is very sophisticated and will improve accuracy. Therefore it will enhance the surgeon`s perspective, but should never replace it.

The use of a computer-assisted navigation leads to reproducible accuracy of implant positioning in all three planes not only in the conventional but also in minimally invasive approaches. In contrast to even the most elaborate mechanical instrumentation system, which relies on visual inspection to confirm the accuracy of the alignment and stability of the TKA, computer-assisted navigation allows the surgeon to objectify every operative osteotomy, the position of trials and finally of the implants. It is well known that there is a definite relationship between the accuracy of implant positioning and longevity and therefore it is imperative to reproduce the implant positioning after a TKA.

Despite the above mentioned advantages and excellent results that may be achieved with computer-assisted navigation, certain factors still cause concern and need to be optimized. As only the cutting guides are navigated, the surgeons may make less than optimal bone resections by bending the saw blade, especially when attempting to cut through sclerotic areas of bone. Differences in cement thickness may also potentially lead to malalignment, even though bone resection was accurate. These latter two problems, which can occur with conventional instrumentation as well, can be obviated only by using the verification plate of the navigation system to verify the correct level and direction of the performed osteotomy.

Computer-assisted technology assists the surgeon to reliably measure kinematics of TKA alignment and stability of the TKA on a screen. Furthermore, surgeons have the opportunity to improve their surgical performance with a direct intra-operative documentation of alignment and orientation of instruments, trials and implants. Additionally computer-assisted navigation allows to verify the final alignment of the implants after component implantation and before the cement hardens to avoid or probably correct considerable error in alignment.

Incorrect positioning of the components may only be a co-factor together with tibiofemoral instability and soft tissue trauma with MIS approach, leading to suboptimal implant loading with early loosening and increased wear. The use of computer-assisted navigation alone will not empower the surgeon to accurately and reproducibly implant a TKA. This might be especially true for the minimally invasive technique. Much technical expertise in the conventional TKA, the skill of the surgeon and their familiarity with the instruments may also be necessary to obtain good results.

4. Competing interests

The authors declare that they have no competing interest.

5. Authors' contributions

We thank Prof. Fabio Catani, Dr. Andrea Ensini, and their collaborator of the Istituti Ortopedici Rizzoli of Bologna, Italy, for their great personal commitment and help with the statistical analysis.

6. Acknowledgements

We appreciate the contribution of Dr. M. Brouwer, Dr. F. Tichler and Dr. M. Stephan, chairmen of the Anesthesiology Department at the Hospital Oberengadin in Samedan, who have contributed to the anesthesiology part of this article, as well. We also acknowledge the great support of the operating room personnel for their cooperation and the Swiss Stryker Company for their permanent remarkable supervision.

No funding or external support was received by any of the authors in support of or in any relationship to the study.

7. References

[1] Callaghan JJ, O'Rourke MR, Iossi MF, Liu SS, Goetz DD, Vittetoe DA, et al. Cemented rotating-platform total knee replacement. A concise follow-up at a minimum of fifteen years. J Bone Joint Surg Am 2005; 87: 1995-1998.

[2] Gill GS, Joshi AB. Long-term results of kinematic condylar knee replacement: An analysis of 404 knees. J Bone Joint Surg Br 2001; 83: 335-358.

[3] Pavone V, Boettner F, Fickert S, Sculco TP. Total condylar knee arthroplasty: A long term follow-up. Clin Orthop Relat Res 2001; 388: 18-25.

[4] Ritter MA, Berend ME, Meding JB, Keating EM, Faris PM, Crites BM. Long-term follow-up of anatomic graduated components posterior cruciate-retaining total knee replacement. Clin Orthop Relat Res 2001; 388: 51-57.

[5] Rodrigues JA, Bhende H, Ranawat CS. Total condylar knee replacement: A 20-year follow-up study. Clin Orthop Relat Res 2001; 388: 10-17.

[6] Insall JN, Binazzi R, Soudry M, Mestriner L. Total knee arthroplasty. Clin Orthop Relat Res 1985; 192: 13-22.

[7] Insall JN, Scuderi GR, Komistek RD, Math K, Dennis D, Anderson DT. Correlation between condylar lift-off and femoral component alignment. Clin Orthop Relat Res 2002; 403: 143-152.

[8] Barrack RL, Schrader T, Bertot AJ, Wolfe MW, Myers L. Component rotation and anterior knee pain after total knee arthroplasty. Clin Orthop Relat Res 2001; 392: 46-55.

[9] Sparmann M, Wolke B, Czupalla H, Banzer D, Zink A. Positioning of total knee arthroplasty with and without navigation support. J Bone Joint Surg Br 2003; 85: 830-835.

[10] Miller MC, Berger RA, Petrella AJ, Karmas A, Rubash HE. Optimizing femoral component rotation in total knee arthroplasty. Clin Orthop Relat Res 2001; 392: 38-45.

[11] Nagamine R, White SE, McCarthy DS, Whiteside LA. Effect of rotational malposition of the femoral component on knee stability kinematics after total knee arthroplasty. J Arthroplasty 1995; 10: 265-270.

[12] Romero J, Duronio JF, Sohrabi A, Alexander N, MacWilliams BC, Jones L, Hungerford D. Varus and valgus flexion laxity of total knee alignment methods in loaded cadaveric knees. Clin Orthop Relat Res 2002; 394: 243-253.

[13] Figgie HE, Goldberg VM, Heiple KG, Moller HS, Gordon NH. The influence of tibial-patellofemoral location on function of the knee in patients with posterior stabilized condylar knee prosthesis. J Bone Joint Surg Am 1986; 68: 1035-40.

[14] Piazza SJ, Delp SL, Stulberg SD, Stern SH. Posterior tilting of the tibial component decreases femoral rollback in posterior-substituting knee replacement: a computer simulation study. J Orthop Res 1998; 16: 264-70.

[15] Ritter MA, Faris PM, Keating EM, Meding JB. Postoperative alignment of total knee replacement. Its effect on survival. Clin Orthop Relat Res 1994; 299: 153-156.

[16] Catani F, Leardini A, Ensini A, Cucca G, Bragonzoni L, Toksvig-Larsen S, Giannini S. The stability of cemented tibial component of total knee arthroplasty: Posterior cruciate-retaining versus posterior-stabilized design. J Arthroplasty 2004; 19(6): 775-782.

[17] Jeffery RS, Morris RW, Denham RA. Coronal alignment after total knee replacement. J Bone Joint Surg Br 1991; 73: 709-714.

[18] Rand JA, Coventry MB. Ten-year evaluation of geometric total knee arthroplasty. Clin Orthop Relat Res 1988; 232: 168-173.

[19] Matziolis G, Krocher D, Weiss U, Tohtz S, Perka C. A prospective, randomized study of computer-assisted and conventional total knee arthroplasty. J Bone Joint Surg Am 2007; 89:236-243.

[20] Lotke PA, Ecker ML. Influence of positioning of prosthesis in total knee replacement. J Bone Joint Surg Am 1977; 59: 77-79.

[21] Nabeyama R, Matsuda S, Miura H, Mawatari T, Kawano T, Iwamoto Y. The accuracy
      of image-guided knee replacement based on computed tomography. J Bone Joint
      Surg Br 2004; 86: 366–371.
[22] Sharkey PF, Hozack WJ, Rothman RH, Shastri S, Jacoby S. Insall Award paper: why are
      total knee arthroplasties failing today? Clin Orthop Relat Res 2002; 404: 7–13.
[23] Stulberg S, Loan P, Sarin V. Computer-assisted navigation in total knee replacement:
      Results of an initial experience in thirty-five patients. J Bone Joint Surg Am 2002;
      84: 90-98.
[24] Chauhan SK, Scott RG, Breidahl W, Beaver RJ. Computer-assisted knee arthroplasty
      versus a conventional jig-based technique. A randomized, prospective trial. J Bone
      Joint Surg Br 2004 Apr; 86(3): 372-7.
[25] Stöckl B, Nogler M, Rosiek R, Fischer M, Kriesmer, Kessler O. Navigation improved
      accuracy of rotational alignment in total knee arthroplasty. Clin Orthop Relat Res
      2004; 426: 180-186.
[26] Bäthis H, Perlick L, Tingart M, Luring C, Zurakowski D, Grifka J. Alignment in total
      knee arthroplasty: A comparison of computer-assisted surgery with conventional
      technique. J Bone Joint Surg Br 2004; 86: 682-687.
[27] Martin A, Wohlgenannt O, Prenn M, Oelsch C, Strempel A. Imageless navigation for
      TKA increased implant accuracy. Clin Orthop Relat Res 2007; 460: 178-184.
[28] Ensini A, Catani F, Leardini A, Romagnoli M, Giannini S. Alignments and clinical
      results in conventional and navigated total knee arthoplasty. Clin Orthop Relat Res
      2007; 457:156-162.
[29] Mielke RK, Clemens U, Jens JH, Kershally S. Navigation in knee endoprosthesis
      implantation: Preliminary experience and prospective comparative study with
      conventional implantation technique. Z Orthop Ihre Grenzgeb 2001; 139: 109-116.
[30] Dalury DF and Dennis DA. Mini-incision total knee arthroplasty can increase risk of
      component malalignment. Clin Orthop Relat Res 2005; 440:77-81.
[31] Insall JN. Choises and compromises in total knee arthroplasty. Clin Orthop Relat Res
      1988; 226:43-48.
[32] Bonutti PM, Mont MA, McMahon M, Ragland PS, Kester M. Minimally invasive total
      knee arthroplasty. J Bone Joint Surg Am 2004; 86: 26-32.
[33] Repicci JA. Mini-invasive knee unicompartmental arthroplasty: bone-sparing
      technique. Surg Technol Int. 2003; 11: 282-286.
[34] Tria AJ, Coon TM. Minimal incision total knee arthroplasty. Clin Orthop Relat Res
      2003; 416: 185-190.
[35] Scuderi GR, Tenholder M, Capeci C. Surgical approaches in mini-incision Total Knee
      Arthroplsty. Clin Orthop Relat Res 2004; 428:61-67.
[36] Hofmann AA, Plaster RL, Murdock LE. Subvastus (southern) approach for primary
      total knee arthroplasty. Clin Orthop Relat Res 1991; 269:70-77.
[37] Engh GA, Holt BT, Parks NL. A midvastus muscle-splitting approach for the total knee
      arthroplasty. J Arthroplasty 1997; 12: 322.
[38] Berger TO, Aglietti P, Mondanelli N, Sensi L. Mini-subvastus versus parapatellar
      approach in total knee arthroplasty. Clin Orthop Relat Res 2005; 440: 82-87.
[39] Dalury DF. Observations of the proximal tibia in total knee arthroplasty. Clin Orthop
      Relat Res 2001; 389:150-155.

[40] Eckhoff DG, Metzger RG, Vandewalle MV. Malrotation associated with implant alignment technique in total knee arthroplasty. Clin Orthop Relat Res 1995; 3211: 28-31.

[41] Labat G. Its Technique and clinical applications: Regional Anesthesia. 2nd edition. Philadelphia, W.B. Saunders, 1924: 45-55.

[42] Winnie AP, Ramamurthy S, Durrani Z. The inguinal paravascular technic of lumbar plexus anesthesia: the '3-in-1 block'. Anesthesia and Analgesia 1973; 52: 989–96.

[43] Biasca N, Wirth S, Bungartz M. Mechanical accuracy of navigated minimally invasive total knee arthroplasty (MIS TKA). The Knee 2009;16 (1): 22–29.

[44] Chin PL, Yang KY, Yeo SJ, Lo NN. Randomized control trial comparing radiographic total knee arthroplasty implant placement using computer navigation versus conventional technique. J Arthroplasty 2005; 20:618-626.

[45] Ewald FC. The Knee Society Total Knee Arthroplasty roentgenographic evaluation and scoring system. Clin Orthop Relat Res 1989; 248: 9-12.

[46] Yoo JH, Chang CB, Shin KS, Seong SC, Kim TK. Anatomical references to assess the posterior tibial slope in total knee arthroplasty: A comparison of 5 anatomical axes. J Arthroplasty 2008; 23(4): 586-592.

[47] Berger RA, Rubash HE, Seel MJ, Thompson WH. Determining the rotational alignment of the femoral component in total knee arthroplasty using the epicondylar axis. Clin Orthop Relat Res 1993; 286: 40-47.

[48] Biasca, N., Bungartz, M.: New on Minimally invasive computer-assisted navigated Total Knee Arthroplasty (MIS TKA). Minerva Orthop Traumat 2010; 1:1-10.

[49] Jenny JY, Boeri C. Navigated implantation of total knee endoprosthesis: A comparative study with conventional instruments. Z Orthop Ihre Grenzgeb 2001; 139: 117-119.

[50] Laskin RS. New techniques and concepts in total knee replacement. Clin Orthop Relat Res 2003; 416:151-153.

[51] Bonutti PM, Neal DJ, Kestler MA. Minimal incision total knee arthroplasty using the suspended leg technique. Orthopedics 2003; 26: 899-903.

[52] Laskin RS. Minimally invasive total knee arthroplasty: The results justify its use. Clin Orthop Relat Res 2005; 440: 54-59.

[53] Karpman RR, Smith HL. Comparison of the early results of minimally invasive vs standard approaches to total knee arthroplasty: A prospective, randomized study. J Arthroplasty 2008, 24(5):681-8.

[54] Catani F, Biasca N, Ensini A, Leardini A, Belvedere C, Giannini S. Tibial and femoral joint line restoration after navigated total knee arthroplasty. J Bone Joint Surg Am 2010, in Review.

[55] Bauwens K, Matthes G, Wich M, Gebhard F, HansonB, Ekkernkamp A, et al. Navigated total knee replacement: A meta-analysis. J Bone Joint Surg Am 2007; 89:261-269.

[56] Mason JB, Fehring TK, Estok R, Banel D, Fahrbach K. Meta-analysis of alignment outcomes in computer-assisted total knee arthroplasty surgery. J Arthroplasty 2007; 22(8): 1097-1106.

[57] Jenny JY, Clemens U, Kohler S, Kiefer H, Konermann W, Miehlke RK. Consistency of implantation of a total knee arthroplasty with a non-image-based navigation system. J Arthroplasty 2005; 20(7): 832-839.

[58] Haaker RG, Stockheim M, Kamp M, Proff G, Breitenfelder J, Ottersbach A. Computer-assisted navigation increased precision of component placement in total knee arthroplasty. Clin Orthop Relat Res 2005; 433: 152-159.
[59] Molfetta L, Caldo D. Computer navigation versus conventional implantation for varus knee total arthroplasty: A case-control study at 5 years follow-up. The Knee 2008; 15: 75-79.
[60] Kim YH, Kim JS, Yoon SH. Alignment and orientation of the components in total knee replacement with and without navigation support. J Bone Joint Surg Br 2007; 89(4): 471-476.
[61] Malik MH, Wadia F, Porter ML. Preliminary radiological evaluation of the Vector Vision CT-free knee module for implantation of the LCS knee prosthesis. The Knee 2007; 14(1): 19-21.
[62] Decking R, Markmann Y, Fuchs J, Puhl W, Scharf HP. Leg axis after computer-navigated total knee arthroplasty: A randomized trial comparing computer-navigated and manual implantation. J Arthroplasty 2005; 20(3): 282-288.
[63] Siston RA, Patel JJ, Goodman SB, Delp SL, Giori NJ. The variability of femoral rotational alignment in total knee arthroplasty. J Bone Joint Surg Am 2005; 87: 2276-2280.
[64] Catani F, Biasca N, Ensini A, Leardini A, Bianchi L, Digennari V, et al. Alignment deviation between bone resection and final implant positioning in computer-navigated total knee arthroplasty. J Bone Joint Surg Am 2008: 90: 765-771.
[65] Hart R, Janecek M, Chaker A, Bucek P. Total knee arthroplasty implanted with and without kinematic navigation. Int Orthop 2003; 27: 366-369.
[66] Oberst M, Bertsch C, Wurstlin S, Holz U. CT analysis of leg alignment after conventional versus navigated knee prosthesis implantation. Unfallchirurg 2003; 106:941-948.
[67] Olcott CW, Scott RD. The Ranawat Award. Femoral component rotation during total knee arthroplasty. Clin Orthop Relat Res 1999; 367: 39-42.
[68] Chauhan SK, Clark GW, Lloyd S, Scott RG, Breidahl W, Sikorski JM. Computer-assisted total knee replacement: A controlled cadaver study using a multi-parameter quantitative ct assessment of alignment (the Perth CT Protocol). J Bone Joint Surg Br 2004; 86-B: 818-23.
[69] Siston RA, Giori NJ, Goodman SB, Delp SL. Surgical navigation for total knee arthroplasty: A perspective. J Biomech 2007; 40: 728-735.
[70] Van Damme G, Defoort K, Ducoulombier Y, Van Glabbeek F, Bellemans J, Victor J. What should the surgeon aim for when performing computer-assisted total knee arthroplasty? J Bone Joint Surg Am 2005; 87(Suppl 2): 52–58
[71] Tokuhara Y, Kadoya, Y, Nakagawa, S., et al. The flexion gap in normal knees: An MRI Study. J Bone Joint Surg [Br] 2004; 86B1: 1133-6
[72] Todo S, Kadoya Y, Moilanen T, et al. Anteroposterior and rotational movement of the femur during knee flexion. Clin Orthop 1999;362: 162-70.
[73] Hill PF, Vedi V, Williams A, et al. Tibiofemoral movement 2: the loaded and unloaded living knee studied by MRI. J Bone Joint Surg 2000;82-B: 1196-8.
[74] Iwaki H, Pinskerova V, Freeman MAR. Tibiofemoral movement 1: the shapes and relative movement of the femur and tibia in the unloaded cadaver knee. J Bone Joint Surg 2000;82-B: 1189-95.

[75] Nakagawa S, Kadoya Y, Todo S, et al. Tibiofemoral movement 3: full flexion in the living knee studied by MRI. J Bone Joint Surg [Br] 2000;82-B: 1199-200.

[76] Moore TH, Meyer MH. Apparatus to position knees for varus-valgus stress roentgenograms. J Bone J Surg Am 1977;59: 984.

[77] Takahashi T, Wada Y, Yamamoto H. Soft tissue balancing with pressure distribution during total knee arthroplasty. J Bone J Surg Br 1997;79: 235-239.

[78] Stahelin T, Kessler O, Pfirmann C, Jacob HAC, Romero J. Fluoroscopy assisted stress radiography for varus-valgus stability assessment in flexion after total knee arthroplasty. J Arthroplasty 2003;18: 513-515.

[79] Oliver JH, Coughlin LP. Objective knee evaluation using the Genucum knee analysis system: Clinical implications. Am J Sports Medicine 1987;15: 571-578.

[80] Wirth S, Biasca N. Joint laxity in navigated total knee arthroplasty. Presented at the 2006 CAOS Annual Meeting, Helsinki, 2006.

[81] Ranawat CS, Insall J, Shine J. Duo-Condylar knee arthroplasty: Hospital for Special Surgery design. Clin Orthop Relat Res 1976; 120: 76-82

[82] Insall JN, Dorr LD, Scott RD, Scott WN. Rationale of the Knee Society Clinical Rating System. Clin Orthop Relat Res 1989; 248: 13-14.

[83] Lingard EA, Katz JN, Wright RJ, Wright EA, Sledge CB. Validity and responsiveness of the Knee Society Clinical Rating System in comparison with the SF-36 and WOMAC. J Bone Joint Surg Am 2001; 83(12): 1856-1864.

[84] Choong PF, Dowsey MM, Stoney JD. Does accurate anatomical alignment result in better function and quality of life? A prospective randomized controlled trial comparing conventional and computer-assisted total knee arthroplasty. J Arthroplasty 2008, 24(4):560-9.

[85] Longstaff LM, Sloan K, Stamp N, Scaddan M, Beaver R. Good alignment after Total Knee Arthroplasty leads to faster rehabilitation and better function. J Arthroplasty 2008, 24(4):570-8.

14

Concepts in Computer Assisted Total Knee Replacement Surgery

M. Fosco[1], R. Ben Ayad[1], R. Fantasia[1],
D. Dallari[1] and D. Tigani[2]
[1]*From First Ward of Orthopaedic Surgery, University
of Bologna, Rizzoli Orthopaedic Institute, Bologna*
[2]*From Department of Orthopaedic Surgery, Santa Maria
alle Scotte Hospital ,Siena
Italy*

1. Introduction

Total knee arthroplasty (TKA) is commonly considered to be a reliable procedure, with implant survival rates higher than 90% at 10 to 15 years of follow-up. The goal of total knee replacement surgery is to relieve pain and obtain better knee function, those achieved by correct patient selection, pre-operative deformity, implant design, correct surgical technique and patient participation in the rehabilitation protocol (Nizard et al, 2002).

Several technical requirements during TKA are important to obtain good results:

- correction of deformities;
- achievement of functional joint motion and stability;
- optimal balancing of soft tissues;
- satisfactory alignment in the frontal, sagittal and horizontal planes.

From literature data alignment in frontal plane must be into 2° or 3° range around a neutral alignment; this thought is demonstrated by Ritter at al who observed that prostheses implanted in varus position had a lower survival rate than prostheses implanted in a neutral or valgus position (Ritter et al, 1994); moreover Jeffery at al observed that when mechanical axis was in 3° valgus-varus range, the loosening rate was 3%, whereas it's 24% when the alignment was out of this range (Jeffery et al, 1991). The alignment in the horizontal plane is of particular importance for extensor mechanism stability, patellar wear, tilted patella, prostheses dislocation or loosening. In a study of Berger et al it was observed that patients with extensor mechanism problems have internal rotation of the femoral and tibial components (Berger et al, 1998).

Technically, there is a definite relationship between the accuracy of implant positioning and long-term durability (Jeffery et al, 1991; Stulberg et al, 2002): the position of prosthetic components and, consequently the alignment of mechanical axis, could be the cause of polyethylene wear due to overload stresses, ending finally by prosthetic loosening. The postoperative mechanical axis of the lower limb should be a straight line passing through the center of the hip, the center of the knee, and the center of the ankle; so that satisfactory position of a TKA prosthesis is commonly accepted to be an alignment within 3° from this neutral axis (Fig. 1).

To improve precision of implant positioning, various mechanical alignment guides are used, both intramedullary and extramedullary, but technical errors with these conventional surgical techniques still occur. Moreover, mechanical alignment and sizing devices presume a standardized bone geometry that may not be applied to all patients. Even the most elaborate mechanical instrumentation systems rely on visual inspection to confirm the accuracy of stability and of limb and implant alignment at the conclusion of the TKA procedure.

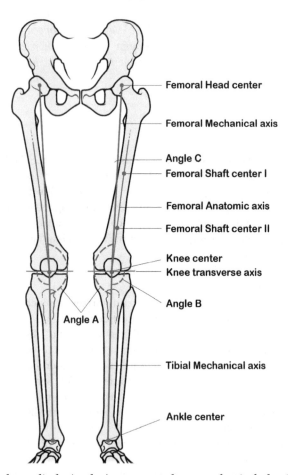

Fig. 1. Axes of the lower limb. Angle A represents knee mechanical physiologic valgus angle of 3°. Angle B represents tibia shaft angle, that is in 3° of varus from knee transverse axis. Angle C corresponds to angle between femoral anatomic and mechanical axis (6° of valgus). Femoral anatomic axis could be easily determined by two points located at the centre of the shaft. Mechanical axis of the lower limb passes near or through knee center and lies from femoral head center to ankle center.

Computer assisted surgery (CAS) for TKA was firstly introduced to improve the accuracy of alignment of the implanted prosthesis, thinking that it could make an inexperienced or occasional TKA surgeon performing more like an expert TKA surgeon, or to address the limitations inherent in mechanical instrumentation systems used for total knee replacement surgery (Jeffery et al, 1991; Stulberg et al, 2002).

During the last Decades CAS instrumentations have been improved in accuracy and various studies have been made to analyse results using this technique in TKA surgery. Advocates of this technique in total knee replacement claim benefits in terms of improving accuracy for alignment of the leg and orientation of the components, as well as a reduction in blood loss and a lower rate of intracranial micro emboli compared with traditional surgery.

The survival rate for modern total knee artroplasty is reported between 80% to 95% after 10 years of follow up (Buechel et al, 2002; Robertsson et al, 2001), and the most important factor of failure is malalignment of mechanical axis (Jeffery et al, 1991; Rand et al, 1988). Recently the introduction of CAS have gained up improvement in post operative mechanical alignment (Bathis et al, 2004; Chauhan et al, 2004; Chin et al, 2005; Decking et al, 2005; Haaker et al, 2005). However, no clear published results associated with superior clinical and patients perceived functional results and consequently longer survival rate (Stulberg et al, 2006).

2. History of CAS and review of literature

The history of CAS for total knee replacement was dated back to the middle nineties (Picard et al, 1997). Intraoperative navigation in total joint replacement began in 1992, when W. Barger, in Sacramento (California) performed the first computer assisted surgery in orthopaedics for total hip replacement, while the first total knee replacement began in France, in January 1997, by F. Picard and D. Saragaglia after a study on cadavers (Picard et al, 1997; Saragaglia et al, 2001; Delp et al; 1998) and then started a prospective randomized study comparing the computer assisted technique to the conventional surgery in 50 patients. The postoperative mechanical axis was 181.2° ± 2.72° in CAS group and 179.04° ± 2.53° in conventional group, with a statistical significant value in favor of CAS group and reduction of outliers. The mechanical axis was in fact between 177° and 183° in 75% of patients in conventional group and in 84% in CAS group (Saragaglia et al, 2001). The Authors concluded their paper saying that computer-assisted surgery for total knee arthroplasty provides remarkably reliable results and that "once the growing pains of this new material have been mastered, all surgeons should be able to expect an improvement in the positioning of prosthetic implantations".

Bathis et al. in a prospective study compared an imageless navigation system to conventional methods using an intramedullary femoral guide and an extra-medullary tibia jig. They reported the postoperative mechanical axis to be within 3° of varus or valgus in 96% of the navigation cases versus 78% of the conventional cases (Bathis et al, 2004).

Other study by Chauman et al. in which they compared a computer-assisted knee arthroplasty with the current conventional jig-based technique in 70 patients randomly allocated to receive either of the methods. All the patients were evaluated postoperatively with computer tomography imaging observing a significant improvement in the alignment of the components using computer-assisted surgery with regard to femoral varus/valgus (p=0.032), femoral rotation (p=0.001), tibial varus/valgus (p=0.047) tibial posterior slope (p=0.0001), tibial rotation (p=0.011) and femoral-tibial mismatch (p=0.037). The Authors reported that computer-assisted surgery took longer time with a mean increase of 13 minutes regarding the conventional technique, but the blood loss was significantly lower (Chauchan et al, 2004).

A significant number of recent randomized controlled trial studies compared the use of imageless CAS with conventional methods; the results of these studies are shown in Table 1.

Authors	Year of publication	M.A >3° (n/N)		M.A >2° (n/N)	
		CAS	Conv	CAS	Conv
Saragaglia	2001	4/25	6/25	10/25	11/25
Sparmann	2003	0/120	16/120	3/120	27/120
Chauhan	2004	5/34	10/30	11/34	11/30
Bathis	2004	3/80	18/80	15/80	32/80
Stulberg	2006	21/38	19/40	30/38	30/40
Pang	2009	2/35	9/35	7/35	17/35
Choong	2009	7/57	21/54	\	\

Table 1. Different RCTs studies comparing post-operative mechanical angle in conventional and imageless CAS knee arthroplasty. CAS=Computer Assisted Surgery, Conv= conventional surgery, M.A= Mechanical Angle, n= number of knees, N= total number of knees.

Most of those meta-analysis studies of the best available evidence indicate significant improvement in component orientation and a better restoration of the mechanical limb alignment when CAS is used (Mason et al, 2007). In review of the past literature, there were only few papers which have indicated that there was no significant difference between computer-assisted navigated TKA and conventional TKA (Mielke et al, 2001).

In the report by Kim et al (Kim et al, 2007), bilateral sequential total knee replacements were carried out by one senior author in 160 patients (320 knees). One knee was replaced using a CT-free computer-assisted navigation system and the other side replaced conventionally without navigation. The Authors studied their cases with both standard radiological and CT imaging to determine the alignment of the components. The results of imaging and the number of outliers for all radiological parameters were not statistically different between the groups (p=0.109 to p=0.920). The post-operative limb alignment (femoral-tibial angle) exceeded 3° of varus/valgus deviation in only 18% (Sparman et al, 2003) of the patients operated by using the conventional technique, and in about 21%(Jenny et al, 2001) of the patients that were operated by navigation system.

3. Different computer navigation systems

Existing computer assisted surgery system must allow the accomplishment of the objectives above described: ensure optimal positioning of the prosthesis in the three planes (frontal, sagittal and horizontal); ensure optimization of the ligament balance; maintain joint stability (Nizard et al, 2002).

Firstly, computer-assisted navigation systems could be distinguished between active and passive computer systems as described by Picard at al. (Picard et al, 2001).

Active computer systems, also named robots, are able to realize the entire surgical procedure after the knee as been exposed through a conventional approach. The use of such complicated systems is viable only if the installation and functions during the surgical procedure can be performed within a reasonable time. The results of such systems have been presented in different studies (Tenbusch et al, 2001).

Passive computer systems do not perform any part of the surgical procedure which remains under direct control of the surgeon, that allowing him to apply and positioning the cutting guides.

Location systems for such CAS procedure crucially require a perfect and permanent fixation to the instrument. Two location systems are currently available, magnetic field detector and optical detector. Magnetic location systems are designed to generate a cylindrical field of about 80cm of diameter, received by collectors called dynamic reference frames (DRFs), which are fixed to the instruments or to the bone. This system does not require any particular position of the surgical team around the patient or between the system and the collectors, so no line of sight issues are present with EM tracking, but this system introduces the problem of metal influence. In fact, their failure is related to the use of ferromagnetic instrument in conventional technique like bone retractors, hammers and drill as well as mobile phones and hand watches. Lionberger (Lionberger et al, 2006) who studied the various problems of electromagnetic technology, pointed out the limited distortion of titanium, cobalt-chrome and some stainless steels. The software is furthermore designed with the possibility to induce an "off-signal" before the externally-generated source of instability or signal inaccuracy can be produced. Potentially, the collectors are linked to the computer system by wires, that could be troublesome during surgery.

Optical systems using infrared light are the most widely employed method of connection between the surgical field and the computer. These consist of two or three infrared camera sensors that detect the position of active or passive trackers implanted on the leg through rigid bodies or special shape instrument, which must all remain within the line of sight (Fig. 2).

The active leg trackers use systems that have light emitting diodes (LED) which sent out light pulsed to the optical localizer (Fig. 3). Opposite passive leg trackers use reflecting spheres mounted to the rigid body; recently new trackers are available consists of reflective discs connected together in angular arrangement (Fig. 4). Potential mistakes of data detection could be due to proximity of two localizers.

The advantage of optical systems is accurate detection without possible distorted information, while main disadvantages are usually due to reflecting spheres wear, the volume of infrared camera in the surgical room and also necessary adaptable positioning of surgical team personal to the system until the collectors have been located by the camera (Table 2).

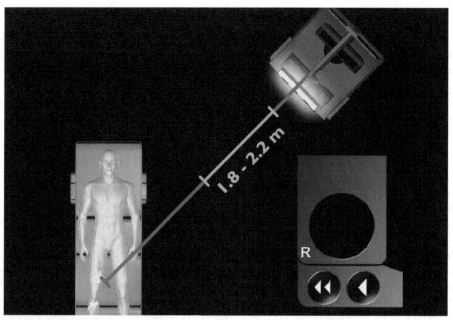

Fig. 2. Working station, consisting on display monitor and infra-red light camera sensors attached to stander, is positioned in a far position. Trackers have to be always within the line of sight with the camera. (Courtesy of B.Braun, Melsungen, D).

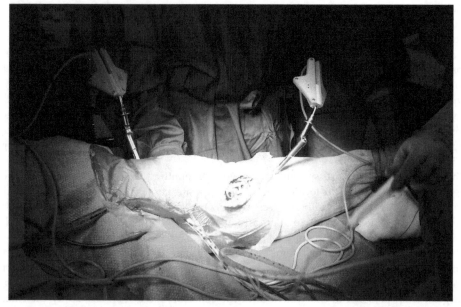

Fig. 3. Active optical trackers and intra-operative alignment of femoral and tibial parts

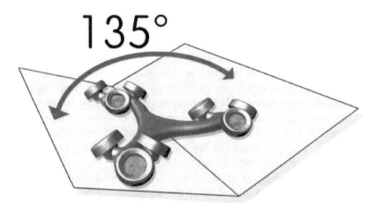

Fig. 4. Disc shape optical passive trackers connected in angular pattern (Courtesy of Zimmer, Warsaw, USA)

NAVIGATION SYSTEM		MAIN DISADVANTAGES
According to Picard et al, 2001	Active computer systems (robots)	Technically complicated and expensive system, very long surgical time
	Passive computer systems	Partially surgeon controlled-dependent results
According to Stulberg et al, 2002	Image-based (CT, MRI, fluoroscopic view)	Irradiation exposure of patient, adjunctive cost for peri-operative imaging procedure
	Image free	Additional surgical time, no clear information concerning the implants rotation
SIGNAL DETECTOR		MAIN DISADVANTAGES
Magnetic field detector		Metal influence needing specific-instrumentation, sometimes distorted information detected
Optical detector		Mistakes of data due to proximity of localizers, bulky camera, adaptable positioning of surgical team personal
TRACKER		MAIN DISADVANTAGES
Active optical trackers		Less detection accuracy due room light interferance
Passive optical trackers		Needing instrument calibration as first step, frequent cleaning of reflecting spheres/discs during surgery

Table 2. Different systems and components of navigation surgery.

3.1 Image-based navigation systems

According to Stulberg et al. CAS for joint replacement can be classified into two categories: image based and image-free navigation systems.

Using imaging devices the preoperative morphological data acquisition is necessary, which is gained by two different sources. The first one is preoperative imaging by a CT scan or MRI; second one is perioperative fluoroscopy imaging, performed in the operating room, during surgery. This imaging requires a specially modified fluoroscopy unit and entails the maneuvering of a relatively bulky and expensive apparatus during surgery.

CT-scan imaging modality which allow 3D reconstruction of bone morphology and bony landmarks, is probably the most time consuming step for the surgeon, while the MRI could be used in order to have information on soft tissue structure, but definition of bony landmarks is far inferior to that of CT-scan.

In such system, the registration and identification of special pointes process during the surgery is needed in order to match it with the image saved on the screen. Programmed software, using a mathematical algorithm, is able to help surgeon to identify these points during the matching process. Main advantage of image based systems is that it can be used in cases with extreme deformities, as seen in post fracture malunion and some bone disease, like Paget disease. It is possible to reconstruct 3D models when ipsilateral hip arthroplasty is present, and also in cases of revision of mono-compartemental knee prostheses or in two stage revision with temporary spacer in situ. However the main disadvantage is mandatory to obtain a preoperative CT-scan which is an additional hospital expense and a source of irradiation for the patients (Nizard et al, 2001).

Although potentially useful for knee reconstructive surgery imaging devices currently employed with CAS have been at present abandoned as requiring additional steps without providing significant benefits.

3.2 Image-free navigation systems

Image-free optical systems using infrared light are currently the most widely employed method of connection between the surgical field and the computer. These systems utilizes either optical (infra-red light), or electromagnetic devices that detect the position of active or passive markers implanted on the leg through rigid bodies or special shape instrument, which must all remain within the line of sight. The most important characteristic of this system is its ability to provide instant information regarding in vivo kinematics of the joint thus allowing the surgeon to quantify data, have dynamic intraoperative feedback or information and obtain more reproducible results..

First step is localization of important bony points: center of femoral head, knee center and ankle center are main points to identify (Fig. 5). Junction between these three points define the mechanical axis of lower limb. Several methods are available to define these points, which include:

- Center of femoral head localized by kinematic analysis of the hip joint; passive mobilization of the hip is needed to determine this center without reference point on the iliac crest.
- Knee center can be defined in two ways, one is based on kinematic analysis which requires passive mobilization of the knee, the other way is based on the definition of anatomic landmark (i.e. intercondylar trochlear notch, anterior tibial plateau eminence) (Yoshioka et al, 1989).

- Ankle center which is also determined by two methods, kinematic analysis of the ankle during passive motion, the other method is acquisition of anatomical points on the medial and lateral malleoli.

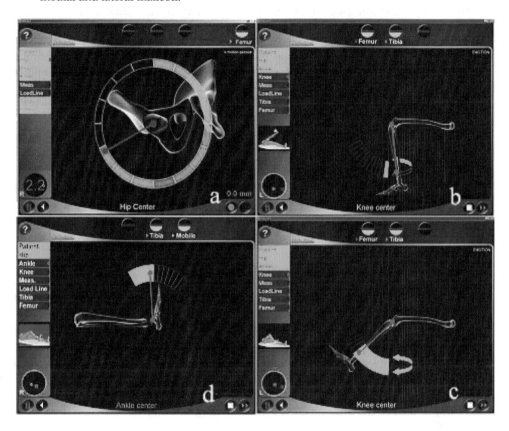

Fig. 5. Localization of hip (A), knee (B,C) and ankle (D) joint center

Two types of information can be given by these image free systems, in two or three dimensions (3D). In two-dimensional systems, only the axes in frontal and sagittal planes are available. In 3D systems, digitization of anatomical structures allows reconstruction of an almost complete distal femur or proximal tibia using either statistically reshaped bony structures or completely redesigned bony structures from direct digitization.

The most important advantage of this system is avoidance of irradiation exposure, while their disadvantages are represented by additional time needed during the operation, and no clear information obtained concerning the rotational position of the implants (Arima et al,1995; Kats et al, 2001; Saragaglia et al, 2001).

The first results reported with these systems are encouraging (Saragaglia et al, 2001; Clemens et al, 2001; Jenny et al, 2001; Kiefer et al, 2001). In a randomized study Saragaglia et al. have compared 25 knees operated with a conventional technique and 25 knees operated with the Orthopilot® navigation system; a satisfactory alignment in the frontal plane, defined as a mechanical axis between 3° varus and 3° valgus alignment, was observed more often with the navigation system (84% versus 75% conventional technique). In a case-control study, Jenny et al. compared 60 prostheses implanted with the Orthopilot® system to 60 prostheses implanted using a conventional technique. With the navigation system 53 out of 60 prostheses were in the 3° valgus-3° varus range, whereas only 43 out of 60 were in this range with conventional system (p<0.05). Tigani et al. analysing 123 patients who underwent TKA with CAS, have retrospectively compared two different techniques of total knee arthroplasty (gap balancing and measured resection) utilizing different computer navigation systems; using inter class correlation ICC and paired t-test, they reported that no difference regarding the joint line level, and significant improvement in the ability to create mechanical alignment at 180°±3° in frontal plane in 95% of the operated patients (Tigani et al, 2010).

4. Indication for CAS in knee surgery

Computer-assisted navigation seems to be helpful in those difficult situations where accurate alignment remains crucial but traditional instrumentation is not applicable. Traditional cutting guides during knee arthroplasty relies on intramedullary (IM) femoral instruments and either intramedullary or extramedullary (EM) tibial instruments to obtain proper axial alignment.

Intramedullary instruments cannot be used in patients with:

- Retained hardware that would be difficult or inadvisable to remove (Fig. 6) or long-stemmed hip implants (Fig. 7) that could obstruct introduction of long IM instruments;
- Severe posttraumatic extrarticular femoral deformity when one is unable to pass an IM guide to accurately make a distal femoral cut (Fig. 8);
- IM guides may increase the infection risk in patients with history of focal diaphyseal osteomyelitis around the knee joint (Fehring et al, 2006);
- Patients with severe cardiopulmonary disease or a history of foramen ovale who may be at risk for embolic dissemination because of femoral IM instrumentation (Berman et al, 1998).

These problems can be avoided with extramedullary jigs on the tibial side, but EM instrumentation is cumbersome on the femoral side, which requires radiographically identifying the femoral head and a freehand technique of pinning the distal femoral resection guide. In cases with retained hardware or prosthesis, the distance from the articular surface is a topic question to take into consideration. The surgeon should be aware that in addition to the 9 to 11 mm of usual resection amount on distal femur a supplementary distance of at least 12 to 17 mm of femoral bone, according to the size and type of prosthesis, is necessary for the central box housing of posterior stabilized prosthesis (Haas et al, 2000).

In cases of extrarticular deformity, simultaneous or staged corrective osteotomy and total knee arthroplasty has been advocated to achieve normal alignment of the long bones and better ligament balancing. However, this technique may be associated with substantial complications, including nonunion at the osteotomy site and arthrofibrosis (Engh et al, 1990; Lonner et al, 2000).

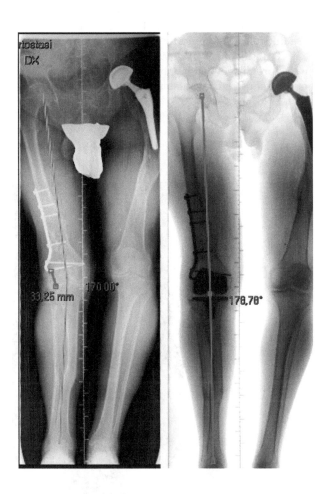

Fig. 6. Patient with blade-plate on distal right femur that prevent use of intramedullary guides. CAS during TKA surgery allow to correct mechanical axis and good positioning of prosthetic components.

An alternative to the combined osteotomy/TKA approach is to perform intraarticular bone resection and soft-tissue balancing. This procedure may be appropriate when the insertion of the collateral ligaments of the knee would not be jeopardized by the intra-articular bone resection (Wolff et al, 1991). The limits of intra-articular correction of an extrarticular deformity have been elucidated by Wang (Wang et al; 2001), who found that intraarticular resection without osteotomy was successful for patients with an average of 20° of coronal plane deformity in the tibia and femur. So that CAS facilitates correction of the deformity and helps avoid massive intra-articular soft tissue release.

Obese patients are another challenging subgroup undergoing TKA. In these cases CAS helps to accurately estimate the center of the femoral head and the overall limb and component alignment, otherwise difficult to be clinically judged with conventional technique. Various authors (Berend et al, 2004; Choong et al, 2009) reported higher incidence of revision when body mass index was more than 30, with only 56% of knees having a final mechanical axis aligned within 3° of neutral using conventional technique, compared to 93% of knees in the navigated group.

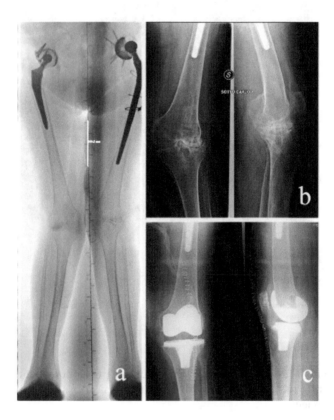

Fig. 7. Valgus osteoarthric knees in patient with long stemmed arthroplasty at left hip. Computer-assisted surgery allow to implant knee prosthesis without use of intramedullary femoral guide.

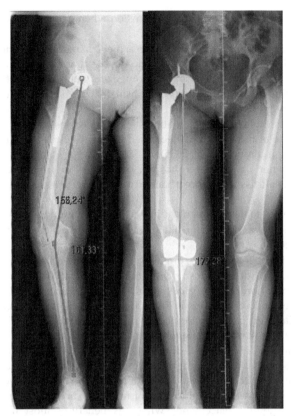

Fig. 8. Knee osteoarthritis with extrarticular femoral post-traumatic deformity(malunion). TKA was performed using computer-assisted technique with intrarticular correction of the deformity.

5. Advantages and disadvantages of CAS

Computer-assisted surgery in TKA offers several advantages against traditional surgery, that can be resumed as follow:

- Better accuracy in bone cutting and positioning of prosthetic components (Martin et al, 2007; Bathis et al, 2004; Aravind et al, 2011). In a study of Martin et al, they found that the mechanical axis of the limb was within 3° varus/valgus in 92% of the patients who had navigated procedures versus 76% of patients who had conventional surgery. The tibial slope showed a rate of inaccuracy of 3° or less for 98 % of the patients in the navigated TKA group versus 80% of the patients in the conventional group (Martin et al, 2007);

- The possibility to do a three-dimensional planning and alignment of the prothesis (Stockl et al, 2004);

- Dynamic assessment of deformity at any angle as opposed to conventional technique where tensioning devices can be used in 0° extension and 90° flexion (Aravind et al, 2011);

- Assessment of soft tissue and collateral tension when gap balancing technique applied (Chauhan et al, 2004);
- Intra-operative range of motion analysis to achieve maximum function, as confirmed by some reports like that of Austin et al, who observed as navigation could be a reliable tool for performing in vivo assessment of range of motion (Austin et al, 2008);
- Decreased incidence of pulmonary embolism in knee surgery, due to using of only extra-medullary guidance (Kalairajah et al, 2005);
- Minimally invasive surgery, which allows lesser blood loss during and after operation, reduces risks at transfusion and decreased hospital admission duration, those gives financial saving (Kalairajah et al, 2005);
- Early rehabilitation and shorter hospital stay, due to improved accuracy in limb alignment and soft tissue balance obtained with computer-assisted TKA (Choong et al, 2009).

Nevertheless, there are some disadvantages by using navigation:

- The surgical time was longer for navigated TKA than for the conventional procedure (Martin et al, 2007);
- Additional incisions for reference pins;
- Increased incidence of fractures or infections related to the pins sites (less than 1% reported complication rate) (Wysocki et al, 2008; Chi-Huan et al, 2008; Manzotti et al, 2008; Bonutti et al, 2008; Jung et al, 2007; Ossendorf et al, 2006). According to literature, larger pins diameter (5 mm), eccentric or repeated drilling and diaphyseal placement may be at greater risk of such complication (Wysocki et al, 2008; Chi-Huan et al, 2008);
- Financial saving by low hospital duration cost effective in health care however is still not realized. Solver et al. applying Moarkov decision model to evaluate the impact of hospital volume on the cost-effectiveness of CAS arthroplasty, have revealed that CAS is less likely to be cost-effective investment in health care improvement in centers with low volume of joint replacements, where its benefit is most likely to be realized; anyway it may be effective in centers with high volume of joint replacements (Solver et al, 2008).

Computer system is very sophisticated and, if used correctly, will improve accuracy. The system enhances the surgeon's perspective but should never replace it. Some pitfalls that can arise by using this technique include:

- Malfunctioning of the navigation system due to: dirty reflectors, camera or rounding errors or dislodgement of the reference pins (low rate of about 0.5%) which is likely due to less secure fixation afforded by unicortical fixation (Richard et al, 2010);
- Stretching against the extensor mechanism by reference pins;
- Inaccurate identification of the anatomic bone landmarks (Robinson et al, 2006);
- Avulsion of the patellae tendon by excessive traction on the patella;
- Inappropriate tibia rotation could be a less frequent pitfall when using imageless systems;
- Data registration inaccuracy; nevertheless causes to this problem must be understood by surgeons who use these devices. At least three potential causes of registration inaccuracy were identified when this image-free navigation system was applied to total knee replacement surgery:

1. Preoperative deformity and instability related to the original pathology of arthritic knee.
2. Computer hardware and software inaccuracy.
3. Surgical technique.

Additional updates of the computer software and surgical hardware are important because they appear to have substantially reduced the registration variations that result from all three causes of this type of inaccuracy in computer-assisted orthopaedic applications.

6. Surgical strategies with CAS

As for standard conventional surgery, two surgical strategies are possible in TKA with CAS (Hungerford et al, 1982): a measured resection approach (Fig. 9), in which bone landmarks are used to guide resections equal to the distal and posterior thickness of the femoral component, or a gap-balancing approach (Fig. 10), in which equal collateral ligament tension in extension and flexion is sought before and as a guide to definitive bone cuts. Both techniques aim to have symmetric flexion and extension gaps in terms of gap size and angular alignment.

In computer aided technique, after the first step of registration and identification of the key anatomic landmarks the computer system will identify the bone position in the space, the pre-requisite for the registration are the trackers which are attached to the bone, thus commonly considered the most fundamental aspect of registration accuracy. After registration process, the computer system kinematically gathers the information regarding joint anatomy, limb alignment, level of bone to be resected and matches knee anatomy with the size and type of the implant. The following implementation and verification step determine cutting blocks position, component to component position and soft tissue balance (Aravind et al, 2011).

Surgical steps in imageless CAS knee arthroplasty, do not require any preoperative plane or image. The initial step is the instrument calibration in passive rigid body systems (Orthosoft- Zimmer®) (Fig. 11), or without calibration in active rigid body systems (Orthopilot®- Aesculap/B-Braun).

This followed by the placement of the femoral and tibial trackers or rigid bodies that should be fixed to bone with precaution, to avoid any injury of adjacent neurovascular structures and the interference with surgical tools. The trackers should be in the field of the infrared camera to remain detectable throughout the procedure. Trackers fixation should be positioned with an angle of almost 90° with respect to diaphysis and on vertical axis 30-45° medially in femur and 45°-60° medially in tibia.

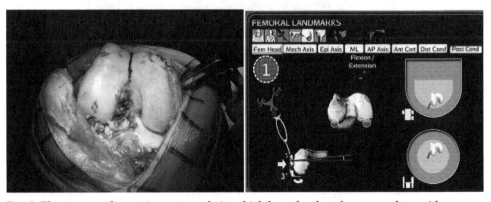

Fig. 9. The measured resection approach, in which bone landmarks are used to guide resections equal to the distal and posterior thickness of the femoral component

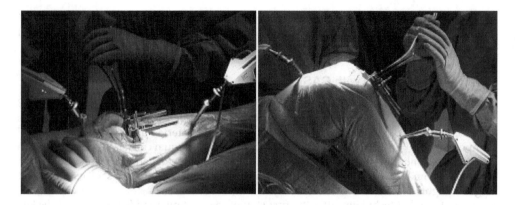

Fig. 10. The gap balancing approach, in which identical collateral ligament tension in extension and flexion is sought before and as a guide to final bone cuts

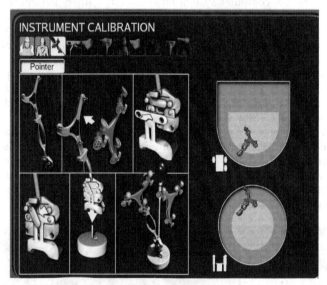

Fig. 11. Passive rigid bodies trackers calibration.

Once the knee is exposed next step consists on registration of the anatomical axis through the localization of the center of the knee, the center of the hip, and the center of the ankle joint using kinematic registration, those visualized on the computer screen (Fig 5).

The other anatomical landmarks located with the pointer or special paddle and necessary for the virtual reconstruction of the lower limb axis are the distal, posterior femoral condyles, medial/lateral tibial plateau and anterior tibial eminence. When soft tissues balance technique is used, it can be performed before or after bone resections with the trial spacer in place or using mechanical retractors both in extension and 90° flexion (Fig. 12).

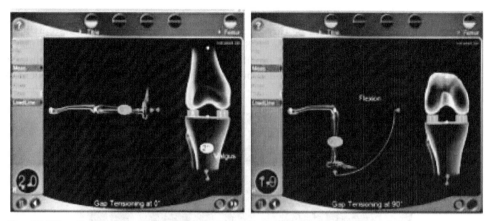

Fig. 12. Visualization of gap after tensioning of soft tissue in extention and flexion.

Now the initial lower limb mechanical axis can be visualized on the screen and in different angles of flexion; in addiction the degree of deformity to be corrected by bone cuts, and the initial knee range of motion can be registered. The most important surgical step in navigating TKA is the planning for 3D reconstruction for bone cuts and prosthesis orientation, through the working screen visible on the monitor (Fig. 13).

During this step, the surgeon by moving the virtual pointer tip, can target any value on the screen, except for the measured gaps. So that, through this procedure all femur cuts and sizes of the components to be implanted can be planned step by step, as well as the notching and the implant rotation.

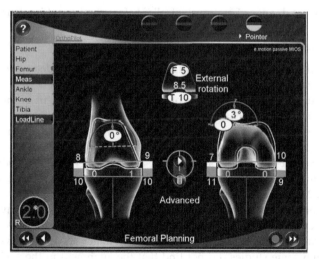

Fig. 13. Planning screen guided by surgeon.

The varus/valgus angle display, resection height display and femoral rotation display can be modified during this step before starting femoral cuts and to achieve equal rectangular gap spaces in both flexion and extention. The tibia display on the screen indicates the gap remaining after all cuts and after the implantation of all components, assuming possible additional soft tissue release will be carried out. Computer-based alignment systems have been developed to address the limitations inherent in mechanical instrumentation, so that it is recommended that before definitive prosthetic components implantation, the limb axis and the knee range of motion be controlled by CAS monitoring with the trail component in place (Fig. 14).

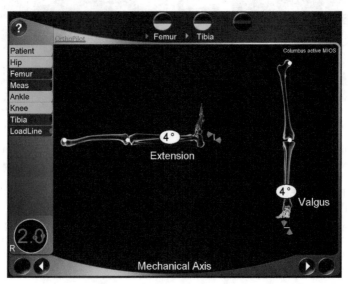

Fig. 14. Limb axis and range of motion controller before component implantation.

7. Conclusions

Total knee prosthetic component implantation using computer aided navigation allows the surgeon to reproduce the mechanical axis measured on full-length of the lower limb radiographs, thus reducing the number of outliers in the alignment of the limb compared with traditional instrument techniques.

Although analysis of alignment and prosthetic component orientation after computer-navigated and conventional implantation shows different results, three recent statistical studies of alignment outcome for computer-assisted knee surgery indicate significant improvement in accuracy of component orientation and mechanical axis restoration (Bauwens et al, 2007; Mason et al, 2007; Tigani et al, 2011).

Furthermore, regarding tibial component orientation, some authors have demonstrated notable improvement in sagittal-tibial component angle (i.e., the tibial slope angle) which can be reconstructed accurately and reproducibly to match the original value of the tibial plateau, although some studies did not find that the alignment in the sagittal plane of the tibial component was improved with navigation guidance (Biasca et al, 2009; Chauhan et al, 2004; Ensini et al, 2007; Matziolis et al, 2007; Sto¨ckl et al, 2004).

Debate about whether a CAS system improves the rotational alignment of the femoral component still exists and as described in the text, several femoral reference landmarks have been proposed to establish proper rotational alignment of the femoral components, although there is no consensus about the best landmarks to gauge that. Siston et al (Siston et al, 2005), in a cadaver study, they found high variability in the rotational alignment of the femoral component. This variability may be explained by the surgeon's greater or lesser ability to identify the medial epicondyle intraoperatively and by the ascending learning curve for the surgeon associated with habitual use of navigation devices, they can minimize the errors in the femoral landmark acquisition.

Although, the rotational mismatch between the tibial and femoral components is decreased with the role of CAS in knee replacement, controversy still exists as to whether navigation systems improve the rotational alignment of the tibial component in the axial plane (Chauhan et al, 2004; Siston et al, 2007). One solution to avoid such complication is the technique describe by Dalury (Dalury et al, 2001) and Eckhoff (Eckhoff et al, 1995) in which the orientation of the tibial tray was determined by allowing it to float into position with respect to the femoral component while the knee was placed through a full arc of motion and in a CT scan postoperative study it was documented an accurate alignment of the tibial component (Biasca et al, 2009).

Other certain factors to be faced intraoperatively, even by experienced surgeon is the patient bone status: in severe osteopenic bone the pins placed to hold the trackers may become loose, making all further measurements inaccurate. Therefore, the surgeon must be very careful when handling pins and trackers. Moreover, attempts to cut through sclerotic areas of bone might create resection errors due to forced bending of the saw blade which can occur with conventional instrumentation as well. Such pitfall can be recognized with the computed-assisted navigation only by using the verification plate of the knee computer system, which allows the surgeon to check-out every cutting procedure during the operation and to verify the correct resection level and also of the programmed joint line level.

Although someone argued that CAS is advised for use for inexperienced surgeons, last researches did not support the assumption of an automatic advantage (Yau et al, 2008). The use of computer navigation technology improve the accuracy in recreation of mechanical alignment in TKA when compared with the conventional jig-based technique. Nevertheless the volume of the operations performed by the surgeon, the experience in using computer navigation technology and severity of the preoperative deformity seems to be major contributing factors.

Knee navigation systems are not yet universally accepted, and their cost/benefit ratio remains a matter for further discussion. In fact, there is an absence of high quality studies demonstrating a longer implant survival rate, better clinical outcome, or enhanced postoperative function.

However CAS has an important value and could be more useful in those particular cases in which standard mechanical instrumentation cannot be used: presence of angular deformities, IM sclerosis, long-stemmed hip implants, or hardware within the femoral canal.

8. Acknowledgment

The authors did not receive any outside funding or grants in support of their research for or preparation of this work.

9. References

Arima J., Whiteside L. A., McCarthy D. S., White S. E. 1995. Femoral rotational alignment, based on the anteroposterior axis, in total knee arthroplasty in a valgus knee. A technical note. *J Bone Joint Surg Am*, Vol.77, No.9 (September 1995), pp. 1331-34, ISSN 1535-1386

Austin, MD Elie Ghanem, MD Ashish Joshi, MD Rachel Trappler, BS Javad Parvizi, MD, FRCS William J. Hozack, MD. (2008). The Assessment of Intraoperative Prosthetic Knee Range of Motion Using Two Methods. *J Arthroplasty*. Vol.23, No.4, (June 2008), pp.515-21, ISSN:0883-5403

Bäthis H, Perlick L, Tingart M, Lüring C, Zurakowski D, Grifka J. (2004). Alignment in total knee arthroplasty. A comparison of computer-assisted surgery with the conventional technique. *J Bone Joint Surg Br*, Vol.86, No.5, (July 2004), pp.682-7, ISSN:0301-620X

Bauwens K, Matthes G, Wich M, Gebhard F, Hanson B, Ekkernkamp A, Stengel D. (2007). Navigated total knee replacement. A meta-analysis. *J Bone Joint Surg Am*, Vol.89, No.2, (February 2007), pp.261-9, ISSN 1535-1386

Berend ME, Ritter MA, Meding JB, Faris PM, Keating EM, Redelman R, Faris GW, Davis KE. (2004). Tibial component failure mechanisms in total knee arthroplasty. *Clin Orthop Relat Res*, Vol.428, (November 2004), pp.26-34, ISSN 1528-1132

Berger RA, Crossett L.S, Jacobs J.J, Rubash H.E. Malrotation causing patellofemoral complications after total knee arthroplasty. *Clin Orthop Relat Res*, Vol.356, (November 1998), pp.144-53, ISSN 1528-1132

Berman AT, Parmet JL, Harding SP, Israelite CL, Chandrasekaran K. (1998). Emboli observed with use of transesophageal echocardiography immediately after tourniquet release during total knee arthroplasty with cement. *J Bone Joint Surg Am*, Vol.80, No.3, (March 1998), pp.389–94, ISSN 1535-1386

Biasca N, Schneider TO, Bungartez M. (2009). Minimally invasive computer-navigated total knee arthroplasty. *Orthop Clin N Am*, Vol.40, No.4, (October 2009), pp.537–63, ISSN 1059-1516

Bonutti P, Dethmers D, Stiehl JB. (2008). Femoral shaft fracture resulting from femoral tracker placement in navigated TKA. *Clin Orthop Relat Res*, Vol.466, No.6, (June 2008), pp.1499-502

Buechel FF. (2002). Long term follow up after mobile-bearing total knee replacement. *Clin Orthop Relat Res*, Vol.404, (November 2002), pp.404:40, ISSN 1528-1132

Chauchan, RG Scott, W Breidhal. (2004). Computer-assisted knee arthroplasty versus a conventional jig-based technique. A randomised, prospective trial. *J Bone Joint Surg Br*, Vol.86, No.3, (April 2004), pp.372-7, ISSN:0301-620X

Chauhan SK, Clark GW, Lioyd S, Scott RG, Breidahl W, Sikorski JM. (2004). Computer assisted total knee replacement. A controlled cadaver study using multi-parametrer quantitative CT assessment of alignment (the Perth CT protocol). *J Bone Joint Surgery Br*, Vol.86, No.6, (August 2004), pp.818-23, ISSN:0301-620X

Chi-Huan L, Tain-Hsiung C, Yu-Ping S, Po-Chou S, Kung-Sheng L, Wei-Ming C. (2008). Periprosthetic femoral supracondylar fracture after total knee arthroplasty with navigation system. *J Arthroplasty*, Vol.23, No.2, (February 2008), pp.304-7, ISSN:0883-5403

Chin PL, Yang KY, Yeo SJ, Lo NN. (2005). Randomized control trial comparing radiographic total knee arthroplasty implant placement using computer navigation versus conventional technique. *J Arthroplasty*, Vol.20, No.5, (August 2005), pp.618-26, ISSN:0883-5403

Choong PF, Dowsey MM, Stoney JD. (2009). Does accurate anatomical alignment result in better function and quality of life? Comparing conventional and computer-assisted total knee arthroplasty. *J Arthroplasty*, Vol.24, No.4, (June 2009), pp.560-569, ISSN:0883-5403

Clemens U., Miehlke R., Jens J. (2001). Computer integrated instrumentation in knee arthroplasty-the first 100 cases with the orthopilot knee navigation system. Poster 6. In: *International CAOS-Symposium*, Davos, 2001

Dalury DF. (2001). Observations of the proximal tibia in total knee arthroplasty. *Clin Orthop Relat Res*, Vol.389, (August 2001), pp.150-5, ISSN 1528-1132

Decking R, Markmann Y, Fuchs J, Puhl W, Scharf HP. (2005). Leg axis after computer-navigated total knee arthroplasty: a prospective randomized trial comparing computer-navigated and manual implantation. *J Arthroplasty*, Vol.20, No.3, (April 2005), pp.282-8, ISSN:0883-5403

Delp SL, Stulberg SD, Davies B, Picard F, Leitner F. (1998). Computer assisted knee replacement. *Clin Orthop Relat Res*, Vol.354, (September 1998), pp.49-56, ISSN 1528-1132

Desai, Asterios Dramis, Danile Kendoff, Tim N. Board. (2011). Critical review of the current practice for computer assisted navigation in total knee replacement surgery: cost-effectiveness and clinical outcome. *Curr Rev Musculoskelet Med*, Vol.4, No.1, (March 2011), pp.11-15, ISSN 1935-9748

Eckhoff DG, Metzger RG, Vandewalle MV. (1995). Malrotation associated with implant alignment technique in total knee arthroplasty. *Clin Orthop Relat Res*,Vol.321, (December 1995), pp.28-31, ISSN 1528-1132

Engh GA,Petersen TL. (1990). Comparative Experience With Intrarnedullary and Extramedullary Alignment in Total Knee Arthroplasty. *J Arthroplasty*, Vol.5, No.1, (March 1990), pp.1-8, ISSN:0883-5403

Ensini A, Catani F, Leardini A, Romagnoli M, Giannini S. (2007). Alignments and clinical results in conventional and navigated total knee arthroplasty. *Clin Orthop Relat Res*, Vol.457, (April 2007), pp.156-62, ISSN 1528-1132

Fehring TK, Mason JB, Moskal J, Pollock DC, Mann J, Williams VJ. (2006). When computer-assisted knee replacement is the best alternative. *Clin Orthop Relat Res*. Vol.452, (November 2006), pp.132-6, ISSN 1528-1132

Haaker RG, Stockheim M, Hamp M, Proff G, Breitenfelder J, Ottersbach A. (2005). Computer assisted navigation increases precision of component placement in total knee arthroplasty. *Clin Orthop Relat Res*, Vol.433, (April 2005), pp.152-9, ISSN 1528-1132

Haas S, C Nelson, R Laskin. (2000). Posterior stabilized knee arthroplasty: an assessment of the bone resection. *Knee*, Vol.7, No.1 (January 2000), pp.25-9, ISSN 1873-5800

Hungerford DS, Kenna RV, Krackow KA. (1982). The porous coated anatomic total knee. *Orthop Clin North Am*, Vol.13, No.1, (January 1982), pp.103-122, ISSN 1558-1373

Jeffery R, Morris R, Denham R. (1991). Coronal alignment after total knee replacement. *J Bone Joint Surg Br*, Vol.73, No.5, September 1991, pp.709-14, ISSN:0301-620X

Jenny J, Boeri C. (2001). Image-free computer-assisted total knee prosthesis implantation: A radiological matched-paired comparison with surgeon-controlled instrumentation. Poster 431. In: *American Academy of Orthopaedic Surgeons*, San Francisco, 2001

Jenny JY, Boeri C. (2001). Navigated implantation of total knee endoprosthesis: a comparative study with conventional instrument. *Z Orthop Ihre Grenzgeb*, Vol.139, No.2, (March-April 2001), pp.117-9, ISSN 0044-3220

Jung HJ, Jung YB, Song KS, Park SJ, Lee JS. (2007). Fractures associated with computer-navigated total knee arthroplasty. A report of two cases. *J Bone Joint Surg Am*, Vol.89, No.10, (October 2007), pp.2280-4, ISSN 1535-1386

Kalairajah Y, Simpson D, Cossey AJ, Verrall GM, Spriggins AJ. (2006). Are systemic emboli reduced in computer-assisted knee surgery? A prospective, randomized, clinical trial. *J Bone Joint Surg Br*,Vol.88, No.2, (February 2006), pp.198-202, ISSN:0301-620X

Katz MA, Beck TD, Silber JS, Seldes RM, Lotke PA (2001). Determining femoral rotational alignment in total knee arthroplasty. Reliability of techniques. *J Arthroplasty*, Vol.16, No.3, (April 2001), pp.301-5, ISSN:0883-5403

Kiefer H, Langemeyer D, Schmerwitz U, Krause F. (2001). Computer aided knee arthroplasty versus conventional technique. First results. Poster 132. In : *International CAOS-Symposium*, Davos, 2001

Kim Y.-H, MD, Kim J.-S, MD and Yoon S.-H, MD. (2007). Alignment and orientation of the components in total knee replacement with and without navigation support. *J Bone Joint Surg Br*, Vol.89, No.4, (April 2007), pp.471-476, ISSN:0301-620X

Lionberger DR. (2006). The attraction of electromagnetic computer-assisted navigation in orthopedic surgery. In: *Navigation and MIS in orthopedic surgery*, Stiehl J, Konermann W, Haaker R, Di Gioia A, (Eds.). pp.44-53, ISBN 978-3-540-36690-4, Springer, Heidelberg

Lonner JH, Siliski JM, Lotke PA. (2000). Simultaneous femoral osteotomy and total knee arthroplasty for treatment of osteoarthritis associated with severe extra-articular deformity. *J Bone Joint Surg Am*, Vol.82, No.3, (March 2000), pp.342-8, ISSN 1535-1386

Manzotti A, Confalonieri N, Pullen C. (2008). Intra-operative tibial fracture during computer assisted total knee replacement: A case report. *Knee Surg Sports Traumatol Arthrosc*, Vol.16, No.5, (May 2008), pp.493-6, ISSN 1433-7347

Martin A, Wohlgenannt O, Prenn M, Prenn M, Oelsch C, von Strempel A. (2007). Imageless navigation for TKA increased implant accuracy. *Clin Orthop Relat Res*, Vol.460, (July 2007), pp.178–84, ISSN 1528-1132

Mason, TK Fehring, R Estok, YD Banel and K Fahrbach. (2007). Meta-Analysis of Alignment Outcomes in Computer-Assisted Total Knee Arthroplasty Surgery. *J Arthroplasty*, Vol.22, No.8, (December 2007), pp.1097-106, ISSN:0883-5403

Matziolis G, Krocher D, Weiss U, Tohtz S, Perka C. (2007). A prospective,randomized study of computer-assisted and conventional total knee arthroplasty. *J Bone Joint Surg Am*, Vol.89, No.2, (February 2007), pp.236-43, ISSN 1535-1386

Mielke. U Clemens, JH Jens, S Kershally. (2001). Navigation in knee endoprosthesis implantation: preliminary experiences and prospective comparative study with conventional implantation technique. *Z Orthop Ihre Grenzgeb*, Vol.139, No.2, (March-April 2001), pp.109-16, ISSN 0044-3220

Nizard R. (2002). Computer assisted surgery for total knee arthroplasty. *Acta Orthopaedica Belgica*, Vol.68, No.3, (June 2002), pp.215-30, ISSN 0001-6462

Nizard R. First experience with a computer-assisted surgery system for total knee arthroplasty. In : *Proceedings of the 5th EFORT Meeting*, Rhodes, 2001

Ossendorf C, Fuchs B, Koch P. (2006). Femoral stress fracture after computer navigated total knee arthroplasty. *Knee* Vol.13, No.5, (October 2006), pp.397-9, ISSN 1873-5800

Picard F., Moody J., Jaramax B., DiGioia A.,Nikou C., LaBarca R. (2001). A classification proposal for computer assisted knee systems. Poster 93. In: *International CAOS-Symposium*, Davos, 2001

Picard, F Leitner, D Saragaglia, P Cinquin. (1997). Mise en place d'une prothèse totale du genou assistée par ordinateur: A propos de 7 implantations sur cadavre. *Rev Chir Orthop Reparatrice Appar Mot*. Vol.83, Suppl.II, (1997), pp.31, ISSN 1776-2553

Rand JA, Coventry MB. (1988). Ten years evaluation of geometric total knee arthroplasty. *Clin Orthop Relat Res*, Vol.232, (July 1988), pp.168-73, ISSN 1528-1132

Richard F., Owens Jr, MD, and Michael L. Swank. (2010). Low incidence of postoperative complications due to pin placement in computer-navigated total knee arthroplasty. *J Arthroplasty*, Vol.25, No.7, (October 2010), pp.1096-1098, ISSN:0883-5403

Ritter M. A, Faris P.M, Keating E.M, Meding J.B. (1994). Postoperative alignment of total knee replacement. It's effect on survival. *Clin Orthop Relat Res*, Vol.299, (February 1994), pp.153-156, ISSN 1528-1132

Robertsson O, Knutson K, lewold S, et al. (2001). The Swedish knee arthroplasty register 1975-1997: an update with special emphasis on 41,223 Knees operated on in 1988-1997. *Acta Orthop Scand* , Vol.72, No.5, (October 2001), pp.503-13, ISSN 0001-6470

Robinson M, Eckhoff DG, Reinig KD, Bagur MM, Bach JM. (2006). Variability of landmark identification in total knee arthroplasty. *Clin Orthop Relat Res*, Vol.442, (January 2006), pp.57-62, ISSN 1528-1132

Saragaglia D, Picard F, Chaussard C, Montbarbon E, Leitner F, Cinquin P. (2001). Computer assisted knee arthropalsty: comparison with a conventional procedure. Results of 50 cases in a prospective randomized study. *Rev Chir Orthop Reparatrice Appar Mot*, Vol.87, No.1, (February 2001), pp.18-28, ISSN 1776-2553

Siston RA, Patel JJ, Goodman SB, Delp SL, Giori NJ. (2005). The variability of femoral rotational alignment in total knee arthroplasty. *J Bone Joint Surg Am*, Vol.87, No.10, (October 2005), pp.2276–80, ISSN 1535-1386

Siston RA, Giori NJ, Goodman SB, Delp SL. (2007). Surgical navigation for total knee arthroplasty: a perspective. *J Biomech*, Vol.40, No.4, (2007), pp.728–35, ISSN 1873-2380

Solver JM, Anna N, Tosteson A, Bozic KJ, Rubash HE, Malchau H. (2008). Impact of the hospital valume on economic value of the computer navigation for total knee replacement. *J Bone Joint Surg Am*, Vol.90, No.7, (July 2008), pp.1492-500, ISSN 1535-1386

Stöckl B, Nogler M, Rosiek R, Fischer M, Krismer M, Kessler O. (2004). Navigation improved accuracy of rotational alignment in total knee arthroplasty. *Clin Orthop Relat Res*, Vol.426, (September 2004), pp.180–6, ISSN 1528-1132

Stulberg SD, Loan P, Sarin B, Sarin V. Computer-assisted navigation in total knee replacement: Results of an initial experience in thirty-five patients. *J Bone Joint Surg Am*, Vol.84, Suppl 2, (2002), pp.90-8, ISSN 1535-1386

Stulberg SD, Yaffe MA, Koo SS. (2006). Computer-Assisted Surgery versus Manual Total Knee Arthroplasty: A Case-Controlled Study. *J Bone Joint Surg Am*, Vol.88, Suppl.4, (December 2006), pp.47-54, ISSN 1535-1386

Tenbusch M., Lahmer A., Wiesel U., Borner M. First results using the Robodoc® system for total knee replacement. Poster 13. In : *International CAOS-Symposium*, Davos, 2001

Tigani D, Sabbioni G, Ben Ayad R, Filanti M, Rani N, Del Piccolo N. (2010). Comparison between two computer-assisted total knee arthroplasty: gap-balancing versus measured resection technique. *Knee Surg Sports Traumatol Arthrosc*, Vol.18, No.10, (October 2010), pp.1304–1310, ISSN 1433-7347

Wang JW, Wang CJ. (2002). Total knee arthroplasty for arthritis of the knee with extra-articular deformity. *J Bone Joint Surg Am*, Vol.84-A, No.10, (October 2002), pp.1769-74, ISSN 1535-1386

Wolff AM, Hungerford DS, Pepe CL. (1991). The effect of extraarticular varus and valgus deformity on total knee arthroplasty. *Clin Orthop Relat Res*, Vol.271, (October 1991), pp.35-51, ISSN 1528-1132

Wysocki WR, Sheinkop B, Virkus WW, Della Valle CJ. (2008). Femoral fracture through a previous pin site after computer-assisted total knee arthroplasty. *J Arthroplasty*, Vol.23, No.3, (April 2008), pp.462-5, ISSN:0883-5403

Yau WP, Chiu KY. Cutting errors in total knee replacement: assessment by computer assisted surgery. (2008). *Knee Surg Sports Traumatol Arthrosc*, Vol.16, No.7, (July 2008), pp.670-3, ISSN 1433-7347

Yau WP, Chiu KY, Zuo JL, Tang WM, and Ng TP. (2008). Computer Navigation Did Not Improve Alignment in a Lower-volume Total Knee Practice. *Clin Orthop Relat Res*, Vol.466, No.4, (April 2008), pp.935–945, ISSN 1528-1132

Yoshioka Y., Siu D., Scudamore R., Cooke T. (1989). Tibial anatomy and functional axes. *J Orthop Res*, Vol.7, No.1, (1989), pp.132-137, ISSN 1554-527X

15

Computer Assisted Orthopedic Surgery in TKA

Eun Kyoo Song and Jong Keun Seon
Chonnam National University Hwasun Hospital
Korea

1. Introduction

Since Campbell and Boyd first developed a mold hemiarthroplasty in 1940, the procedure for a total knee arthroplasty has advanced greatly with the development of new materials and the increasing understanding of the knee joint biomechanics. And accurate alignment of the component and soft tissue balancing has been cited as the essential for the success of total knee arthroplasty. Although mechanical alignment guides have been designed to improve alignment accuracy, there are several fundamental limitations of this technology that will inhibit additional improvements. The long-term survival rate of a total knee arthroplasty after a 10-year follow up was reported to be 80% to 95% (Knutson et al., 1986; Ranawat et al., 1993; Scuderi et al., 1989). Various factors affect this long-term survival, the most closely related factor being the physiologic recovery of the leg alignment (Laskin, 1984; Ritter et al., 1994). Upon a follow-up study of more than 8 years, the loosening rate was only 3% in those patients with a correctly recovered leg alignment, but was 24% in those with an incomplete recovery of the leg alignment(Stulberg et al., 2002). There are limits on improving the alignment accuracy using a conventional total knee arthroplasty. Teter et al. (Teter et al., 1995) found that when a tibial extramedullary alignment guide was used, approximately 8% of the cuts were deviated 4 degrees of the ideal 90 degrees cut (perpendicular to the mechanical axis). However, this finding was based on coronal imaging, and the rate of malalignment may be considerably greater when the sagittal imaging is considered. Computer-assisted surgery(CAS) was introduced to overcome these difficulties and errors. Computer-assisted total knee arthroplasty has gained increasing acceptance among orthopedic surgeons as a technique to improve surgical precision and patient outcomes.

2. The history of computer assisted TKA

Computer-assisted surgery was first introduced in the neurosurgical field in 1980s to find surgical sites in the brain or spinal cord accurately. In orthopedic surgery, the American veterinarian Howard Paul and the orthopedic surgeon William Bargar first sought to improve femoral stem incorporation during total hip arthroplasty(THA), and devised a new drill to achieve a precise match for femoral prostheses. In fact, this concept was the basic idea that drove the development of medical robot. In 1986, Davis started a joint project between IBM(International Business Machine Corp.) and the University of California to develop the ROBODOC®(Integrated Surgical Systems, Davis, CA) system. As a resultant, Integrated Surgical Systems (ISS) was founded by IBM in 1990, and subsequently, the first robot-assisted THA was performed on a human in 1992 in California using the ROBODOC system, which was later approved by the European Union in 1994. In 1997, Saragaglia developed a navigation system called Orthopilot®(Aesculap, Tuttlingen, Germany), which allows surgeons to perform surgery without any other imaging technique.

These Computer-assisted Orthopedic Surgery (CAOS) techniques were developed to minimize errors due to malalignment and inappropriate prosthesis insertion. The navigation system produced good results clinically and radiologically, but other factors, such as, the subtle movements of cutting blocks and the vibration of oscillating saws were then focused on as potential causes of inaccurate bone cutting, and these efforts resulted in the developments of robot systems. The ROBODOC and CASPAR systems were introduced almost simultaneously in Germany in 2000, and used to conduct the first robotic TKA in the same year. In 2007, ISS was purchased by the South Korean company Curexo, and in 2008 the FDA approved ROBODOC for THA. However, the FDA has not yet to approve ROBODOC for TKA. Nevertheless, 10 institutions in South Korea and 60 institutions worldwide use the ROBODOC system for TKA.

3. Navigation-assisted TKA

3.1 Classification

Many manufacturers produce navigation-assisted surgery systems and it is difficult to classify. However they can be divided into two groups based on their dependence to imaging; image based systems and image free systems.

3.1.1 Image based system

Image based navigation systems use the data acquired from computed tomography or fluoroscopy to determine operating factors, such as, joint centers, the movement tracks of surgical tools, and the alignments of prostheses. These systems require the registration of a CT image acquired prior to surgery, or the registration of fluoroscopic data during surgery, where registration means not only inputting CT or fluoroscopic data, but also matching imaging data to joint kinematic information acquired during surgery and bone dimensional information acquired using indexes and calipers. By using kinematic and surface registration data, the system determines in real-time the location of the bone resection site, placement and alignment of the cutting block, and joint alignment for the prosthesis concerned. Surgery is then performed according to the data produced.

Accordingly, the registration process is perhaps the most critical for image based systems. The accuracy of registration can be detrimentally affected when border lines on CT images are blurred or segmented, cortical fixation screws are loose, or when computer hardware or software is defective. All image based systems can perform fluoroscopic registration automatically during surgery. However, this can be inconvenient because the fluoroscope is needed during operation.

3.1.2 Image free system

Although image based systems are useful during preoperative planning and postoperative evaluation, the image-acquiring process can be time-consuming and troublesome, and consequently, image free systems are becoming more popular. These systems track the sizes, shapes, locations, and alignments of musculoskeletal structure based on a standard human frame in real-time during surgery, and then register and guide bone resection using navigation. Image free systems need tracking cameras and markers, the latter of which are referred to as rigid bodies, because they are fixed onto bones (at least four sites) with a pin or clamp. In addition, the tools and calipers used also have tracing markers that used by the system to guide the operative procedure. Optical systems use infrared lights and electromagnetic systems use electromagnets to detect markers. Systems based on the use of ultrasound are also under development, and have been reported to have errors of < 1mm or 1° of error range.

3.1.2.1 Optical systems

Both active and passive optical systems are available. Active systems have an LED (light-emitting diode) attached to each rigid body that emits infrared signals that are captured by a camera, whereas passive systems have a reflecting sphere attached to each rigid body, and the system senses the reflection of light emitted from an LED source mounted on the camera. It should be noted that signal interpretation depends on the amount of light detected, and thus, the active type requires a cable type or a battery type probe, and the passive type requires that the reflecting spheres are meticulously cleaned. For the active type, surgery starts with the attachment of a rigid body to the tibia and femur; the infrared LEDs are then attached using a cortical screw. When the hip, knee, and ankle joint are moved in sequence, LEDs emit infrared and the optical localizer monitors and calculates the joint centers and the movement ranges of the three joints 3-dimensionally to determine the location of the mechanical axis (kinematic registration). During surgery, the surgeon uses a pointer to mark the bony and articular landmarks and notes useful surgical information, such as, the locations and orientations of the femur and tibia. Using this information, the surgeon can promptly identify the optimal bone cutting line, and decide on its direction and position.

The ligament tensioner can be used to balance the ligament by tensioning the internal and external lateral ligament, and the internal and external knee joint gaps can then be measured in extension and flexion, which allows the external rotation range to be adjusted in accordance with flexion and extension intervals during distal femur anterior and posterior side dissections. In addition, It can assess implant size and location, which enables the surgeon to consider individual joint properties.

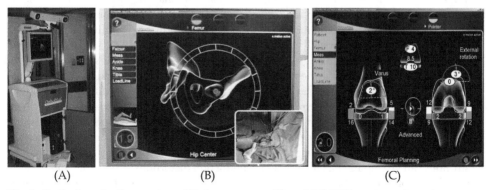

(A) (B) (C)

Fig. 1. Optical navigation system. (A) Appearance, (B) and (C) Different monitor views.

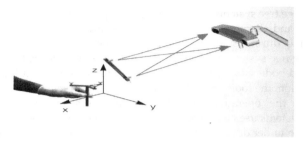

Fig. 2. Optical camera

The optical system of image free systems is fast and highly accurate, but operators should be careful about individual positioning to ensure visualization of the surgical field. The field can also be influenced by illumination intensity, and according to Tria(Tria et al, 2006), this system uses a large transmitter, which requires additional skin incision and a larger drill hole to hold the transmitter.

3.1.2.2 Electromagnetic Computer System (EMC)

As its name implies the EMC system is based on the detection of a weak magnetic field by sensors, transformed to digitalized voltage by receivers, and then transmitted to a computer. The magnetic field is produced by a localizer using direct or variable currents, although direct currents operation provides a more stable magnetic field. The localizer contains at least three generator coils and the coil numbers to a large extent dictate the performance of system because precision is dependent on the coil number. On the other hand, larger capacity computers are required for high coil numbers. EMC systems use dynamic reference frames(DRFs), which function as trackers, and resulting movement information can be used during surgery.

The early computer-based navigation systems had some disadvantages, such as, limited camera field of view, the requirement for sterilization, damage and tethering of soft tissue, and disruption of the surgical field by large surgical instruments. To avoid these disadvantages, researchers attempted to use non-line-of sight signals, which represented the beginning of EMC.

The EMC system was first applied in the pediatric neurologic surgical and ENT fields. In the orthopedic field, it was used secondary to conventional navigation due to signal instabilities, metallic interference, and its slower speed, which was caused by positional changes. However, after the coil number was increased and by enabling it to be attached to soft tissue, it has been more widely used.

The EMC system has the advantage of convenience during surgery, because it is not affected by the surgeon's position. Furthermore, gap balance is easily matched because the real shape of bone and dimensional data can be seen simultaneously. In addition, when a bone excision is incorrect, it can be corrected promptly, and because surgical instruments were small, it can easily be used during 'Minimal Invasive Surgery'. However, the EMC system suffers from distortion and low speed, and its safety has not been proven in humans. Furthermore, costs are high because the coil can only be used once.

Distortions can be classified as being due to conduction distortions and ferrous interference. When distortions are present, data may be incorrect or the monitor screen freezes or displays 'no reading'. Conduction distortions can be caused by most metals, including aluminum, and carbon based materials, although titanium causes less distortion. Metal disturbances are more problematic when the ferrous content is high, and thus, efforts must be made to eliminate ferrous content from the proximity of the unit system, for example, a 'fluoroscopy-possible' operating table should be used and EMC instruments should be located near the surgical field. In addition, it should be added that surgeons require training and experience of the EMC system.

However, EMC represents advancement over other navigation systems because gap balance can be easily adjusted, incorrect bone dissection can be corrected promptly, and because its small size is useful for minimally invasive surgery.

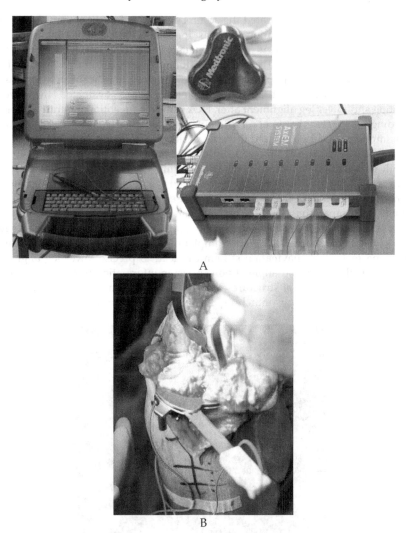

Fig. 3. Electromagnetic navigation system. (A) A structure; monitor, detector. (B) Intraoperative instrument.

According to Seon and Song(Seon and Song, 2004), the above two navigation systems showed more than a 3° malalignment in 15% of patients. It was suggested that this was caused by anatomical point ambiguity in real patients and registration failure. Furthermore, when registration failure occurs, EMS determined mechanical axis are more affected, and thus, these two authors concluded that EMS is more inaccurate than optical system.

3.2 Advantages and disadvantages navigation-assisted TKA
3.2.1 Advantages
3.2.1.1 Limb alignment

Many researchers have demonstrated the accuracy of lower leg alignment and the excellent implantation offered by navigation systems for TKA. Bathis et al.(Bathis et al., 2004) prospectively compared 80 TKAs performed using a navigation system with 80 TKAs performed using a conventional method, and found that varus and valgus angles of the mechanical axis and femur implantation in the coronal plane were more precise in the navigation group. Sterlbug et al. (Sterlbug et al., 2002) evaluated the precision of implantation and lower leg alignment after TKA using a conventional intramedullary guide. Their findings suggested that femoral implants tend to be varus, flex, internally rotate, and that tibia implants tend to be placed in varus position . There was no misalignment of more than 3°, and only 4 of 20 cases showed less than 3° alignment in the coronal or axial plane.

This result supports the previously reported argument that conventional TKA tends to cause varus, and that the margin of error between femur and tibia implantation could be less than 1°, which reduces the overall alignment error and can enhance surgical accuracy. According to comparative studies on navigation and conventional surgery groups, navigation systems showed statistically better results in terms of mechanical axis recovery, far fewer outliers, and more precise femur implantation in the coronal and axial planes.

The following features of navigation system can lead to precise lower leg alignment. The surgeon obtains thickness and angle of bone excision information in real time, and patients with an abnormal anatomical structure can be operated on correctly. During operation of total knee joint arthroplasty, matching flexion and extension intervals and ligament

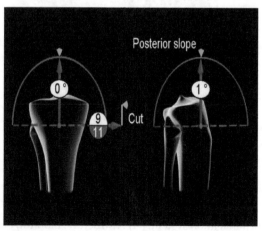

Fig. 4. Real-time monitoring

balancing are difficult due to damaged soft tissue, but navigation system can check flexion and extension intervals and ligament balancing instantly. Haaker et al.(Haaker et al., 2005) reported that real-time correction is possible after evaluating and collecting exact osteotomy data, implantation and soft tissue stability status promptly.

3.2.1.2 Functional results

The use of navigation systems during TKA produces accurate limb alignment, but the effect of this accuracy on functional outcome is still under dispute. However, Choong et al.(Choong et al., 2009) reported patients that underwent navigation assisted surgery showed precise limb alignment (<3°), and concluded that accuracy improved new knee function and quality of life. Lehnen et al. (Lehnen et al., 2010) reported, in a 1-year follow up study, that Western Ontario and McMaster University (WOMAC) scores and Knee Society scores of 43 navigation assisted surgery patients were notably higher than those of 122 patients that underwent conventional surgery. Patient satisfaction was 91% in the navigation assisted group, but only 70% in the conventional surgery group.

3.2.1.3 Bleeding

In navigation assisted total knee arthroplasty, the intramedullary jigs are not needed, and therefore, less bleeding can be expected as compared with conventional methods. Chauhan et al.(Chauhan et al., 2004) performed a randomized prospective study on 70 patients randomly allocated to computer-assisted surgery or conventional surgery. Mean amounts of bleeding were compared, and whereas the computer surgery group lost an average of 252mL (25-620), the conventional surgery group lost 446mL (100-1100). Furthermore, this low bleeding amount reduced the incidence of blood transfusions, and was useful when operating on patients in whom blood transfusion was problematic. Schnurr et al.(Schnurr et al., 2010) studied blood losses and transfusion amounts for 500 TKA operations. Average blood loss in their conventional and navigation groups were 1375mL and 1242mL, respectively. Furthermore, mean transfusion ratio was 0.23 in the conventional group and 0.12 in the navigation assisted group.

3.2.1.4 Embolisms

Conventional TKA uses intramedullary jigs, which increase intramedullary pressure and increase the risk of fat embolism. Chauhan et al.(Chauhan et al., 2004) compared navigation guided TKA and conventional TKA and reported that acute confusional states caused by transient fat embolisms occurred more frequently in conventional TKA patients. On the other hand, the risk of fat embolism in TKA patients is remarkably reduced when navigation systems or extramedullary alignment guides are used. Kalairajah et al. (Kalairajah et al., 2006) reporting on a study based on noninvasive monitoring, navigation assisted surgery stated fewer embolisms in the systemic circulation during operation than during conventional surgery.

3.2.1.5 Miscellaneous

Navigation assisted surgery, unlike conventional surgery, provides accurate records and comprehensive data on operations performed, which can be helpful during future investigations. Surgical wound healing characteristic are known to be similar for the two methods. Browne et al.(Browne et al., 2010) in a meta-analysis of 101,596 TKA patients, found that patients who underwent navigation guided surgery had a lower risk of cardiovascular complications than patient who underwent conventional surgery.

3.2.2 Disadvantages

3.2.2.1 Pin fixation

In a navigation assisted surgery, pins are fixed on to the bones to acquire real-time information of the limb alignment. Potential complications involving the pin fixations have been reported. Some investigators reported that additional 4cm of incision was needed for the pin fixations during navigation surgery, and this could cause delayed soft tissue healing and increased risk of infection. The additional incision of the quadriceps femoris muscle were needed in order to install the femoral tracking array can cause delayed healing of the muscle during the early stage of rehabilitation. The fracture of the pin fixation site for the reference array could also occur. Sikorski et al.(Sikorski et al., 2004) reported that the accuracy of the navigation assisted surgery can be impaired in osteoporotic patients due to the loosening of the pinning site. Song et al.(Song et al., 2006) reported that inappropriately registered data in navigation assisted surgery can change the outcome of the operation creating an incorrect mechanical axis.

3.2.2.2 Prolonged operation time

Operation time differ between authors, but generally, navigation assisted TKA takes 15 to 30 minutes longer than conventional TKA. The type of prosthesis used and the skills of the operator can affect operation time, it has been reported that the learning curve requires 10~20 procedures. Bauwen et al(Bauwen et al., 2004) reviewed computer-assisted TKA related articles between 1990 and 2008, and reported that the accuracy of mechanical axis alignment was the same as that of conventional TKA and that operation times were 23% longer.

3.2.2.3 Cost

Newer techniques require new equipment, and thus, costs inevitably increases. However, several authors have concluded that navigation assisted surgery extends the life spans of prostheses and reduces the potential risk of revision surgery, and that it is less costly in the long term.

3.2.2.4 Errors of the navigation system

Many investigators have reported that navigation assisted TKA produces more accurate results. Seon et al.(Seon et al., 2004) reported that the accuracies of optical and electromagnetic navigation systems are affected by the registration of anatomical locations. Mullaji et al.(Mullaji et al., 2007) reported in a comparative study of navigation assisted TKA and conventional TKA that the accuracies of navigation systems depends on joint deformity, instability, computer hardware, computer software, and the surgical techniques used. In addition, they found that patients with 20~30° of varus deformity before TKA had more varus mechanical axes after surgery than patients with 10~20°of varus deformity before operation. Furthermore, the former patients showed significantly higher rates of varus locations of femoral and tibial prostheses. These findings indicate that radiographs should be used to determine the degree of varus deformity when placing sensors.

3.3 Operative procedure (Orthopilot® Version 4.0 or 4.2)

The following text concerns that of the Orthopilot Version 4.0 or 4.2 (Aesculap, Tuttlingen, Germany) navigation system which is an image-free system.

Operation was performed using the gap technique with navigation. Using a medial parapatellar approach, the knee joint was exposed and the hip, knee, and ankle centers were navigated. Anatomical landmarks were registered by hand using a pointer to define the joint line and the mechanical axis of the leg. The mechanical axis was then restored to neutral (±2°) at full extension by stepwise meticulous medial soft tissue release and osteophyte removal (Fig. 5). Proximal tibial bone cutting was performed under real-time navigation system control and the posterior cruciate ligament was preserved and confirmed to be functionally intact. Flexion and extension gaps were measured at full extension and at 90° of flexion using a tensioning device (V-STAT tensor, Zimmer) and a special torque wrench set at 200N before femoral bone cutting (precutting flexion and extension gaps) (Fig. 6). Gap differences were classified as; balanced, tight in flexion, or tight in extension. A balanced gap was defined as one having a flexion/extension gap difference of within 3mm, a tight flexion gap as a gap with an extension gap of at least 3mm more that the corresponding flexion gap, and a tight extension gap as one with a flexion gap of at least 3mm more that the corresponding extension gap. Levels of distal and posterior femoral cuts and amounts of femoral component rotations were determined based on extension-flexion and medial-lateral gap differences (Fig. 7). Following final bone cuts and soft tissue release completion, flexion, and extension gaps were reassessed (final flexion and extension gaps) (Fig. 8). And if soft tissue balance is adequate, the prosthesis are inserted.

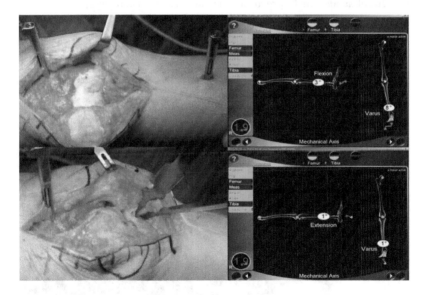

Fig. 5. After performing anatomical and kinematic registrations, the mechanical axis was restored to neutral (±2°) at full extension by incremental meticulous medial soft tissue release and osteophyte removal.

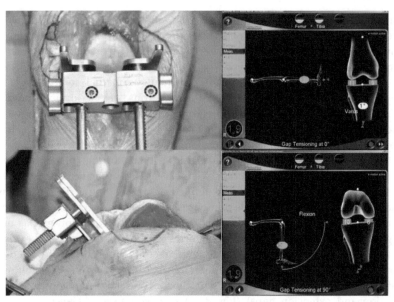

Fig. 6. After proximal tibial bone cutting while preserving the posterior cruciate ligament under navigation and before femoral bone cutting, flexion, and extension gaps were measured at full extension and at 90° of flexion using a tensioning device and a special torque wrench set at 50lb/inch (precutting flexion and extension gaps).

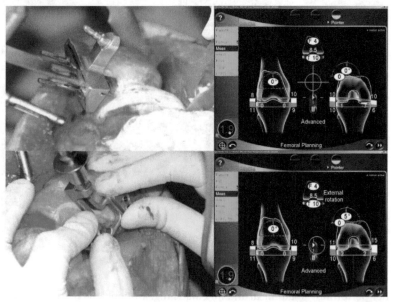

Fig. 7. Levels of distal and posterior femoral cuts and amounts of femoral component rotation were planned based on extension-flexion and medial-lateral gap differences.

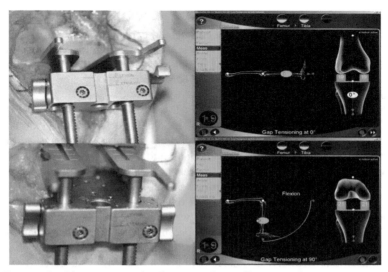

Fig. 8. Following final bone cuts and soft tissue release, flexion and extension gaps were reassessed (final flexion and extension gaps).

3.4 Clinical outcomes

Many reports have concluded that computer-assisted TKA produces consistent results, reduces malalignment and inappropriate prosthesis placement, and promotes rapid recovery and rehabilitation after surgery. Rosenberger et al.(Rosenberger et al., 2008) investigated 100 patients, and found that 50 patients who underwent navigation assisted TKA showed an average varus angle of 0.28°, whereas patients who underwent conventional TKA showed 1.88° in the coronal plane. The ideal prosthesis location was achieved in 16 cases (32%) in the conventional TKA group, and in 31 cases (62%) in the navigation assisted TKA group. These results show that navigation assisted surgery is a straightforward, stable, useful procedure for total knee arthroplasty.

Seon and Song et al.(Seon et al., 2009) investigated 43 cases in a 2-year follow up study, and found that Hospital for Special Surgery(HSS) and Western Ontario and McMaster University (WOMAC) scores were increased in both the navigation assisted and conventional groups, the scores were non-significantly different in both groups. Ranges of knee joint movement were also similar, but limb and prostheses alignments were better in the navigation assisted group.

However, others have reported that the conventional and navigational methods are no different with respect to pain, range of motion, ankylosis knee scores, and patient satisfaction. Spencer et al.(Spencer et al., 2007) reported that after a 2-year follow up of 71 patients with navigation assisted TKA group showed better alignment, but other factors such as functional assessments failed to reveal any significant difference.

4. Robotic-assisted TKA

4.1 Introduction to robot systems

Robotic surgery systems can be classified according to level of function, into three groups, that is, as passive types, active types, or semi-active types, and further devided into image based or image free systems. Passive types guide the surgeon through the fixation and cutting block resection stages – the actual cutting and drilling processes are executed by the surgeon. Navigation systems are passive types. Whereas active robotic types prepare and execute the operation process entirely or in part, and perform the bone cutting. Initially, these robots were custom-made in small numbers, but many others originated from larger industrial robots.

The ROBODOC® (Integrated Surgical Systems, Davis, CA), and the CASPAR® (URS Ortho Rastatt, Germany) are typical commercial TKA robotic systems. ROBODOC was the first of its kind, and is the only system used in South Korea. The system is composed of two main parts; Orthodoc, a supercomputer which plans and executes surgery, and ROBODOC, which has robot arms and performs the surgery (Fig. 9). Orthodoc uses pre-operative CT images to analyze anatomy, to choose a prosthesis of the right size, a prosthesis location, to plan cutting, drilling, and finally to register the data in ROBODOC for execution.

The development of the CASPAR® system was inspired by the commercial success of ROBODOC in Germany, and was first developed by OrtoMaquet (a subsidiary of Maquet). This system uses infrared cameras and reflective trackers to track limb positions. The system is designed to stop if excessive limb movement is detected during surgery. Care is required during operation to ensure that bone debris or fluid spatter on reflective tracker is removed; splash-guards may be needed. However, the ROBODOC system uses bone motion detectors fixed about 5mm deep in bone, which are not compromised by debris or fluid.

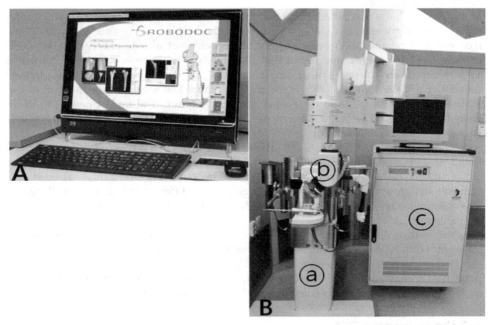

Fig. 9. ROBODOC ® system (Integrated Surgical Systems, Davis, CA) is composed of two primary components. (A) CT-based preoperative planning using ORTHODOC, and (B) Robot-assisted surgery using the ROBODOC surgical assistant (ⓐ = robot base, ⓑ = robot arm, ⓒ = the control computer)

Semi-active systems are a combination of the passive and active types, whereby a robot guides the cutting tools within specific ranges, and the operator controls robot arms within these ranges to process bone. The Acrobot® system (Acrobot Co. Ltd., London) and the MAKO Tactile Guidance System (TGS) (MAKO Surgical Corp., Fort Lauderdale, Fla)(Fig. 10) are semi-active types, and are often used for conducting unicompartmental knee arthroplasty.

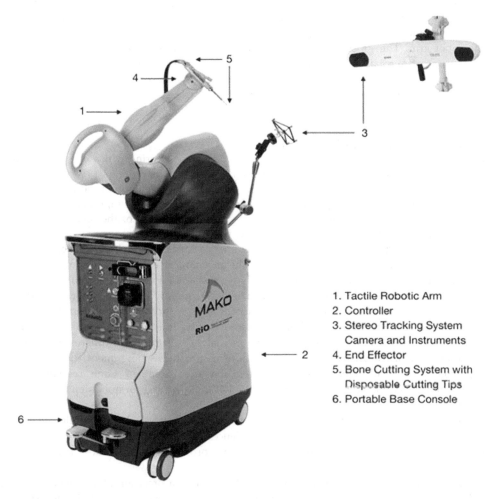

1. Tactile Robotic Arm
2. Controller
3. Stereo Tracking System
   Camera and Instruments
4. End Effector
5. Bone Cutting System with
   Disposable Cutting Tips
6. Portable Base Console

Fig. 10. MAKO Tactile Guidance System (TGS) (MAKO Surgical Corp., Fort Lauderdale, Fla)

The Acrobot system was developed at Imperial College (London) and was the first of its kind in the TKA field. According to this semi-active system, cutting tools are located within the dimensional range of bone to be cut. The tools are controlled by an Active Constraint Control™ system. At first Acrobot was used for TKA, but now it is more often used for unicompartmental knee arthroplasty. The robot software limits the movements of cutting tools within a pre-set range, and the operator resects bone to the planned extent in this range. The developers of the Acrobot system believe that it will be more attractive to surgeons than active systems like ROBODOC or CASPAR. The Acrobot® system consists of two robots; a large robot which functions as a gross positioning device, and a smaller robot which controls the active constraint function; technically, Acrobot refers to the smaller robot. The Acrobot has a spherical kinematic design that contains two rotational axes (yaw and pitch) and one prismatic axis (extension). The handle is equipped with a sensor that measures the force applied by the operator and controls the power output of the robot arm. The gross positioning device holds the limb in a manner that enables positioning of Acrobot near the cut volume. A six-axis gross positioning device is used for TKA, and a three-axis device for UKA. Anatomical data is registered using pre-op CT images; the operator marks 20-30 dots on the bone surface, and matching of the 3D-CT image and actual bone is then performed.

4.2 Surgical procedure (ROBODOC®)
Robotic TKA is composed of two steps; pre-op preparation (during which operation plans are determined based on CT images) and robot-assisted surgery.
CT images are acquired with the knee joint flexed at 15~20°. A calibration rod is attached to the limb, and CT scans are acquired at five different levels (the foot joint, mid tibia, the knee joint, mid femur, and the femoral head). When acquiring images of the distal femur and proximal tibia, slice thickness is reduced to 0.625 mm to improve accuracy.
Orthodoc reconstructs sagittal images and 3D images (surface models of the tibia and the femur) from acquired coronal CT images. The mechanical axis of the virtual 3D bone models is then set using the centers of hip, knee, and ankle joints. The virtual femur and tibia are then set parallel to the mechanical axis. Subsequently, suitable femoral and tibial prostheses, in terms of extent of resection, prosthesis size, and degree of external rotation, are then placed. The tibial prosthesis is placed on the line between the center of the posterior cruciate ligament's origin and the medial 1/3 of the tibial tuberosity. Finally, Orthodoc performs virtual surgery to confirm prosthesis alignment (Fig. 11). A supercomputer then determines exact sites and the extent of bone resection, the information saved on a disc, is delivered to ROBODOC. This preparatory step takes about 15~30 minutes.
The operation begins by fixing the robot to the subject knee, and this is followed by a verification process, during which correspondences are determined between anatomical bone surfaces and virtual bone. Bone resection and prosthesis insertion are then executed (Fig. 12).
Before surgery, a calibration process is initiated to achieve a precision of less than 0.2 mm. Robotic surgery is conducted, like conventional surgery, using a medial parapatellar approach. The approach is conducted by the surgeon. The patella is then everted to expose the knee joint, and the joint is fixed at 90~120°. The robot then inserts a Schanz pin in the proximal tibia and in the distal femur, and two straight beams are used to connect the limb. Traction devices (two curved S pins) are then attached to pull soft tissue and achieve maximum exposure. These devices are placed so as not to interfere with movement of the cutting arm. Next, the recovery markers, a screw and a pin, are fixed to the femur and tibia

respectively. These markers enable the robot to sense unwanted limb movements (if movement exceeds 2 mm the robot will stop). This connecting step takes about 5-10 minutes (Fig. 13).

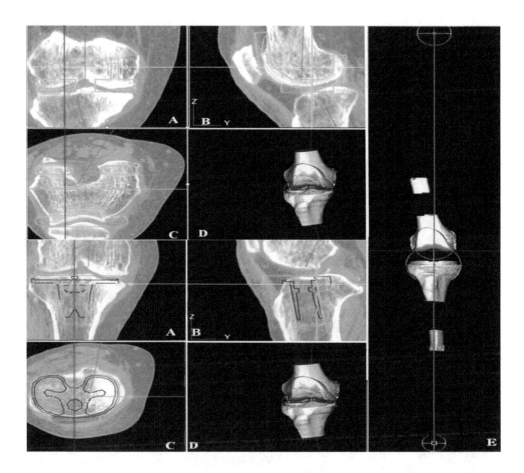

Fig. 11. Preoperative planning of the insertion of a femoral and tibial prosthesis using ORTHODOC. A= frontal plane; B= sagittal plane; C = transverse plane; and D= three-dimensional bone model of the femur and tibia; E= virtual surgery was conducted to verify femoral and tibial alignments and sizes with respect to the established femoral and tibial mechanical axes

Registration then performed. Actual knee joint bone surfaces are matched to the data saved in ROBODOC. This process is involves making the ball probe of the robot contact each of 97 contact points in 28 different locations as indicated by the computer program. After this process has been completed, which takes 5-10 minutes, the robot can recognize anatomical landmarks and bone spatial details.

After verifying data, physiological saline is applied continuously for cooling and irrigation, and the robot begins milling the femur and the tibia. The milling sequence proceeds in the following order; distal femur, anterior femur, posterior medial condyle, and posterior lateral condyle. At the tibia, milling begins at the tibial plateau, and after milling, pilot holes are drilled. The saw is replaced with a smaller one to make the peg holes and tibial flanges. The whole milling process takes about 20 minutes. The robot's job ends here.

The surgeon proceeds with trimming of the resection margin. Soft tissue is then relaxed and balanced. The knee is flexed and extended, from 0° to 90° to check for soft tissue stretching, and if soft tissue balance is adequate, the prostheses are inserted.

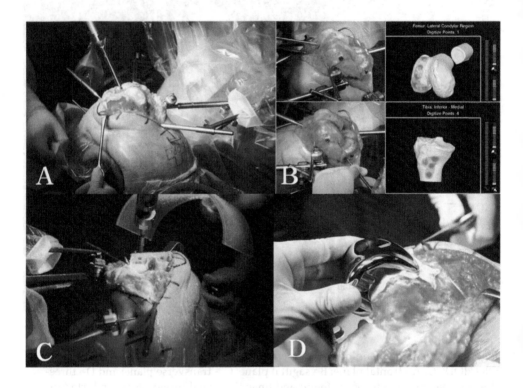

Fig. 12. Photographs showing the ROBODOC surgical procedure; Fixation between the patient's leg and surgical robot (A), Registration (B), Milling by the surgical robot (C), Implantation (D). During pinless registration (B), the digitizer arm is guided by the surgeon to certain points on the distal femur or proximal tibia. Digitized points are shown on the computer monitor. A correct hit is indicated when the point concerned turns green.

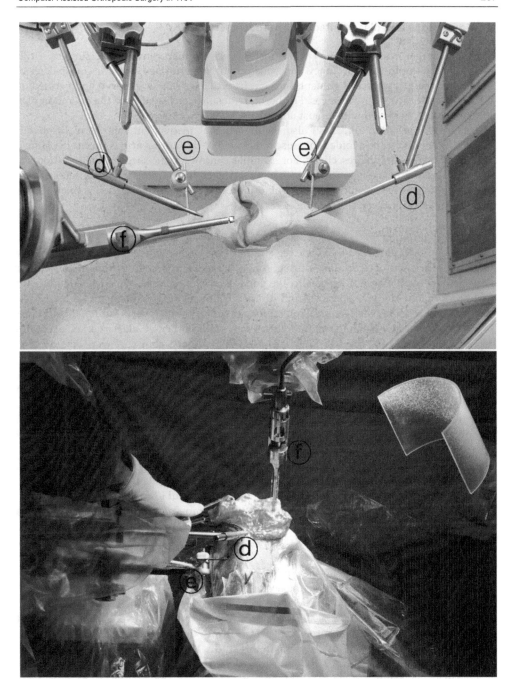

Fig. 13. The ROBODOC surgical robot. ⓐ, ⓑ, ⓒ (see Fig. 9), ⓓ = bone-motion detector, ⓔ = femoral and tibial fixators, ⓕ = the bone milling cutter.

4.3 Advantages and disadvantages of robotic-assisted TKA
4.3.1 Advantages

The robot surgery can be planned with greater precision than conventional surgery. Drills are guided with pin-point accuracy and bone milling is performed without any shaking or vibration. Ideal prostheses alignments and mechanical axes can be achieved and verified on CT or weight-bearing x-ray images. Furthermore, results consistent with the operation plan are consistently achieved with almost no outliers.

Siebert et al. (Siebert et al., 2002) also mentioned that inadvertent injuries of ligaments, vessels, or nerves can be avoided, because movement of the cutting arm is precisely planned and calculated, as are the resections. For example, during robotic surgery, the insertion site of the posterior cruciate ligament always remains intact. In addition, milled surfaces almost perfectly fit prostheses, and the amount of resected bone is minimized, which makes potential revision surgery less complicated.

4.3.2 Disadvantages

Coon(Coon, 2009) remarked that bone registration, burr exchanging, and a long milling time limit the efficiency of workflow during robot-assisted surgery. In addition, the author criticized the robot's design, especially the unnecessarily long arms, which make it difficult to appropriately deploy, sterilize, and drape. Bellmans et al. (Bellmans et al., 2007) discontinued robot-assisted surgery due to longer surgery time (over 30 min.), the need for highly experienced personnel, and higher costs, and Borner et al.(Borner et al., 2010) reported of the first 100 cases of ROBODOC assisted surgery, about 5% were converted to conventional surgery due to technical problems, such as, digitization error, calibration error, or bone motion.

Park and Lee(Park & Lee, 2007) found that the large pins required and the wide radius of robot arm movements made robot surgery unsuitable for minimally invasive surgery. They reported that of the first 32 patients that underwent robot surgery, 6 experienced complications, such as, superficial infections, rupture of the patellar ligament, dislocation of the patella, supracondylar fracture, or peroneal nerve injury.

Decking et al. (Decking et al., 2004) commented that before it could be viewed as an integrated method for total arthroplasty, robot surgery should be quicker, cheaper, smaller, and include an integrated soft tissue balancing process without losing its integrity.

Currently, we lack evidence that superior accuracy improves clinical outcomes, and thus, more investigations are required.

4.4 Clinical outcomes

Little information is available on the clinical outcomes of robot-assisted TKA. In a cadaver-based study undertaken to evaluate the accuracy of a robot system, alignment errors of the mechanical axis averaged 1° and ranged up to 2°, and average prosthetic displacement was 1mm with a maximum of 2mm. 3D CT pre-operative planning and the precision of the robot made ideal prosthesis placement possible. Decking et al.(Decking et al., 2004) acquired similar results using the CASPAR system. In this study, 13 patients underwent TKA and CT images acquired preop and 10 days postop were compared. Average mechanical axis discrepancy, as compared with preop images, was 0.2°. The accuracies of prostheses alignments in the coronal, sagittal, and axial planes were ±1.2°, whereas accuracies of linear alignments (anteroposterior, mediolateral, and craniocaudal) were ±1.1 mm. The authors concluded that robot-assisted TKA enables much more precise placement of prostheses. However, the authors added that the robotic procedure should include soft tissue balancing, and that robotic surgery should be quicker and less expensive to ensure its adoption.

Siebert et al. (Siebert et al., 2002) reported that in 70 cases of robot-assisted surgery, the average mechanical axis error was 0.8° and that the average operation time was 135 minutes. Furthermore, the conventional method had an average axis error of 2.6°, whereas robot surgery was more accurate. The authors mentioned that surgical precision (based on comparisons with pre-op CT images) was a strong point, but that the insertion and placement of markers, the longer operation time, and higher costs were weak points of the technique.

Borner et al.(Borner et al., 2004) reported 100 cases of ROBODOC assisted TKA. Mechanical axis errors were all within 3° and operations took only 90~100 minutes after sufficient experience. Precision beyond that achieved by the conventional technique has not been proven to be a requirement of TKAs, but it appears reasonable to believe that long term outcomes will surpass those of conventional surgery. Although most TKAs are viable for at least 15 years, robot-assisted surgery provides better axis alignment, and thus, minimizes prostheses wear and bone osteolysis, which should prolong the life spans of replaced knees.

Bellmans et al. (Bellmans et al., 2007) investigated 25 patients who underwent robotic TKA using the CASPER system. In this average 5-year follow up study, mechanical axis errors, alignments of prostheses in the coronal/sagittal planes, and rotation angles of femoral prosthesis were all < 1°.

Park and Lee(Park & Lee, 2007) compared 30 cases treated using the conventional method with 32 cases of ROBODOC assisted surgery and concluded that the robotic system offers – accurate procedural planning, precise resection of bone, and accurate alignments and locations of prostheses and axes. They also mentioned that big pins and the robot's wide arm radius are not suitable for minimally invasive surgery.

Song et al.(Song et al., 2009) found in a minimum 3-year follow up study of 50 ROBODOC-surgery patients that mechanical axes were corrected 0.49° varus on average, and that they were within 2° in 46 patients and within 3° in the remaining four. Average angles of femoral and tibial prostheses in the coronal plane were 89.5° and 90.1°, respectively, and average gradients in the sagittal plane were 1.06° and 85.56° respectively. The accuracies of coronal and sagittal plane were within 2°.

In a later study, Song et al.(Song et al., 2011) investigated 30 cases of bilateral degenerative arthritis of the knee in a randomized, prospective, comparative trial of robot-assisted and conventional surgery. One knee was operated on using ROBODOC, and the other was treated conventionally. Patients were followed up for at least 2 years. Clinical scores and ranges of movement were not significantly different in the two groups. Moreover, when patients were surveyed for pain, joint stability, joint weakness, snapping, swelling, and unexplained discomfort, 11 preferred the ROBODOC operated knee, 13 expressed no preference, and 6 preferred the conventionally operated side. However, in terms of mechanical axis alignments, whereas as the conventional method had 7 outliers, ROBODOC had none, and in terms of tibial prosthesis alignments, there were six outliers in the conventional group, and none in the ROBODOC group. The authors concluded that robot-assisted surgery produces better clinical and radiologic outcomes.

4.5 Future directions

Computer assisted orthopedic surgeries are being rapidly developed, and the future of navigation assisted surgery appears bright. In particular, if the physical sizes of these systems could be reduced they would be more useful for minimally invasive surgery. Furthermore, accuracies will undoubtedly be improved and errors will become infinitesimal.

The ROBODOC and CASPAR systems have achieved commercial success, and are now used in more than 100 European institutes. Furthermore, in South Korea, 10 institutions now routinely use the ROBODOC system. As was mentioned above, neither the ROBODOC nor the CASPAR system reduce operation costs, although robot supporters claim that by not using manual instrumentation the expenses of sterilization are saved, and that the superior clinical outcomes (lower revision operation rates, faster recovery, return to society, and others) offer across the board savings. However, there is insufficiency of the objective, and currently, it cannot be said that the superior accuracy provided by robot systems leads to better clinical outcomes.

5. Conclusion

In the orthopedic surgery field, navigation assisted surgery provides real-time alignment values, and allows the intra-operative evaluation and adjustment of prosthesis placement. Furthermore, computer-assisted surgery methods are expected to improve the qualities of surgical procedures. The majority of orthopedic surgeons believe that a computer system is needed during TKA to provide axis alignment, whereas others believe that computer-assisted surgery provides results that are effectively similar to those of conventional surgery. However, navigation assisted TKA provides precise information about femoral and tibial prostheses, enables optimal prosthesis sizes to be chosen for individual patients, and provides better range of knee movement after surgery. Furthermore, it improves the surgical experience for both the surgeon and patient.

In the operation room, robots have no limits regarding bone resection, which is why robot systems have been adopted in the orthopedic surgery field. In the TKA field, currently available robotic systems require more operative time and are more expensive than conventional surgery, but even at this stage of development they offer much more precise pre-operative planning.

6. Index

Knee joint, Osteoarthritis, Navigation, Kinematic registration, Surface registration, Infra-red, Optical system, Electromagnetic system, Light-emitting diodes, Ligament balancing, Tensioner, Real-time information, Robot, ROBODOC, ORTHODOC, Preoperative planning, Computer tomography, Passive system, Active system, Milling, Verification, Calibration, Bone motion, Mechanical alignment method, Anatomical alignment method

7. References

Bathis H, Perlick L, Tingart M, Luring C, Zurakowski D, Grifka J. Alignment in total knee arthroplasty. A comparison of computer-assisted surgery with the conventional technique. J Bone Joint Surg Br. 2004;86(5):682-687.

Bellemans J, Vandenneucker H, Vanlauwe J. Robot-assisted total knee arthroplasty. Clin Orthop Relat Res. 2007;464:111-116.

Borner M, Wiesel U, Ditzen W. Clinical experience with Robodoc and the Duracon Total Knee. In: Stiehl J, Konermann W, Haaker R(eds). Navigation and Robotics in Total joint and Spine Surgery. Berlin, Germany: Springer-Verlag. 2004:362-366.

Browne JA, Cook C, Hofmann AA, Bolognesi MP. Postoperative morbidity and mortality following total knee arthroplasty with computer navigation. Knee. 2010;17(2):152-156.

Chauhan SK, Scott RG, Breidahl W, Beaver RJ. Computer-assisted knee arthroplasty versus a conventional jig-based technique. A randomized, prospective trial. J Bone Joint Surg Br. 2004;86(3):372-377.

Choong PF, Dowsey MM, Stoney JD. Does accurate anatomical alignment result in better function and quality of life? Comparing conventional and computer-assisted total knee arthroplasty. J Arthroplasty. 2009;24(4):560-569.

Coon Thomas M. Integrating robotic technology into the operating room. Am J Orthop. 2009;38(2 Suppl):7-9.

Decking J, Theis C, Achenbach T, Roth E, Nafe B, Eckardt A. Robotic total knee arthroplasty: the accuracy of CT-based component placement. Acta Orthop Scand. 2004;75(5):573-579.

Ensini A, Catani F, Leardini A, Romagnoli M, Giannini S. Alignments and clinical results in conventional and navigated total knee arthroplasty. Clin Orthop Relat Res. 2007;457:156-162.

Fadda M, Marcacci M, Toksvig-Larsen S, Wang T, Meneghello R. Improving accuracy of bone resections using robotics tool holder and a high speed milling cutting tool. J Med Eng Technol. 1998;22(6):280-284.

Haaker RG, Stockheim M, Kamp M, Proff G, Breitenfelder J, Ottersbach A. Computer-assisted navigation increases precision of component placement in total knee arthroplasty. Clin Orthop Relat Res. 2005(433):152-159.

Kalairajah Y, Cossey AJ, Verrall GM, Ludbrook G, Spriggins AJ. Are systemic emboli reduced in computer-assisted knee surgery?: A prospective, randomised, clinical trial. J Bone Joint Surg Br. 2006;88(2):198-202.

Knutson K, Lindstrand A and Lidgren L. Survival of knee arthroplasties, a nation-wide multicenter investigation of 8,000 cases. J Bone Joint Surg. 1986; 68-B: 795-803.

Laskin RS. Alignment of total knee components. Orthopedics. 1984; 7:62.

Lehnen K, Giesinger K, Warschkow R, Porter M, Koch E, Kuster MS. Clinical outcome using a ligament referencing technique in CAS versus conventional technique. Knee Surg Sports Traumatol Arthrosc. 2010.

Matziolis G, Krocker D, Weiss U, Tohtz S, Perka C. A prospective, randomized study of computer-assisted and conventional total knee arthroplasty. Three-dimensional evaluation of implant alignment and rotation. J Bone Joint Surg Am. 2007;89(2):236-243.

Mullaji A, Kanna R, Marawar S, Kohli A, Sharma A. Comparison of limb and component alignment using computer-assisted navigation versus image intensifier-guided conventional total knee arthroplasty: a prospective, randomized, single-surgeon study of 467 knees. J Arthroplasty. 2007;22(7):953-959.

Park SE, Lee CT. Comparison of robotic-assisted and conventional manual implantation of a primary total knee arthroplasty. J Arthroplasty. 2007;22(7):1054-1059.

Plaskos C, Hodgson AJ, Inkpen K, McGraw RW. Bone cutting errors in total knee arthroplasty. J Arthroplasty. 2002;17(6):698-705.

Ranawat CS, Flynn WF, Saddler S, Hansraj KH, Maynhard MJ. Long-term results of total condylar knee arthroplasty. A 12-years survivorship study. Clin Orthop. 1993; 286: 94-102.

Ritter MA, Faris PM, Keating EM, Meding JB. Postoperative alignment of total knee replacement its effect on survival. Clin Orthop. 1994;299: 153-156.

Rosenberger RE, Hoser C, Quirbach S, Attal R, Hennerbichler A, Fink C. Improved accuracy of component alignment with the implementation of image-free navigation in total knee arthroplasty. Knee Surg Sports Traumatol Arthrosc. 2008;16(3):249-257.

Schnurr C, Csecsei G, Eysel P, Konig DP. The effect of computer navigation on blood loss and transfusion rate in TKA. Orthopedics. 2010;33(7):474

Scuderi GR, Insall JN, Windsor RE, Moran MC. Survivorship analysis of cemented knee replacement. J Bone Joint Surg. 1989;71-B:798-809

Seon JK, Park SJ, Lee KB, Li G, Kozanek M, Song EK. Functional comparison of total knee arthroplasty performed with and without a navigation system. Int Orthop. 2009;33(4):987-990.

Seon JK, Song EK. The Accuracy of Lower Extremity Alignment in a Total Knee Arthroplasty Using Computer-Assisted Navigation System. J of Korean Orthop Assoc 2004;39:566~571.

Siebert W, Mai S, Kober R, Heeckt PF. Technique and first clinical results of robot-assisted total knee replacement. Knee. 2002;9(3):173-180.

Sikorski JM. Computer-assisted revision total knee replacement. J Bone Joint Surg Br. 2004;86(4):510-514.

Song EK, Seon JK, Park SJ, Jung WB, Park HW, Lee GW. Simultaneous bilateral total knee arthroplasty with robotic and conventional techniques: a prospective, randomized study. 1. Knee Surg Sports Traumatol Arthrosc. 2011 Feb 11. [Epub ahead of print]

Song EK, Seon JK, Park SJ, Park JK, Park CH. Robotic Total Knee Arthroplasty - Minimal Follow-up of 3 Years - J Korean Knee Soc 2009;21:251~257.

Song EK, Seon JK, Yoon TR, Park SJ, Bae BH, Cho SG. Functional results of navigated minimally invasive and conventional total knee arthroplasty: a comparison in bilateral cases. Orthopedics. 2006;29(10 Suppl):S145-147.

Spencer JM, Chauhan SK, Sloan K, Taylor A, Beaver RJ. Computer navigation versus conventional total knee replacement: no difference in functional results at two years. J Bone Joint Surg Br. 2007;89(4):477-480.

Stulberg SD, Loan P, Sarin V. Computer-assisted navigation in total knee replacement: results of an initial experience in thirty-five patients. J Bone Joint Surg Am. 2002;84-A Suppl 2:90-98.

Teter KE, Bregman D, Colwell CW, Jr. Accuracy of intramedullary versus extramedullary tibial alignment cutting systems in total knee arthroplasty. Clin Orthop Relat Res. 1995(321):106-110.

Tria AJ, Jr. The evolving role of navigation in minimally invasive total knee arthroplasty. Am J Orthop (Belle Mead NJ). 2006;35(7 Suppl):18-22.

Van Ham G, Denis K, Vander Sloten J, Van Audekercke R, Van der Perre G, De Schutter J, Aertbelien E, Demey S, Bellemans J. Machining and accuracy studies for a tibial knee implant using a force-controlled robot. Comput Aided Surg. 1998;3(3):123-133.

16

Computer Assisted Total Knee Arthroplasty – The Learning Curve

Jean-Claude Bové

Multispecialties Private Hospital Clinique du Val de Sambre Maubeuge
France

1. Introduction

Over the last decades, orthopedic surgery has encountered a growing development that remains unfailing today.

Particularly in the field of total joint replacement, it is indeed a functional surgery aimed at a rather elderly population whose functional demand is increasing.

It is undeniable that a senior aged 60 in 2011 is very different from the senior suffering physical or psychological constraints caused by the ageing of his body about thirty years ago.

Nowadays, many seniors are willing to have an active lifestyle or even practice sport on a regular basis.

In the field of total joint replacement, that demand generates steady progress, which can come up to that expectation.

Among all orthopedic interventions that marked the twentieth century, total hip and knee arthroplasties are the most important.

Total hip replacement has even been labeled "intervention of the century."

Many forms specifically aiming to improve the quality of life have been incorporated into the various protocols for total prostheses monitoring (SF 16, HSS).

They accurately reflect the increasing demand of patients, which currently consists of simply forgetting the presence of the prosthetic joint.

This growing demand requires the constant search for improved joint replacement outcomes. That improvement is necessary to gradually reduce the rate of complications or imperfect results found in the literature.

Although few interventions have so much improved the quality of life for patients, much progress is still needed in order to increase the percentage of patients satisfied with their prosthesis.

The goal of arthroplasty is to obtain a joint which will be and remain mobile and painless as long as possible.

However, some studies [1-3] estimate that more than ten percent of the number of total knee prostheses do not fully come up to the patients' expectations, particularly in terms of residual pain.

The ideal thing would be to replace in due course the osteoarthritic joint (joint whose cartilage is worn) with the prosthesis and to obtain a prosthesis which would be functional all throughout the patient's life.

In other words, total joint replacement would be performed once and for all, and its sufficient longevity would prevent all prosthetic revision imposed by the failure or wear of the implant.

However, it is clear that the current average lifespan [4-5] of prostheses does not allow to avoid that revision among relatively young patients, that is to say patients who are younger than 50 years old.

Considering the gradual increase in the population's life expectancy and the more intensive use of the prosthesis among younger patients, one or two prosthetic changes are frequently required in such cases.

At the beginning of the twenty-first century, improving prosthetic longevity is still an absolute necessity.

This improvement in the lifespan of the implant must be combined with an improvement in the functional outcomes of arthroplasty, making some daily life activities easier to carry out thanks to the increase in prosthetic knee flexion, the opportunity to squat or kneel, to drive or practice some more demanding sport activities.

But how can that prosthetic function be improved as well as the prosthetic longevity of the implant?

First by working on the prosthetic design in order to increase its functional capabilities.

Much progress has been made in prosthetic design (design of the total hip prosthesis femoral stem, femoral offset, metaphyseal filling, anti-rotation wings,etc., radii of curvature of the total knee prosthesis femoral condyles, femoral offset, posterior slope of the tibial component, trochlear design, etc.).

Therefore we are currently moving towards an almost uniform design, gradually tending towards an almost unanimous prosthetic shape.

Progress will probably be made in that field in the coming years but the major part seems to have been done.

Similarly, many studies have been conducted to improve prosthetic anchorage (cemented prosthesis or not, press-fit effect, screwed prostheses, etc.) and many others will still have to be conducted in the future.

It is in the field of tribology, that is to say the science of the materials used in friction couples, that discussions are still lively, especially between the advocates of "hard-hard" and those of "hard-soft".

After decades of "hard-soft" corresponding to the first years of total joint replacement, roughly to the polyethylene-metal friction couple, the hard-hard friction couple appeared in the 1980s and 1990s (mainly alumina ceramic/alumina ceramic, metal/metal), those friction couples permitting to reduce the volume of wear debris, which are responsible for the so-called "aseptic" loosening.

Indeed the regular production of wear particles (cement, polyethylene, metal) will initiate a macrophage reaction of resorption, which when increasing, will compromise the prosthetic anchoring.

A certain number of complications of 'hard/hard' couples (breakage of ceramics, dissemination of metal ions in the body) has made the debate a little more lively but it is still not resolved. Some operators prefer so-called "hybrid" couples (alumina ceramic/polyethylene).

Improving the manufacturing techniques of various materials used is certainly an argument in the debate (maximum purity of ceramics limiting the risk of breakage, cross-linked polyethylene for superior mechanical resistance, etc.).

As it can be noted, contrary to the field of prosthetic design, significant progress is still desirable in the field of tribology.

The improvement in the technical realization of total joint replacement remains a key-issue.

This improvement in the insertion technique is a major factor to lengthen prosthetic longevity.

In the field of total knee arthroplasty, improving the accuracy of bone cuts is bound to have consequences on prosthetic stability (ligament balancing) and overall alignment of the lower limb on which prosthetic longevity depends [6-7].

Improving the arthroplasty's accuracy means improving the equipment used for the implantation of the prosthesis, which is called "ancillary equipment".

Over the last decade, new ancillaries have emerged, which allow to carry out knee arthroplasty minimizing the damage to soft tissues and exposure of bone ends, in a view to simplify the postoperative course. These techniques are known as "minimally invasive" [8-9].

The length of surgical incisions was significantly reduced, limiting the aggression of the surrounding soft tissues (skin, subcutaneous cellular tissue, muscles and tendons). Some operators limit their incision to a few centimeters (approximately half a conventional incision).

Clinical improvement was described in the immediate aftermath of these minimally invasive techniques. Studies are currently being carried out to confirm such progress.

Computer-assisted surgery is the second line of research to improve the ancillary equipment.

The computer appeared in operating rooms in the early 1990s under the leadership of neurosurgeons. The precursor surgical intervention was the computer-assisted transpedicular spine surgery, then, in the mid-1990s, it was followed by the computer-navigated total knee arthroplasty performed in France by the Grenoble university surgical team [10].

From the beginning, two systems were used, one using pre-operative imaging (CT), the other one using "bone-morphing" TM.

At the time, the computer created practical difficulties because of its volume and the numerous cables required by a complex connection.

An immediate preoperative tedious calibration of the ancillary equipment considerably lengthens operating time.

For simplicity, concerning total knee arthroplasty, computer-assisted surgery must be regarded as a tool aiming to bring improved accuracy in the realization of bone cuts, leading to a better ligament balancing of the prosthetic knee and a global alignment of the lower limb being more frequently close to the vertical (the ideal range of the angle between the femoral mechanical axis and the tibial mechanical axis extending from 3 degrees of varus to 3 degrees of valgus).

The so-called femoral mechanical axis is the line joining the center of the femoral head and the center of the knee; the tibial mechanical axis connects the middle of the tibial plateaus and the center of the ankle joint.

Thanks to that regularity in the alignment, the unexplained outliers of the overall mechanical axis of the lower limb are scarce.

With the help of a stereoscopic infrared camera, the rays being reflected by optically reflective balls, it is possible to obtain a virtual anatomical reconstruction of the operated knee. The software, using an extensive database, then guides the various bone cuts via a graphical user interface (screen) and benchmarks for instant viewing of the various cutting blocks.

This is seen as an aid to surgery and not a robot automation of the surgical gesture. The surgeon remains the master of the surgical gesture, following on the screen the computer's visual indications to guide and set the different cutting blocks.

As mentioned above, this improvement in cutting accuracy induces a better ligament balancing and an alignment of the lower limb more consistently correct, which should increase prosthetic longevity.

However no study has so far clinically demonstrated any lengthening of the lifespan of a so-called "navigated" total knee prosthesis.

The follow-up is too short, which explains this gap. Indeed, computer navigation is still, in terms of its regular practice, in its infancy.

Therefore the success is less massive than expected with the improvements achieved during surgery. Among the reasons for this limited development, the cost of materials [11] is mentioned, given its limited distribution. Longer operative time with the addition of specific technical steps required by the computer, leading to an increased septic risk, and finally difficulty of learning the technique, even for a trained operator. Given his experience and the excellent results of the so-called conventional prosthetic surgery, the operator is not always convinced that new technique is really useful.

It seemed interesting to mention our personal experience of learning computer-assisted surgery in the field of total knee replacement.

Indeed, the obstacles seemed to be overcome without great difficulty. Using more user friendly and easier systems, we were even able to modify our practice as our experience grew.

A comparison of operating times enabled us to demonstrate the permanent aspect of learning by making our adaption to a totally new and unknown computer system easier and easier.

2. Materials and methods

In February 2003 we achieved our first computer-assisted total knee arthroplasty.

Two implantations were performed during the same operating session in the Val de Sambre clinic in Maubeuge.

At the time, concerning the primary knee arthroplasty, the author exclusively used the Natural Knee II TM sliding prosthesis (Zimmer, Warsaw, Indiana, USA).

The provision on a trial basis of the Navitrack Navigation System TM (Orthosoft, Zimmer) allowed those first two projects.

It is an imageless system requiring the calibration of computer tools (pointer, and cutting blocks) (Fig. 1) during the operation and not involving the bone morphing TM.

It was actually a simplified bone morphing including deposition of "computer chips" on the screen allowing to adjust cutting thickness (Fig. 2).

The graphical user interface not being interactive, the use of keyboards and pedals in the immediate vicinity or in direct contact with the operative field was a source of congestion and increased the risk of lack of asepsis.

After those two trials which were considered conclusive, the decision to purchase the equipment was made and, from September 2003, all primary knee arthroplasties were performed by the author using that system.

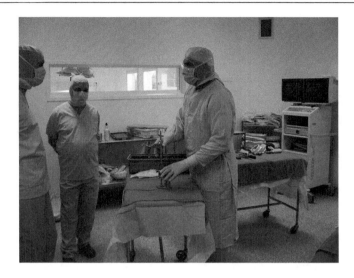

Fig. 1.

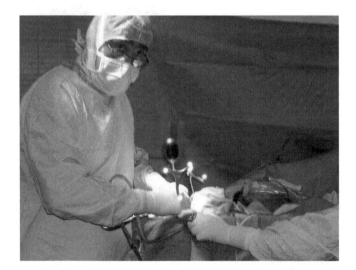

Fig. 2.

Computer-assisted surgery has been exclusively used whereas conventional surgery was only used for revision arthroplasty surgery.

Thus more than 200 total knee prostheses were implanted with a system that may now seem outdated, but which, at that time, gave entire satisfaction from September 2003 to July 2006.

The duration of the intervention and more specifically the time of tourniquet were studied [12] at the beginning and end of the user experience (Fig. 3) of this system.

In July 2006, we decided to use a more user-friendly system including a touch screen covered with a sterile drape allowing us to avoid cumbersome cables and pedals. It is also

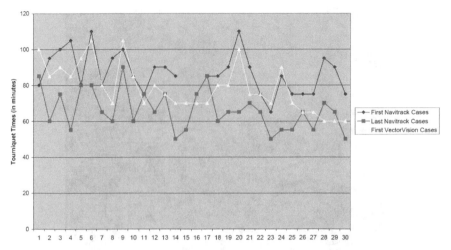

Fig. 3. Tourniquet Time

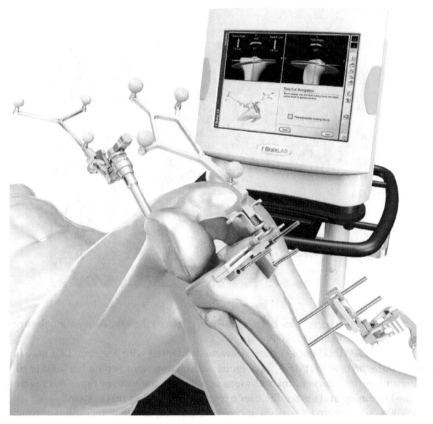

Fig. 4.

an imageless system based on a standardized bone morphing carried out using a pointer fitted with reflective balls and not requiring time-consuming instrumental calibration (VectorVision, Brainlab, Munich, Germany) (Fig. 4).

A "coloring" of the reference bone surfaces using a computer pointer (stylus provided with reflective balls) permits to transmit essential anatomical data to the computer. The data allows the operator to choose a knee anatomical model being as close as possible to the operated knee in a huge database.

More than 300 arthroplasties have been carried out so far using that system, which is still used in the service now.

3. Results

When using the computer system, an average lengthening of time tourniquet of 18 minutes has been noticed (range 0-45 minutes), which is likely to increase the septic risk. That average lengthening refers to the average tourniquet time of "conventional" total knee arthroplasties performed by the author during the previous five years.

The more detailed analysis of the curves indirectly shows the technical difficulties experienced by the operator since, for an average tourniquet time of 87 minutes during the very first use of navigation (first 30 implantations with the Navitrack system), we observe that in 4 out of the first 10 cases, 100 minutes are reached or exceeded.

This period of 100 minutes is critical because it jeopardizes the achievement of the entire knee arthroplasty under pneumatic tourniquet, because the latter cannot be maintained more than 120 minutes or it can cause complications. The tourniquet release before the setting of cement may compromise the prosthetic anchorage, although for some operators the procedure is performed without any tourniquet.

When examining the curves, we can notice a progressive decrease in the time of tourniquet as the operator's experience and mastery of the technique develops.

Last but not least, a comparison of tourniquet time in the series performed using the second system has identified a more rapid decrease in additional operative time induced by the use of the computer ancillary, which supports the working hypothesis of the study, namely the maintenance of the operator's knowledge.

That situation could be compared to driving : the successive adaptation to a different vehicle is done gradually with less difficulty as the driving technique improves.

Over the last eight years, no specific complication to navigation has been deplored, except, at the beginning of our practice, some cases of transitory inflammation or suppuration of the holes of the tibial antenna fixation pins.

These were probably caused by the excessive overheating of the drilling, which caused neighboring bone necrosis. The problem was solved by the use of tibial fixation rods with a 3.5 mm diameter.

We observed no supracondylar fracture on way to the fixing pin of the femoral rigid body and a single non-displaced tibial fracture, which rapidly consolidated.

Particular care is brought to the precise location of the fixing rods to reduce the risk of fracture [13].

Similarly, the average rate of postoperative prosthetic sepsis (less than one percent in the literature and personal experience) has not been modified by the lengthening of operating time.

The functional results and the possible and expected lengthening of computer-assisted arthroplasty longevity will be clinically studied as soon as the mean perspective of the series will be sufficient to be scientifically exploited.

4. Discussion

As seen, after studying of the duration of the learning curve, we can consider this learning difficulty as easily surmountable.

The reluctance of some practitioners, experienced in the practice of orthopedic joint replacement, to perform computer-assisted surgery is mainly due to the supposed difficulty of learning an innovative technology, with all the constraints that it brings, and not to the duration of the learning curve itself.

In addition, the computer ancillary equipment itself, tends to annoy or frighten those trained operators who only consider that equipment as an additional constraint.

Actually the major obstacle now seems to be the cost of equipment and particularly in France since the supervisory bodies consider that the benefit induced by the technique is not sufficient to support the extra cost induced by the purchase and use of computer equipment. That benefit will only be found and admitted through the rigorous exploitation of satisfactory scientific studies. To be useful, such studies must always have sufficient perspective (10-year-follow-up minimum), but computer-assisted surgery started being used on a regular basis about 12 years ago. In the coming years, exploitable series should appear.

Similarly, the proliferation of studies on the comparative functional results of conventional arthroplasties versus navigated arthroplasties should rapidly lead to interesting conclusions.

It is mainly in the private sector that the financial aspect has the greatest impact. Indeed, in a context of economic crisis, the health system severely suffers from the decline of its funding due to a reduction in social contributions, if only because of rising unemployment.

The financial investors involved in the management of the private health care system in France are increasingly careful with potential investments such as the purchase of a new ancillary equipment.

The need for learning computer-assisted surgery, considered by some operators as tedious, with the costs incurred by the purchase of computer equipment (hardware and software), is currently a major obstacle to the further development of that promising technique.

However, that development will itself lead to a consequent decrease in acquisition costs through the diffusion of technology.

Similarly, the different national science societies for computer-assisted surgery will have to continue their efforts of representation, for educational purposes, including in university education.

5. Conclusion

In our view, and especially in the field of total hip and knee arthroplasties, computer-assisted surgery represents a promising technique, able to bring significant progress in terms of function and prosthetic longevity.

These improvements will meet the needs of elderly patients, who are more and more numerous, more and more demanding about maintaining a good quality of life and sometimes wishing to practice sport on a regular basis.

Similarly, younger and younger patients will take advantage of that technical progress.

To allow further development of computer navigated surgery, a reduction of costs is necessary and will only be obtained thanks to the diffusion of the technique and the improved support of those costs by supervisory bodies, once they have been convinced of the reality of the benefit provided by the computer.

To achieve this goal, the proliferation of scientific studies is essential. Those studies must be very serious, have a sufficient perspective, and be rigorously statistically exploited.

In those conditions, the expected improvement in terms of longevity and prosthetic function will be clearly demonstrated and allow the financial support of supervisory bodies.

As for the supposed inconvenience of learning time, our study has shown that it is minimal. On the one hand, a limited number of implantations is necessary to that learning (about 30 cases) and on the other hand, the growing experience allows the operator to adapt more easily to any new computer ancillary.

Finally, the educational value of the material is undeniable. Young operators should not be trained to the exclusive practice of computer-aided prosthetic surgery but their introduction to that technique should enable them to have a more rigorous, thoughtful and interactive approach of the different stages of arthroplasty surgery, which could improve their reasoning.

6. References

[1] Sun ZH, Liu J, Tian MQ, Zhang Y, Zhao HW, Zhu RS. Management of post operative pain after total knee arthroplasty. Zhonghua Wai Ke Za Zhi. 2011 Mar 1; 49 (3): 222-6.

[2] Jacofsky DJ, Della Valle CJ, Meneghini RM, Sporer SM, Cercek RM. Revision total knee arthroplasty: what the practicing orthopaedic surgeon needs to know. Instr Course Lect. 2011; 60: 269-81.

[3] Bonnin MP, Basiglini L, Archbold HA. What are the factors of residual pain after uncomplicated TKA? Knee Surg Sports Traumatol Arthrosc. 2011 May 20 [Epub ahead of print].

[4] Keeney JA, Eunice S, Pashos G, Wright RW, Clohisy JC. What is the evidence for total knee arthroplasty in young patients?: a systematic review of the literature. Clin Orthop Relat Res; 2011 Feb; 469 (2): 574-83.

[5] Ritter MA, Meneghini RM. Twenty-year survivorship of cementless anatomic graduated component total knee arthroplasty. J Arthroplasty. 2010 Jun; 25(4): 507-13.

[6] Rosenberger RE, Hoser C, Quirbach S, Attal R, Hennerbichler A, Fink C. Improved accuracy ofcomponent alignment with the implementation of image-free navigation in total knee arthroplasty. Knee Surg Sports Traumatol Arthrosc. 2008 Mar; 16(3): 249-57.

[7] El Masri F, Rammal H, Ghanem I, El Hage S, El Abiad R, Kharrat K, Dagher F. Computer-assistedsurgery in total knee replacement. Preliminary results: report of 60 cases. Rev Chir Orthop Reparatrice Appar Mot. 2008 May; 94(3): 261-67.

[8] Watanabe T, Muneta T, Ishizuki M. Is a minimally invasive approach superior to a conventional approach for total knee arthroplasty? Early outcome and 2 to 4 year follow-up. J Orthop Sci. 2009 Sep; 14(5): 589-95.

[9] Tria AJ Jr. Minimally invasive total knee arthroplasty: past, present and future. Am J Orthop (Belle Mead NJ). 2007 Sep; 36 (9 Suppl): 6-7.

[10] Saragaglia D. Computer-assisted total knee arthroplasty: 12 years experience in Grenoble. Bull Acad Natl Med. 2009 Jan; 193 (1): 91-104; discussion 104-5.

[11] Rivkin G, Liebergall M. Challenges of technology integration and computer-assisted surgery. J Bone Joint Surg AM. 2009 Feb; 91 Suppl 1: 13-6.

[12] Bové JC. Computer-assisted total knee arthroplasty. Comparison of two successive systems. Learning curve. Rev Chir Orthop Reparatrice Appar Mot. 2008 May; 94(3): 252-60.

[13] Beldame J, Boisrenoult P, Beaufils P. Pin track induced fractures around computer-assisted TKA. Orthop Traumatol Surg Res; 2010 May; 96(3): 249-55.

Permissions

The contributors of this book come from diverse backgrounds, making this book a truly international effort. This book will bring forth new frontiers with its revolutionizing research information and detailed analysis of the nascent developments around the world.

We would like to thank Dr. Samo K. Fokter, MD, for lending his expertise to make the book truly unique. He has played a crucial role in the development of this book. Without his invaluable contribution this book wouldn't have been possible. He has made vital efforts to compile up to date information on the varied aspects of this subject to make this book a valuable addition to the collection of many professionals and students.

This book was conceptualized with the vision of imparting up-to-date information and advanced data in this field. To ensure the same, a matchless editorial board was set up. Every individual on the board went through rigorous rounds of assessment to prove their worth. After which they invested a large part of their time researching and compiling the most relevant data for our readers. Conferences and sessions were held from time to time between the editorial board and the contributing authors to present the data in the most comprehensible form. The editorial team has worked tirelessly to provide valuable and valid information to help people across the globe.

Every chapter published in this book has been scrutinized by our experts. Their significance has been extensively debated. The topics covered herein carry significant findings which will fuel the growth of the discipline. They may even be implemented as practical applications or may be referred to as a beginning point for another development. Chapters in this book were first published by InTech; hereby published with permission under the Creative Commons Attribution License or equivalent.

The editorial board has been involved in producing this book since its inception. They have spent rigorous hours researching and exploring the diverse topics which have resulted in the successful publishing of this book. They have passed on their knowledge of decades through this book. To expedite this challenging task, the publisher supported the team at every step. A small team of assistant editors was also appointed to further simplify the editing procedure and attain best results for the readers.

Our editorial team has been hand-picked from every corner of the world. Their multi-ethnicity adds dynamic inputs to the discussions which result in innovative outcomes. These outcomes are then further discussed with the researchers and contributors who give their valuable feedback and opinion regarding the same. The feedback is then collaborated with the researches and they are edited in a comprehensive manner to aid the understanding of the subject.

Apart from the editorial board, the designing team has also invested a significant amount of their time in understanding the subject and creating the most relevant covers. They scrutinized every image to scout for the most suitable representation of the subject and create an appropriate cover for the book.

The publishing team has been involved in this book since its early stages. They were actively engaged in every process, be it collecting the data, connecting with the contributors or procuring relevant information. The team has been an ardent support to the editorial, designing and production team. Their endless efforts to recruit the best for this project, has resulted in the accomplishment of this book. They are a veteran in the field of academics and their pool of knowledge is as vast as their experience in printing. Their expertise and guidance has proved useful at every step. Their uncompromising quality standards have made this book an exceptional effort. Their encouragement from time to time has been an inspiration for everyone.

The publisher and the editorial board hope that this book will prove to be a valuable piece of knowledge for researchers, students, practitioners and scholars across the globe.

List of Contributors

Luca Amendola
Department of Orthopedic and Traumatology, Maggiore Hospital, Bologna, Italy

Domenico Tigani
Department of Orthopaedic Surgery, Santa Maria alle Scotte Hospital, Siena, Italy

Matteo Fosco and Dante Dallari
First Ward of Orthopaedic Surgery, Rizzoli Orthopaedic Institute, Bologna, Italy

Fabio Orozco and Alvin Ong
Atlanticare Care Regional Medical Center, Pomona, New Jersey, USA
Joint Replacement, Rothman Institute, Thomas Jefferson, USA
University, Philadelphia, Pennsylvani, USA

Nahum Rosenberg and Michael Soudry
Orthopaedic Surgery "A" Dept., Rambam – Health Care Campus, Haifa, Israel
Ruth and Bruce Rappaport Faculty of Medicine, Technion – Israel Institute of Technology, Haifa, Israel

Arnan Greental
Orthopaedic Surgery "A" Dept., Rambam – Health Care Campus, Haifa, Israel

Joern Bengt Seeger
Center for Musculoskeletal Surgery, Charité - Universitätsmedizin Berlin,Campus Charité Mitte (CCM), Berlin, Germany

Michael Clarius
Department of Orthopaedic and Trauma Surgery, Vulpius Klinik GmbH, Bad Rappenau, Germany

Tomoyuki Matsumoto Seiji Kubo, Masahiro Kurosaka and Ryosuke Kuroda
Department of Orthopaedic Surgery, Kobe University Graduate School of Medicine, Kobe Japan

Hirotsugu Muratsu
Department of Orthopaedic Surgery, Nippon Steel Hirohata Hospital, Himeji, Japan

Ta-Wei Tai, Chyun-Yu Yang and Chih-Wei Chang
Department of Orthopedics, National Cheng Kung University Hospital, Tainan, Taiwan

Hakan Boya
Başkent University, Faculty of Medicine, Department of Orthopaedics and Traumatology, Zübeyde Hanım Hospital, İzmir, Turkey

Orlando M. de Cárdenas Centeno and Felix A. Croas Fernández
"Frank País" International Scientific Orthopedic Complex, Medical Sciences University, Havana, Cuba

K. Kolb
Department of Trauma Surgery Klinikum am Steinenberg, Reutlingen, Germany

P.A. Grützner
Department of Trauma Surgery Unfallklinik Ludwigshafen, Germany

F. Marx
Department of Trauma Surgery, Friedrich-Schiller-University, Jena, Germany

W. Kolb
Department of Trauma and Orthopaedic Surgery, Bethesda Hospital, Stuttgart, Germany

Domenick J. Sisto
Los Angeles Orthopaedic Institute, Sherman Oaks, California, USA

Ronald P. Grelsamer
Mount Sinai Medical Center, New York, New York, USA

Vineet K. Sarin
Kinamed Incorporated, Camarillo, California, USA

M. Spina
Department of Orthopaedics and Traumatology Surgery, Ospedale Borgo Trento, Azienda Universitaria Integrata, Verona, Italy

G. Gualdrini, M. Fosco and A. Giunti
First Department of Orthopaedics and Traumatology Surgery, Istituto Ortopedico Rizzoli, Bologna, Italy

František Okál, Adel Safi, Martin Komzák and Radek Hart
Department of Orthopaedics & Traumatology, General Hospital Znojmo, Czech Republic

Nicola Biasca
Orthopedic Clinic Luzern AG, Hirslanden Clinic St. Anna, Luzern, Switzerland

Matthias Bungartz
Klinik für Orthopädie und Unfallchirurgie, Lehrstuhl für Orthopädie der Friedrich-Schiller-Universität Jena, Waldkrankenhaus „Rudolf Elle" Eisenberg, Germany

M. Fosco, R. Ben Ayad, R. Fantasia and D. Dallari
From First Ward of Orthopaedic Surgery, University of Bologna, Rizzoli Orthopaedic Institute, Bologna, Italy

D. Tigani
From Department of Orthopaedic Surgery, Santa Maria alle Scotte Hospital, Siena, Italy

Eun Kyoo Song and Jong Keun Seon
Chonnam National University Hwasun Hospital, Korea

Jean-Claude Bové
Multispecialties Private Hospital Clinique du Val de Sambre Maubeuge, France

CPSIA information can be obtained at www.ICGtesting.com
Printed in the USA
LVOW01*1137260215

428336LV00004BB/58/P